Interventional Pulmonology

Guest Editor

ATUL C. MEHTA, MB, BS, FACP, FCCP

CLINICS IN CHEST MEDICINE

www.chestmed.theclinics.com

March 2010 • Volume 31 • Number 1

SAUNDERS an imprint of ELSEVIER, Inc.

W.B. SAUNDERS COMPANY
A Division of Elsevier Inc.

1600 John F. Kennedy Boulevard • Suite 1800 • Philadelphia, Pennsylvania 19103

http://www.theclinics.com

CLINICS IN CHEST MEDICINE Volume 31, Number 1
March 2010 ISSN 0272-5231, ISBN-13: 978-1-4377-1202-5

Editor: Sarah E. Barth
Developmental Editor: Theresa Collier

Clinics in Chest Medicine (ISSN 0272-5231) is published quarterly by Elsevier Inc., 360 Park Avenue South, New York, NY 10010-1710. Months of issue are March, June, September, and December. Periodicals postage paid at New York, NY and additional mailing offices. Subscription prices are $274.00 per year (domestic individuals), $432.00 per year (domestic institutions), $133.00 per year (domestic students/residents), $300.00 per year (Canadian individuals), $530.00 per year (Canadian institutions), $373.00 per year (international individuals), $530.00 per year (international institutions), and $186.00 per year (international and Canadian students/residents). International air speed delivery is included in all Clinics subscription prices. All prices are subject to change without notice. **POSTMASTER:** Send address changes to Clinics in Chest Medicine, Elsevier Health Sciences Division, Subscription Customer Service, 3251 Riverport Lane, Maryland Heights, MO 63043. **Customer Service: Telephone: 1-800-654-2452** (U.S. and Canada); **1-314-447-8871** (outside U.S. and Canada). **Fax: 1-314-447-8029. E-mail: journalscustomerservice-usa@elsevier.com** (for print support); **journalsonlinesupport-usa@elsevier.com** (for online support).

Reprints. For copies of 100 or more of articles in this publication, please contact the Commercial Reprints Department, Elsevier Inc., 360 Park Avenue South, New York, NY 10010-1710. Tel.: 212-633-3812; Fax: 212-462-1935; E-mail: reprints@elsevier.com.

Clinics in Chest Medicine is covered in *MEDLINE/PubMed (Index Medicus), Current Contents/Clinical Medicine, EMBASE/ Excerpta Medica, Science Citation Index,* and *ISI/BIOMED.*

Printed and bound in the United Kingdom
Transferred to Digital Print 2011

Contributors

GUEST EDITOR

ATUL C. MEHTA, MB, BS, FACP, FCCP
Professor of Medicine, Chief Medical Officer,
Sheikh Khalifa Medical City Managed by
Cleveland Clinic, Abu Dhabi, UAE; Staff
Physician, Respiratory Institute, Cleveland
Clinic, Cleveland, Ohio

AUTHORS

SANJAY AGRAWAL, MD, FCCP
Department of Respiratory Medicine,
Glenfield Hospital, University Hospitals of
Leicester NHS Trust, Leicestershire, United
Kingdom

**DEVANAND ANANTHAM, MBBS,
MRCP, FCCP**
Consultant, Department of Respiratory
and Critical Care Medicine, Singapore
General Hospital; Instructor in Medicine,
Duke-NUS, Graduate Medical School,
Singapore

FUMIHIRO ASANO, MD, FCCP
Director, Department of Pulmonary Medicine
and Bronchoscopy, Gifu Prefectural General
Medical Center, Gifu, Japan

HEINRICH D. BECKER, MD
Head, Department of Interdisciplinary
Endoscopy, Thoraxklinik at Heidelberg
University, Heidelberg, Germany

**JONATHAN A. BENNETT, BS, MD,
DM, FRCP**
Department of Respiratory Medicine,
Glenfield Hospital, University Hospitals
of Leicester NHS Trust, Leicestershire,
United Kingdom

ROBERTO F. CASAL, MD
Department of Pulmonary Medicine, The
University of Texas M.D. Anderson Cancer
Center, Houston, Texas

ROBERT J. CERFOLIO, MD
Professor of Surgery, Chief of Section of
Thoracic Surgery at University of Alabama
at Birmingham; Department of Surgery,
University of Alabama, Birmingham, Alabama

HENRI G. COLT, MD
Professor of Medicine, Director of Clinical
Programs, University of California, Irvine
Medical Center, Pulmonary Division, Orange,
California

GERARD COX, MB, FRCP(C), FRCP(I)
Professor of Medicine, McMaster University,
Firestone Institute for Respiratory Health,
St Joseph's Healthcare Hamilton, Hamilton,
Ontario, Canada

GEORGE A. EAPEN, MD
Associate Professor, Department of Pulmonary
Medicine, The University of Texas M.D.
Anderson Cancer Center, Houston, Texas

RALF EBERHARDT, MD
Department of Pneumology and Critical Care
Medicine, Thoraxklinik, University of
Heidelberg, Heidelberg, Germany

ARMIN ERNST, MD
Chief, Interventional Pulmonology; Director,
Clinical, Sponsored and Translational
Research Interventional Pulmonology/Thoracic
Surgery, Beth Israel Deaconess Medical
Center; Associate Professor of Medicine
(Pediatrics) and Surgery, Harvard Medical
School, Boston, Massachusetts

DAVID FELLER-KOPMAN, MD, FCCP
Director of Bronchoscopy and Interventional Pulmonology, Associate Professor of Medicine, Division of Pulmonary and Critical Care, The Johns Hopkins Hospital, Baltimore, Maryland

CATHERINE M. FREE, MD, DM, MRCP
Department of Respiratory Medicine, Glenfield Hospital, University Hospitals of Leicester NHS Trust, Leicestershire, United Kingdom

XAVIER GONZALEZ, MD
Chief Scientific Officer, Spiration, Inc, Redmond, Washington

CHRISTOPHER A. HERGOTT, MD, FRCPC
Interventional Pulmonary Medicine Fellow, Division of Respiratory Medicine, University of Calgary, Calgary, Canada

FELIX J.F. HERTH, MD, DSc, FCCP
Department of Pneumology and Critical Care Medicine, Thoraxklinik, University of Heidelberg, Heidelberg, Germany

ELIF KUPELI, MD
Department of Pulmonary Medicine, Mesa Hospital, Ankara, Turkey

PYNG LEE, MD
Department of Respiratory and Critical Care Medicine, Singapore General Hospital, Singapore

ANDREW R.L. MEDFORD, BS, MD, DM, MRCP, Dip(Clin Risk Mgt)
Department of Respiratory Medicine, Glenfield Hospital, University Hospitals of Leicester NHS Trust, Leicestershire; Consultant Respiratory Physician, North Bristol Lung Centre, Southmead Hospital, Avon, United Kingdom

ATUL C. MEHTA, MB, BS, FACP, FCCP
Professor of Medicine, Chief Medical Officer, Sheikh Khalifa Medical City Managed by Cleveland Clinic, Abu Dhabi, UAE; Staff Physician, Respiratory Institute, Cleveland Clinic, Cleveland, Ohio

SEPTIMIU D. MURGU, MD
Assistant Professor of Medicine, University of California, Irvine Medical Center, Pulmonary Division, Orange, California

YEHUDA SCHWARZ, MD, FCCP
Director of Pulmonary Medicine, Department of Pulmonology, Tel-Aviv Sourasky Medical Center; Sackler Faculty of Medicine, Tel Aviv University, Tel-Aviv, Israel

STEVEN C. SPRINGMEYER, MD
Vice President and Medical Director, Spiration, Inc, Redmond, Washington; Clinical Professor of Medicine, Division of Pulmonary and Critical Care Medicine, University of Washington, Seattle, Washington

ALDA L. TAM, MD
Assistant Professor, Department of Diagnostic Radiology, Section of Interventional Radiology, The University of Texas M.D. Anderson Cancer Center, Houston, Texas

ALAIN TREMBLAY, MDCM, FRCPC, FCCP
Associate Professor of Medicine, Division of Respiratory Medicine, University of Calgary, Calgary, Canada

DOUGLAS E. WOOD, MD
Professor and Chief, Division of Cardiothoracic Surgery, Endowed Chair of Lung Cancer Research, University of Washington; University of Washington Medical Center, Seattle, Washington

Contents

multiple stages from squamous metaplasia to dysplasia, followed by carcinoma in situ (CIS), progressing to invasive cancer. It would be ideal to be able to detect and treat preinvasive bronchial lesions defined as dysplasia and CIS before progressing to invasive cancer. Great efforts have been made to develop new mucosal imaging techniques. Bronchoscopic imaging techniques capable of detecting preinvasive lesions and currently available in clinical practice include autofluorescence bronchoscopy (AFB), high magnification ronchovideoscope, and narrow band imaging (NBI). For a more precise evaluation of newly detected preinvasive lesions, endobronchial ultrasound (EBUS) and optical coherence tomography (OCT) can be used.

The past decade has witnessed the application of many advanced bronchoscopic modalities to improve access to the solitary pulmonary nodule (SPN). Although many of the techniques are applied on a regular basis by bronchoscopists, which technique—or which combination of techniques—will offer the best performance and cost-effectiveness remains to be determined. The authors anticipate that bronchoscopic approaches to the SPN will continue to proliferate as technologic advances and clinical data accumulate. Research should focus on combinations of techniques, cost-effectiveness, and incorporation of these tools in diagnostic algorithms for lung nodules/masses.

Electromagnetic navigation bronchoscopy using overlaid CT Images is a safe procedure. It improves the diagnostic yield of the flexible bronchoscopy for peripheral lesions and also allows sampling of the mediastinal lymph nodes. Additionally, the system provides several other advantages: there is no additional radiation, and it has a short learning curve. It can also be used for fiducial marker placement for brachytherapy or stereotactic radiosurgery. It plays a complementary role to other modalities such as ultrathin bronchoscopy or an endobronchial ultrasonography.

Virtual bronchoscopic navigation (VBN) is a method for the guidance of a bronchoscope to peripheral lesions using virtual bronchoscopy (VB) images of the bronchial path. Irrespective of the bronchoscopist's skill level, the bronchoscope can be readily guided to the target in a short time. A system to automatically search for the bronchial path to the target has been developed and clinically applied; this system produces VB images of the path to the fourth- to twelfth- (median, sixth-) generation bronchi, and displays the VB images simultaneously with real bronchoscopic images. In this article, the author discusses VBN and the automatic VBN system, reviews the published literature, and describes its usefulness and limitations.

Technologic advances in bronchoscopy continue to improve the ability to perform minimally invasive, accurate evaluations of the tracheobronchial tree and to perform an ever-increasing array of diagnostic, staging, therapeutic, and palliative interventions. The role of both old and new diagnostic bronchoscopy will continue to evolve as further improvements are made in bronchoscopes, accessory equipment, and imaging technologies. The major challenge is the adoption of the many new bronchoscopic techniques into routine clinical practice. There is a need for well-designed studies to delineate the appropriate use of these interventions and to better define their limitations and cost effectiveness.

Interventional Bronchoscopy from Bench to Bedside: New Techniques for Central and Peripheral Airway Obstruction

Septimiu D. Murgu and Henri G. Colt

This article discusses how basic scientific concepts, based on a greater understanding of airway physiology, support the development and dissemination of multidimensional classification systems for tracheal stenosis, expiratory central airway collapse, and innovative interventional bronchoscopic procedures for patients with asthma and chronic obstructive pulmonary disease.

Endoscopic Management of Emphysema

Armin Ernst and Devanand Anantham

Lung volume reduction surgery has proven benefits in emphysema. However, high postoperative morbidity and stringent selection criteria for suitable candidates are limitations in clinical practice. Endoscopic approaches to lung volume reduction have used a range of different techniques such as endobronchial blockers, airway bypass, endobronchial valves, biologic sealants, and airway implants to address the limitations of surgery. The underlying physiologic mechanisms of endoscopic modalities vary, and homogeneous and heterogeneous emphysema are targeted. Currently available data on efficacy of bronchoscopic lung volume reduction are not consistently conclusive, and subjective benefit in dyspnea scores is a more frequent finding than improvements on spirometry or exercise tolerance. The safety data are more promising, with rare procedure-related mortality, fewer complications than lung volume reduction surgery, and short hospital length of stay. The field of bronchoscopic lung volume reduction continues to evolve as ongoing prospective randomized trials aim to clarify the efficacy data from earlier feasibility and safety studies.

Bronchoscopic Management of Prolonged Air Leak

Douglas E. Wood, Robert J. Cerfolio, Xavier Gonzalez, and Steven C. Springmeyer

Prolonged pulmonary parenchymal air leaks are an important clinical problem. Standard treatment of prolonged air leaks include continued chest tube drainage, pleural sclerosis, or surgery. Approaches that are less invasive than bedside sclerosis or surgery are desirable but bronchoscopy approaches tried over the years have had limited success. In 2001, an American College of Chest Physicians (ACCP) consensus statement concluded there was no role for bronchoscopy for the treatment of prolonged air leaks. The development of bronchial valves for treatment of emphysema allowed the use of these devices for air leaks under compassionate use regulations. Multiple reports of successful bronchial valve treatments, along with the US Food and Drug Administration's (FDA) humanitarian use approval of a bronchial valve for certain postsurgical air leaks, provide new evidence that there is likely a role for endobronchial treatment of prolonged air leaks in selected patients.

Bronchial Thermoplasty

Gerard Cox

Asthma, by definition is a variable disease. When there is more than normal natural variation in airflow, asthma can be provoked by a wide range of stimuli that include infectious, allergic, and environmental agents. Bronchoconstriction determines much of the short-term variability in airflow that characterizes asthma. Current treatments do not redress the excess smooth muscle mass that is present in the remodeled airway in chronic asthma. Thus, it is intriguing to consider the potential contribution of bronchial thermoplasty (a procedure that involves controlled heat treatment to reduce the mass of the airway smooth muscle) as an effective therapy for poorly controlled asthma.

Stents are used for palliation of symptoms of central airway obstruction caused by either malignant or benign conditions. Stents may be applied for maintaining airway patency after dilatation of postinflammatory and infectious strictures, for airway dehiscence after lung transplantation, and for the management of tracheobronchomalacia. Fistulas between trachea or bronchi and the esophagus and dehiscence of pneumonectomy stump can be protected with covered stents. Choice of stent depends on careful patient selection, characteristics of airway stenosis, physician's expertise, and availability of equipment. Placement of tube stents requires rigid bronchoscopy and dilatation of strictures beforehand, whereas metal stents can be applied using a flexible bronchoscope. Advantages and disadvantages of commonly used airway stents are discussed.

Lung cancer is the commonest cause of cancer-related mortality throughout the world. Only 25% of patients are diagnosed early and are candidates for surgical resection with curative intent. Many early-stage patients are medically inoperable owing to comorbidities. For these patients, and for selected patients with pulmonary metastases, radiofrequency ablation is a minimally invasive therapeutic alternative. Radiofrequency ablation can be performed percutaneously, under conscious sedation, and as an outpatient or with a short hospital stay. Outcomes are similar or even superior to those obtained with more aggressive procedures, with lower complication rates. Human studies describing the feasibility, safety, and outcomes of radiofrequency ablation for the treatment of primary and secondary lung malignancies are the focus of this article.

Medical pleuroscopy (MP) offers a safe and minimally invasive tool for interventional pulmonologists. It allows diagnosis of unexplained effusion, while at the same time allowing drainage and pleurodesis. It can also help in the diagnosis of diffuse interstitial disease or associated peripheral lung abnormality in the presence of effusion. It can have a therapeutic role in pneumothorax and hyperhidrosis or chronic pancreatic pain. This article reviews the technical aspects and range of applications of MP.

Clinics in Chest Medicine

RELATED INTEREST

Gastrointestinal Endoscopy Clinics Volume 20, Issue 1, Pages 1–168 (January 2010)
Endoluminal Therapy for Esophageal Disease
Edited by Herbert C. Wolfsen

Radiologic Clinics of North America Volume 48, Issue 1, Pages 1–212 (January 2010)
Thoracic MDCT Comes of Age
Edited by Sanjeev Bhalla

THE CLINICS ARE NOW AVAILABLE ONLINE!

Access your subscription at:
www.theclinics.com

Preface

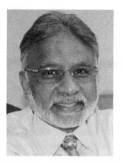

Atul C. Mehta, MB, BS, FACP, FCCP
Guest Editor

It is with great excitement and satisfaction that I submit to readers this issue of *Clinics in Chest Medicine* with a focus on interventional pulmonology. This is my fourth opportunity to be an editor on related topics, which gives me a chance to compare my notes from over the past 10 years. I'm glad to report that we have been on the right path.

Over the last decade, not only have we honored our past, but we have also become cognizant of the potential of our subspecialty. The pioneering work of Drs Killian, Jackson, Jackson, and Ikeda has been fully recognized and has been placed into a "time capsule." The World Association for Bronchology has established an award in the name of Dr Gustav Killian for his valuable contributions to the field and the legacy continues in its recipients. As the interest in the field has grown, several fellowship programs have come into being around the world and are playing roles in creating able, young bronchoscopists. This new generation continues to further the field in all different directions, seeming to take up the challenge of eliminating nondiagnostic bronchoscopy. Newer diagnostic tools, such as electromagnetic navigation, endobronchial ultrasound, autofluorescence bronchoscopy, and narrow-band imaging, have emerged, significantly improving the diagnostic utility of bronchoscopy. Pulmonologists have joined hands with radiologists, gastroenterologists, and thoracic surgeons to eliminate unnecessary mediastinoscopy and thoracotomy. Such innovations have improved the quality of life of patients suffering with terminal illnesses.

The therapeutic potentials of bronchoscopy, beyond laser applications and stent placement, are also being recognized. Research continues to confirm benefits of lung-volume reduction via endoscopic approaches. It is likely that, in the future, patients will no longer need to undergo major surgery for bronchopleural fistulas. "Bronchial thermoplasty" represents a new facet for treatment and shines a ray of hope in the management of bronchial asthma. At this juncture in the developing phase of interventional pulmonology, I claim that there is no pulmonary disease that a little bronchoscope can't either diagnose, palliate, or cure. As long as there are pulmonary ailments, the bronchoscope will continue to contribute to patients' welfare. Meanwhile, international societies now are welcoming the contributions of our subspecialty. Consensus statements and guidelines are being established for safe and judicious applications related to the subspecialty.

Of course, challenges remain. Technology is too expensive where it is most needed. The industry and physicians must seek out less expensive options. In certain areas of the world, including North America, remuneration falls far behind the cost and the value of procedures. This discrepancy needs to be adjusted. Meanwhile, charitable foundations need to step up to the plate to support bronchoscopy activity. Even today, some pulmonologists try to learn tricks of the trade without formal training (ie, "bronchoscopy by the books"). I compliment them for their enthusiasm and efforts. Nevertheless more training programs and courses should be created to disseminate the art and the science of interventional pulmonology. I also believe that success of our discipline requires that we be highly discriminating in the application of these advanced, expensive, and invasive procedures. As others

Clin Chest Med 31 (2010) xi–xiii
doi:10.1016/j.ccm.2009.12.001

have said: Because it can be done doesn't mean that it should be done. None of these tools should be used strictly to maintain skills or for secondary gains if other less invasive options exist.

My coauthors and I and other contributors to this volume of *Clinics in Chest Medicine* have tried to address some of these issues in a most comprehensive, state-of-the-art, yet concise fashion. I'm very thankful to this diverse group of international experts for helping me formulate a balanced perspective on interventional pulmonology. I sincerely hope readers appreciate and approve our efforts.

Atul C. Mehta, MB, BS, FACP, FCCP
Sheikh Khalifa Medical City Managed by
Cleveland Clinic, Abu Dhabi, UAE
Respiratory Institute, Cleveland Clinic
Cleveland, OH 44195, USA

E-mail address:
amehta@skmc.gov.ae

Dedication

To today's students and
Tomorrow's bronchoscopists.

Erratum

In the article, "Screening and Preventive Therapy for Tuberculosis" by Ben J. Marais, MMed Paed, FCPaed(SA), PhD, Helen Ayles, MB BS, PhD, Stephen M. Graham, MB BS, FRACP, DTCH, Peter Godfrey-Faussett, BA, MB BS, DTM&H, FRCP, which appeared in the December 2009 issue of *Clinics in Chest Medicine* (Vol. 30, No. 4), several of the author degrees were incorrect. The correct author degrees are listed herewith.

Clin Chest Med 31 (2010) xv
doi:10.1016/j.ccm.2010.01.001
0272-5231/10/$ – see front matter © 2010 Published by Elsevier Inc.

Bronchoscopy: The Past, the Present, and the Future

Heinrich D. Becker, MD

KEYWORDS

• Bronchoscopy • Endoscopy • History • Pioneers

In 1897, Kollofrath, assistant to Gustav Killian at the Poliklinik of Freiburg University, Germany, in the introduction to his report on the first broncho-scopic extraction of a foreign body, "Entfernung eines Knochenstücks aus dem rechten Bronchus auf natürlichem Wege und unter Anwendung der directen Laryngoskopie" in *Münchener Medicinische Wochenschrift*, wrote, "On March 30th of this year I had the honor to assist my admired principal, Prof. Killian in extraction of a piece of bone from the right bronchus. This case is of such peculiarity with respect to its diagnostic and therapeutic importance that a more extensive description seems justified."[1] In order to understand this statement, the state of the art of airway inspection at that time should be considered.[2]

THE PRE-ENDOSCOPIC ERA

Access to the airways in a living patient had been tried by Hippocrates (460–370 BC), who advised the introduction of a pipe into the larynx in a suffocating patient. Avicenna of Buchara (approximately AD 1000) used a silver pipe for the same purpose. Vesalius' observations (approximately 1542) reported that the heartbeat and pulsation of the great vessels stopped when he opened the chest of an experimental animal but returned again after he introduced a reed into the airway and inflated the lungs using bellows, mistakenly leading him to assume that the trachea was part of the circulation system, thereby carrying the name *tracus* (Greek for "rough") or *arteria aspera* (Latin for "the rough artery").[3,4]

Desault (1744–1795) advised nasotracheal intubation for the treatment of suffocation and removal of foreign bodies. For ages, the inhalation of a foreign body in more than half of accidents caused death or chronic illness from purulent infection, abscess or fistula formation, and malnutrition. Diverse instruments were designed to remove these foreign bodies blindly from the airways via the larynx or a tracheotomy, then called *bronchotomy*. The latter was also used for the treatment of subglottic stenosis, such as that caused by diphtheria.

As late as the second half of the nineteenth century, tracheotomy had a high mortality of more than 50%[5] and methods were developed for blind intubation. When he presented his "Treatise on the Diseases of the Air Passages," Horace Green in 1846 was blamed by the Commission of the New York Academy of Medical Sciences as presenting "...a monstrous assumption, ludicrously absurd, and physically impossible...an anatomical impossibility and unwarrantable innovation in practical medicine" and was removed from the society,[6,7] yet Joseph O'Dwyer agreed with Green, remained steadfast, and introduced the method for emergency intubation in children suffering from diphtheria.

THE DEVELOPMENT OF ENDOSCOPY

Although instruments for inspection of the body cavities, such as the mouth, nose, ear, vagina, rectum, urethra, and others, had been in use for ages, Porter in 1838 stated, "There is perhaps no kind of disease covered by greater darkness or posing more difficulties to the practitioner than those of the larynx and the trachea."[6] Until that point, the larynx could be only insufficiently inspected by forcible depression of the tongue with a spatula, a so-called Glossokatochon, and nobody had ever looked into the living trachea. It

Department of Interdisciplinary Endoscopy, Thoraxklinik at Heidelberg University, Amalienstrasse 5, D-69126, Heidelberg, Germany
E-mail address: hdb@bronchology.org

Clin Chest Med 31 (2010) 1–18
doi:10.1016/j.ccm.2009.11.001

was only after the advent of three major inventions that direct inspection of the airways and visually controlled treatment became possible: (1) instruments for inspection, (2) suitable light sources, and (3) adequate anesthesia.

The Laryngeal Mirror

Experiments for inspection of the larynx with the help of mirrors had been performed, among others, by Latour (1825), Senn (1829), Belloc (1837), Liston (1840), and Avery (1844). It was not a physician, however, but a singing teacher in London, Manuel Garcia, who in 1854 first observed his own larynx with the help of a dental mirror that he had bought from the French instrument maker, Charriére, in Paris.[8–10] Without knowing his work, almost at the same time, in 1856, a laryngologist, Ludwig Türck, in Vienna, performed his first experiments with a similar device. He gave away his device to a physiologist, Czermak, from Budapest, when in winter the illumination was no longer sufficient for continuation of his studies. Czermak reported his findings before Türck, which resulted in a long fight over rights of priority, the so-called Türkenkrieg (Turks war).[11,12]

Using these instruments, diagnosis and treatment of laryngeal diseases became much easier, so that Gibb in 1862 stated, "It has fallen to my lot to see cases of laryngeal disease...that have existed for ten or twenty years, and submitted to every variety of treatment, without the slightest benefit, at the hands of some of the foremost amongst us, wherein the symptoms have depended upon a little growth attached to one or both vocal chords, which was recognized in as many seconds as the complaints had existed years. The nature of the malady thus being made out, the plan of treatment to be pursued became obvious."[13] Also in 1862, the German surgeon, von Bruns, in Tübingen, with the help of this laryngoscopic mirror was able for the first time to remove a polyp from a vocal chord in his own brother. Without suitable anesthetics, the procedure needed weeks of preparation by gradual desensitization on the patient's part and much training on anatomic/surgical preparations and living larynx of volunteers. His report was rejected as "...a daring deed that should not be imitated and the practical importance of which seems less as there would be hardly another opportunity for its repetition." One of the major problems was the indirect and reverse view of the image, which added to the difficulties.[14]

The First Endoscopes and Light Sources

In contrast to other fields of endoscopy, where daylight or candlelight could be introduced for inspection of the vagina, rectum, urethra, and so forth, it was only after Bozzini (**Fig. 1**), a general practitioner in Frankfurt, developed an "illuminator" in 1805 that a suitable light source for inspection of the trachea came within sight. This somewhat clumsy device consisted of a box containing a candle, the light of which was reflected by a hollow mirror into a "conductor," a split metallic tube that could be spread by a simple mechanism. For organs that could not be visualized by direct inspection, he used a tube with a mirror for reflection of the light and image.[15]

The first recognized successor of this technology was Desormeaux, who in 1853 introduced the word, *endoscope*, for his instrument to inspect body cavities. It was with Desormeaux's endoscope that Kußmaul could perform the first esophagoscopies in 1867–1868.[16] The illumination by Gazogen, however, was insufficient for inspection of the stomach. The first suitable gastroscope was introduced in 1881 by von Mikulicz and Leiter. It was made up of a closed optics with lenses and prisms that were electrically illuminated at the distal end by a glowing platinum wire; the latter had to be cooled off by a constant flow of water and thus was not suitable for application in the airways.[17]

Esophagoscopy was performed mainly by the use of hollow tubes and spatulas that were connected to a proximal illumination sources. The Viennese endoscope maker, Leiter, also produced, in 1886, the first so-called panelectroscope, a tube that was connected to a handle that contained an electric bulb and a prism for illumination. The instrument was modified by many, including Gottstein, who was the first to attach a metal tube to this device, in 1891. Rosenheim accidentally passed the instrument into the trachea and Kirstein from Berlin intentionally started to intubate the larynx with the esophagoscope. After his initial experiments in 1894, Kirstein began systematic, direct inspection of the airways, which he referred to as "autoscopy" (*autos* is Greek for himself, thus *autoscopy* means directly without help of a mirror). "...I convinced myself...that one can pass the vocal chords intentionally with a middle sized esophagoscope into the cocainized trachea and right down to the bifurcation; this experience should be eventually fructified." But as "The region of the lower trachea is a very dangerous place!...The rhythmic protrusion of its wall is...a regular and awe inspiring phenomenon, which gives cause for utmost care in introducing rigid instruments." He unfortunately did not "fructify"(ie, expand his experiments).[18] The rhinolaryngologist, Killian (**Fig. 2**), in 1895, attended Kirstein's lecture in Heidelberg at the second Congress of

1805

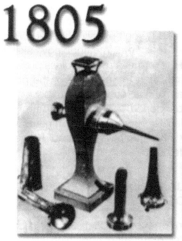 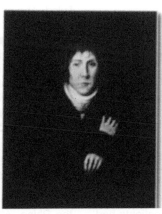 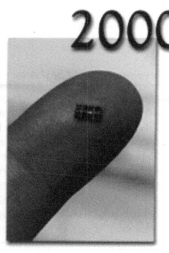

2000

Fig. 1. Philipp Bozzini, practitioner in Frankfurt, Germany (*center*), inventor of the first illuminator for endoscopes in 1805 (*left*). The heat of the candle within the wooden box escapes via a vent on the top. The light is reflected by a mirror to a side port, to which different devices for inspection of body cavities can be attached. When he presented his prototype at the medical faculty of Vienna university in 1807, it was dismissed as "merely a toy," useless for clinical application. The physicians at the Military Academy of Emperor Joseph II, however, were enthusiastic and greeted it as, "the eye at the fingertip" of the physician, which today, with chip technology, has proved correct (*right*).

the Southern German Laryngologists and immediately recognized the importance of Kirstein's observation for the diagnosis and treatment of laryngotracheal diseases and began his experiments with this new method.

In 1877, a urologist, Nitze, of Dresden, and the manufacturer Leiter, of Vienna constructed the

first optic lens in which electric illumination was performed by a glowing platinum wire at the distal end. Once again, the platinum wire had to be cooled off by a constant flow of water when not used inside the urinary bladder, similar to von Mikulicz' first gastroscope. Only after 1879, when Edison invented the electric bulb, which was

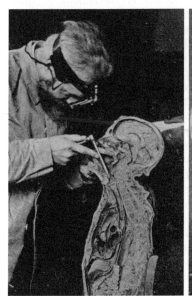 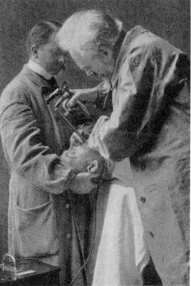

Fig. 2. Gustav Killian, inventor of bronchoscopy. After exploring the possibility of introducing a rigid tube for inspection of the airways by direct access via the oropharyngeal route on frozen corpses, he ventured to examine patients. Here he is seen introducing the rigid bronchoscope, which is attached to the Casper's electroscope handle while an assistant is holding the patient's head.

further miniaturized by Mignon, could distal electric illumination be applied to endoscopy of the airways.

The Development of Local Anesthesia

In his first report on the invention of direct bronchoscopy, Killian wrote, "Whether one stops inspection with the rigid tube at the bifurcation or passes on for some distance into a major bronchus does not matter for the patient. If he is sufficiently cocainized he does not even realize it."[19] Before the discovery of cocaine, many attempts had been made to anesthetize the airways by the use of potassium bromide, ammonia, belladonna, iodine solution, chloroform, morphine, and so forth. Nothing proved adequate and patients had to be desensitized with weeks of rehearsing touching the pharynx and the vocal chords by themselves before a procedure could be performed. The examiner had to be extremely skilled and swift as operations had to be performed within seconds before the view disappeared. von Bruns advised training on an excised larynx and on a head that had been severed from a corpse and hung from a hook before training on a volunteer "…who certainly could be found rather easily for a little amount of money and would suffer such not really pleasant but not at all painful or dangerous experiments."[14]

Although Morton in Boston had introduced general anesthesia by chloroform in 1848, its use was so dangerous that it was only rarely applied in laryngoscopic operations. In 1882, a young scientist at the Pharmacological Institute in Vienna, Sigmund Freud, experimented with cocaine, a sample of which he had bought from Merck.[20] He was eager to make a fortune with a breakthrough invention in science and be able to marry his fiancée. But to his later dismay his experiments in withdrawing morphinists from their addiction resulted in disaster. Although he had advised his colleague, Koller, an eye specialist, to use cocaine solution for pain relief when he suffered from severe conjunctivitis, he failed to recognize the importance of his observation himself that cocaine caused numbness when he put it to his tongue. Koller, however, immediately realized the potential of this observation and after feverishly experimenting with this new "miracle drug" on rabbits and patients he inaugurated local anesthesia in his lecture on September 15, 1884, at the annual Congress of German Ophthalmologists in Heidelberg. At the same time, a Viennese laryngologist, Jellinek, introduced cocaine as local anesthetic for inspection of the airways: "By eliminating the reflexes of the pharynx and the larynx it

was possible to perform some of the operations in which even the most skillful artists in surgery had failed. The procedure completely changed. Virtuosity gave way to careful methodology, skill to exactness and the former almost endless preparation that so often tried the patience of the physician as well as of the patient could be almost completely abandoned."[6] Thus the path was paved for Killian to pursue his experiments with bronchoscopy after he had attended Kirstein's lecture in Heidelberg.

GUSTAV KILLIAN AND THE INVENTION OF BRONCHOSCOPY

Killian was born on the June 2, 1860, at Mainz on the Rhine. After graduation from high school in 1878, he began to study medicine at the University of Strassburg, where one of his teachers was Adolf Kussmaul. After 1880 he continued clinical education at Freiburg, Berlin, and Heidelberg (Germany), where he passed his final examination in 1882. He started practical work at the municipal hospital of Mannheim, close to Heidelberg, and later in Berlin to get special education in otorhinolaryngology by Hartmann and Fraenkel. As he could not find other employment, Killian settled down as practitioner in Mannheim in 1887, yet within 4 months he was offered a position as head of the section of rhinolaryngology at Freiburg, a part of the large faculty of internal medicine, which he gladly accepted.[3,21]

At the meeting of the South German Laryngological Society in Heidelberg in 1889, he gave a short report on a new technique for examination of the dorsal wall of the larynx. Killian learned about Kirstein's new technique at the meeting of the Laryngological Society in Heidelberg in 1895. Because of the experiences of Pieniazek at Krakau, who had introduced direct lower tracheoscopy via tracheostomy without any complications,[22] Killian realized the potential of this new method of direct inspection of the trachea and in 1896 began his own experimental work. In tracheotomized patients, he passed the bifurcation with the bronchoscope, a somewhat modified esophagoscope of Rosenheim and noticed that the bronchi were elastic and flexible and he was "stopped only when the diameter of the tube was surpassing that of the bronchi." After confirming his findings in corpses without tracheotomies, he performed the first direct endoscopy via the larynx in a healthy volunteer. He noticed the flexibility of the trachea and how easy he could adjust it to the angle of the main bronchi and introduce the endoscope down to the lobar airways. "I think I have made an important discovery," he noted afterwards. Thus the bronchoscopy was born. During the same year, 1897, he removed the first foreign body via the translaryngeal route, which was elegantly reported by his coworker, Kollofrath.[1]

After further experiences and removal of two more foreign bodies Killian felt safe to present his new method of "direct bronchoscopy" at the sixth meeting of the South German Laryngological Society at Heidelberg in 1898. During the same year, his first publication on direct bronchoscopy was also published.[19] The following years at Freiburg were full of technical improvements of the new method, with the quest for more and more indications for its use. He published 34 papers concerning discovery, technique, and clinical application of his invention. In 1900 he received an award from *Wiener Klinische Wochenschrift* for his article, "Bronchoscopy and its Application in Foreign Bodies of the Lung." As a result of his publications and many lectures he became famous and Freiburg became a mecca for bronchoscopy. Hundreds of physicians came from all over the world (the list of participants notes 437 foreign guests from all continents, including more than 120 from the United States) and up to 20 training courses had to be held every year. He was invited as a popular speaker all over Europe and patients were sent to him from as far as South America for treatment of foreign bodies, as his son, Hans Killian, a famous surgeon himself, later reported.[23]

In order to fully understand the importance of endoscopic removal of foreign bodies the state of thoracic surgery during Killian's era should be considered. Most patients fell chronically ill after the aspiration of a foreign body, suffering from atelectasis, chronic pneumonia, and hemorrhage, to which half of them succumbed if left untreated. Surgical procedures were restricted to "pneumotomy," when the bronchus was occluded by extensive solid scar tissue and the foreign body could not be reached by the bronchoscope, which had a high mortality rate. Lobectomy or pneumonectomy could not be performed at that time. Brunn and Lilienthal developed the surgical techniques for lobectomy in 1910 and Nissen, Haight, and Graham introduced pneumonectomy in 1930, as until that time techniques of safe closure of the bronchial stump were nonexistent.[24] Thus, for those who were confronted with these patients, it must have seemed like a miracle that, shortly after the introduction of bronchoscopy, almost all patients could be cured. According to a statistical analysis by Killian's coworker Albrecht on 703 patients with aspiration, between the years 1911 and 1921, in all but 12 the foreign body could be removed bronchoscopically. In many of these patients, the foreign bodies were of prolonged duration despite a success rate of 98.3%.[25] In light

of this situation, Killian's triumphant remarks become understandable when he stated, "One has to be witness when a patient who feels himself doomed to death can be saved by the simple procedure of introducing a tube with the help of a little cocaine. One must have had the experience of seeing a child that at 4PM aspirated a little stone, and that, after the stone has been bronchoscopically removed at 6PM, may happily return home at 8PM after anesthesia has faded away. Even if bronchoscopy was ten times more difficult as it really is, we would have to perform it just for having these results."[21]

In addition to this major innovation, Killian introduced many instruments for foreign body extraction and other devices, such as a dilator and even the first endobronchial stent.[26] Although the development of bronchoscopy was Killian's main interest in the years at Freiburg, he also pushed ahead in other fields. He developed the method of submucosal resection of the septum and a new technique for the radical surgery for chronic empyema of the nasal sinuses with resection of the orbital roof and creation of an osseous flap.[27] In approximately 1906 he began intensive studies of the anatomy and the function of the esophageal orifice and found the lower part of the cricopharyngeus muscle to be the anatomic substrate of the upper esophageal sphincter. According to his observations, it was between this lower horizontal part and the oblique upper part of the muscle that Zenker's pulsion diverticulum developed, where the muscular layer was thinnest. One of his scholars, Seiffert, later developed a method of endoscopic dissection of the membrane formed by the posterior wall of the diverticulum and the anterior wall of the esophagus. In 1907, he received an invitation by the American Laryngological, Rhinological and Otological Society and it was on this triumphant journey through the United States that he gave a lecture on these findings at the meeting of the German Medical Society of New York, which was also published in *Laryngoscope* during the same year.[28] His lectures were followed by practical demonstrations of his bronchoscopic and surgical techniques and by banquets at night. On his trip he also visited Washington, DC, and had a brief meeting with President Theodore Roosevelt. In Pittsburgh, he met Chevalier Jackson (**Fig. 3**), already an outstanding pioneer of esophagobronchology at the University of Pennsylvania. He was awarded the first honorary membership of the American Laryngological, Rhinological and Otological Society, became an honorary member of the American Medical Association, and received a medal in commemoration of his visit.[21]

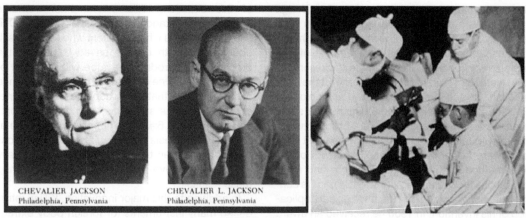

CHEVALIER JACKSON
Philadelphia, Pennsylvania

CHEVALIER L. JACKSON
Philadelphia, Pennsylvania

Fig. 3. Chevalier Jackson and his son and successor, Chevalier L. Jackson, were the pioneers of bronchoscopy in the United States. With the patient in supine position, an assistant still had to hold the head, which was hanging free over the edge of the examination table.

Killian was the most famous laryngologist in Germany and in 1911 when Fraenkel at Berlin retired, he became the successor to the most important chair of rhinolaryngology. Although bronchoscopy seemed to have reached its peak, he believed that visualization of the larynx was unsatisfactory. Using Kirstein's spatula, Killian realized that inspection of the larynx in a hanging position of the head was much easier. This made him design a special laryngoscope that could be fixed to a supporting devise by a hook, a technique he called *suspension-laryngoscopy*, by which he could use both hands for manipulation.[29] His coworker, Seiffert, improved the method by using a chest rest, a technique that later was brought to perfection by Kleinsasser and is still used for endolaryngeal microsurgery.

In 1911 Killian was nominated as a professor at the Kaiser Wilhelm Military Academy of Medicine. During World War I he had to treat laryngeal injuries at the front line in France. He was joined by his two sons, who were assigned to the same front. After his return, he founded a center for the treatment of injuries of the larynx and the trachea. During this era he was also concerned with reconstruction of these organs by plastic surgery. He referred to work by Dieffenbach and Lexer, two of the most outstanding plastic surgeons of that time, who had also worked in Berlin. The article on the injuries of the larynx was his last scientific work before he death in 1921 from gastric cancer.

During his last years, Killian prepared several publications on the history of laryngotracheobronchoscopy.[30] For teaching purposes, in 1893 he began illustrating his lectures by direct epidiascopic projection of the endoscopic image above the patient's head. Phantoms of the nose, the larynx, and the tracheobronchial tree were constructed according to his suggestions.[31] Because of his always cheerful mood, he was called *semper ridens* (always smiling) and in his later years, his head being framed by a tuft of white hair, his nickname was Santa Claus. He created a school for laryngologists and his pupils dominated the field of German laryngology and bronchology for years. Albrecht and Brünings published a textbook on direct endoscopy of the airways and esophagus in 1915.[25] Like von Eicken at Erlangen and Berlin and Seiffert at Heidelberg, they had become heads of the most important departments of otorhinolaryngology in Germany. It was to his merit that the separate disciplines of rhinolaryngology and otology were combined. After Killian died in 1921, his ideas spread around the world. Everywhere, skilled endoscopists developed new techniques, and bronchoscopy became a standard procedure in diagnosis of the airways. His work was also the foundation for the new discipline of anesthesiology, providing the idea and instruments (laryngoscope by Macintosh) for the access to the airways and endotracheal anesthesia.

Throughout his professional life, Killian continued to improve and invent instruments and look for new applications. He applied fluoroscopy, which had been detected by Roentgen of Würzburg (Germany) in 1895, for probing peripheral lesions and foreign bodies.[32,33] To establish the x-ray anatomy of the segmental bronchi, he introduced bismuth powder.[34] Killian drained pulmonary abscesses and instilled drugs for clearance via the bronchial route and he even used the bronchoscope for "pleuroscopy" (thoracoscopy) and transthoracic "pneumoscopy" when abscesses had drained externally.[32] Foreign bodies that had been in place for a long time and had been imbedded by extensive granulations were successfully extracted after treatment of the stenosis by a metallic dilator and, in cases of restenosis, metallic or rubber tubes were introduced as stents. Although cancer was a relatively rare disease (31 primary and 135 secondary cancers in 11,000 postmortem examinations), he pointed out the importance of pre- and postoperative bronchoscopy.[34] In 1914 Killian described endoluminal radiotherapy in cancer of the larynx by mesothorium[35] and in the textbook of his coworkers, Brünings and Albrecht, published in 1915, there is the first description of successful curation of a tracheal carcinoma after endoluminal brachyradiotherapy.[25] Killian took special interest in teaching his students to maintain high standards in quality management by constantly analyzing the results of their work and always keeping in mind that they were standing on the shoulders of excellent pioneers. He always tried he keep up with the tradition of the excellence of the most respected physicians in his profession, such as Billroth of Vienna. In his inaugural lecture in Berlin in 1911, Killian pointed out that it was internal medicine from which the art spread to the other faculties, that patience and empathy should be the main features of physicians, and that they should remain persistent in following their dreams because "to live means to fight." He ignited the flame of enthusiasm in hundreds of his contemporaries who spread the technique of bronchoscopy to other specialties, thus establishing the roots of contemporary interventional procedures, such as microsurgery of the larynx (Kleinsasser) and intubation anesthesia (Macintosh, Melzer, and Kuhn).

RIGID BRONCHOSCOPY IN THE TWENTIETH CENTURY
Main Schools

Because of the enthusiastic activities of Killian and his assistants in teaching and spreading the new technique, hundreds of specialists all over the world learned bronchoscopy and many improvements were added to the instrument. Thus by 1910 Killian had collected and reviewed 1116 articles—410 on esophagoscopy, 34 on gastroscopy, and 672 on laryngotracheobronchoscopy—in order to write his comprehensive review of the history of bronchoscopy and esophagoscopy.[30] At that stage, it was evident that it was not possible to follow all traits in every continent and several schools of thoughts started to emerge.

Killian's coworkers—von Eicken, Albrecht, Brünings, Seiffert, and others—for decades held the chairs of all important departments in Germany. They improved Killian's instruments and introduced new methods, such as endoscopic treatment of Zenker's diverticulum by Seiffert. Seiffert also developed a chest rest for suspension laryngoscopy in 1922, which was perfected by Kleinsasser in 1964 as the currently used device for microlaryngoscopy. Unfortunately, after World War II the development of rigid bronchoscopy took separate paths, until recently. In Western Germany, Huzly in Stuttgart was the most prominent proponent of rigid bronchoscopy and in 1961 edited his photographic atlas of bronchoscopy.[36] Riecker introduced relaxation by curare in 1952, which was replaced by succinylcholine by Mündnich and Hoflehner in 1953. Maassen introduced bronchography via double-lumen catheter in 1956. Two companies, Storz and Wolf, became the most important instrument makers in Germany and introduced new technologies, such as the Hopkins telescope and television cameras. Currently, Dierkesmann, Freitag, Häußinger, Macha, and Becker are the proponents of rigid bronchoscopy for the development and performance of interventional procedures, such as laser treatment, stenting, and photodynamic laser therapy. In East Germany, Friedel developed the first ventilation bronchoscope (1956), which was modified by Brandt (1963), who edited an extensive textbook on endoscopy of the air and food passages, in 1985, in which he reported on more than 100 successful treatments by endobronchial stenting, which he had began in the early 1970s.[37] In the same year that Schiepatti of Buenos Aires wrote about transtracheal puncture of the carinal lymph nodes, Euler reported on pulmonary and aortic angiography by transbronchial puncture in 1948–1949, and later, in 1955, he reported on the technique of rigid transbronchial needle aspiration (TBNA) for mediastinal masses, which was further perfected by Schießle in 1962.[38]

In the United States, Coolidge, in 1898, performed the first lower tracheobronchoscopy at Massachusetts General Hospital.[4] Jackson in Philadelphia, whom Killian had met on his visit to the United States in 1907, together with the Pillings Manufacturing Company, made many improvements to instruments for bronchoscopy and esophagoscopy and was recognized as the Father of American Bronchoesophagology. During his training to become a laryngologist, he visited London in 1886, where he was shown the "impractical device designed by Morel Mackenzie in an effort visually to inspect the esophagus."[39] In 1890 he constructed the first endoscope "worthy of the name" for esophagoscopy and in 1904 he constructed the first "American Bronchoscope." After Einhorn in New York added an integrated light conductor and Ingals of Chicago introduced distal illumination to the esophagoscope, Jackson equipped his bronchoscope with a light carrier with a miniaturized electric mignon bulb at the distal end and with an additional suction channel. Confronted by many patients suffering from aspiration of foreign bodies, he invented many instruments for their retrieval. In 1907 he published the first systematic textbook on bronchoesophagology, which he dedicated to Killian, the Father of Bronchoscopy. In this book, he addressed modern issues of quality management, such as analysis and prevention of complications; rationale for the construction of bronchoscopy suites; and arrangement of equipment and staffing of such facilities (**Fig. 4**). As a philanthropist, he constantly refused to have his inventions patented as he wanted them to be used as widely as possible, and through his persistence with the government, he pushed forward a law for the prevention of accidents by ingestion of caustic agents. He was a perfectionist in technique and convinced that teaching had to be performed on animals before treating patients. Therefore, he always refused to go back to England where animal rights activists prevented such training courses. In 1928, in recognition of his "conspicuous achievements in the broad field of surgical science," he was awarded the Bigelow Medal by the Boston Surgical Society, presented to him by Cushing "for his eminent performances and creative power by which he opened new fields of endeavor" and in acknowledgement of his "indefinable greatness of personality."[40] He simultaneously held five chairs of laryngology at different hospitals in his hometowns of Pittsburgh and Philadelphia. His son, Chevalier L. Jackson, also became a laryngologist and was his successor at the Temple University of Philadelphia. He was the founder of the Pan American Association of Otorhinolaryngology and Bronchology and of the International Bronchoesophagological Society

and cofounder of the World Medical Association. With his father, he edited the last issue of a textbook in otorhinolaryngology.[41] Their school extends into the modern era, as many of today's specialists teachers were trained by the Jacksons, including Broyles in Baltimore, who, after additional training by Haslinger in Vienna, introduced the optic telescope for bronchoscopy in 1940, the optical forceps in 1948, and fiber illumination for the rigid bronchoscope in 1962. His scholar, Tucker, became professor at Thomas Jefferson University in Philadelphia, where he trained Marsh, who maintained the tradition with Norris, Hollinger, and Brubaker, who became specialists in pediatric bronchoscopy and introduced color photography in the 1940s. Hollinger's son today is a famous pediatric laryngologist. Andersen was the first to perform bronchoscopic transbronchial lung biopsy via the rigid bronchoscope in 1965. Sanders in 1967 introduced jet ventilation for rigid bronchoscopy.

After spending some time with Killian in Freiburg, it was Kubo of Kyushu University in Fukuoka who introduced bronchoscopy to Japan in 1907. He was joined by Chiba, who, after training with Brünings, stayed in Tokyo from 1910 on. Ono, who was trained by Jackson in 1934, founded the Japan Broncho-Esophagological Society in 1949. Ikeda (**Fig. 5**), who later developed the flexible fiberscope, introduced fiberglass illumination for the rigid bronchoscope in 1962. When Ikeda, who found rigid bronchoscopy under local anesthesia in the sitting position on Killian's chair cumbersome, introduced the flexible bronchoscope, he used it in combination with a flexible tube that could be straightened by a locking mechanism so that he was still able to introduce the rigid endoscope in the same session. In the era of expanding interventional procedures, this method of combining the rigid and the flexible endoscope has regained attention.

Technical Developments

Illumination
After the advent of the electric bulb, illumination became sufficient for the airways. Initially the lamps were installed separately on statives or fixed to a headrest from which the light was reflected into the endoscope. Connection of the light source to the endoscope improved handling considerably. Killian and his coworkers preferred to use Casper's panelectroscope, which integrated the light bulb into the handle from which it was reflected by a prism to the endoscope because it was not as easily soiled by secretions. Jackson, however, used distal illumination via a light guide with a mignon bulb at its tip. In the

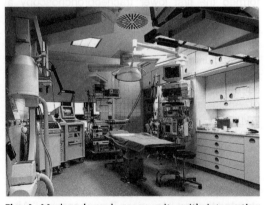

Fig. 4. Modern bronchoscopy suite with integration of all advanced diagnostic and interventional instruments.

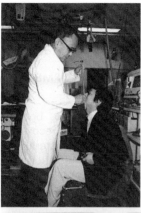

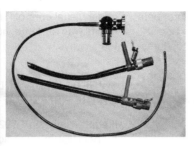

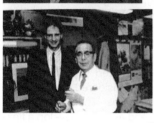

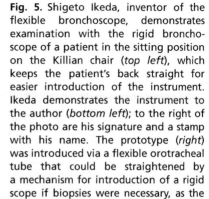

Fig. 5. Shigeto Ikeda, inventor of the flexible bronchoscope, demonstrates examination with the rigid bronchoscope of a patient in the sitting position on the Killian chair (*top left*), which keeps the patient's back straight for easier introduction of the instrument. Ikeda demonstrates the instrument to the author (*bottom left*); to the right of the photo are his signature and a stamp with his name. The prototype (*right*) was introduced via a flexible orotracheal tube that could be straightened by a mechanism for introduction of a rigid scope if biopsies were necessary, as the flexible scope lacked a biopsy channel.

late 1880s, von Schrötter in Vienna developed a rigid light guide made up of glass, which Storz improved by introducing quartz. After Tyndall's first description of the optical properties of glass fibers in 1872, patents for glass fibers as a transport medium were almost simultaneously given to Baird in England (1926), Hansell in the United States (1927), and Marconi in England (1930). The first prototype of a fiberscope was presented by Lamm in Munich (1930). After Hansen in Denmark described the first fiber bundles for light transportation in 1930, van Heel in the Netherlands and O'Brian in the United States developed the first endoscopes for bronchoscopy and gastroscopy in 1953 and 1954, respectively. The rod lens and fiberoptic lighting device by Hopkins in London was adopted by Storz as cold light illumination source for his rigid endoscopes in 1963. The transition to fully flexible endoscopes with image transport by glass fibers was performed by Hirschowitz and the American Cystoscope Makers company in 1958 after Curtiss of Ann Arbor, Michigan, had described the first medical fiber instrument in 1955.

Pictures, films, and video documentation

The first (even stereoscopic) endophotographies were performed by Czermak using a giant laryngeal mirror. Stein in Frankfurt used magnesium illumination for his photographic apparatus, the "heliopictor" (in approximately 1875), technically the predecessor of the Polaroid Land camera of 100 years later. Stein's camera was further improved by Nitze and Kollmann. In 1907 Benda introduced color photography, which was first introduced by Hollinger to bronchoscopy in 1941. Soulas (1949) and Hollinger (1956) also introduced endoscopic film documentation. The first television transmission of a bronchoscopy was performed by de Monternaud in 1955. Wittmoser constructed an angulated optic for improvement of image transfer and produced the first video documentation in 1969.

Prospects

With the advent of the flexible bronchoscope after 1966 two developments took place. First, bronchoscopy rapidly spread beyond otorhinolaryngologic and specialized thoracic clinics and the overall number of rigid bronchoscopies declined rapidly until the late 1980s and early 1990s because flexible bronchoscopy was much easier to perform. Once again, however, an increasing number of interventional techniques demanded use of the rigid bronchoscope for safety reasons. Special rigid devices were developed by Dumon for application of the Nd:YAG laser and placement of his dedicated stent. Consensus task forces of the Scientific Section of Endoscopy of the German

Society of Pulmonology and of the European Respiratory Society/American Thoracic Society agreed that for many interventional procedures bronchoscopists and staff should at least be trained in the technique of rigid bronchoscopy and should have the instrument at hand in case of an emergency (**Fig. 6**). Thus, in training courses all over the world handling of the rigid instrument is being taught once again.

Flexible Bronchoscopy

Broad application of bronchoscopy took place only after the development of flexible instruments that could be easily introduced under local anesthesia. The pioneer of this technique was Ikeda at the National Cancer Center Hospital in Tokyo, Japan. After Kubo and Ono had introduced rigid bronchoscopy and related technologies to Japan, Ikeda became the proponent of bronchoscopy and pioneer in flexible bronchoscopy.[42,43] Fiberoptic technology had been introduced to gastrointestinal endoscopy some time earlier. Glass fiber bundles were used for illumination by cold light to replace bulbs at the tip of endoscopes, which produced considerable heat and potential damage. In addition, the instruments themselves became flexible and made inspection of the organs easier. The first application was in connection with gastrocameras that had a small photographic lens system at their tip with miniature films that could be analyzed by viewing with a projector. With progress of reduction in fiber size and improvement of fiber arrangement, imaging via optic fiber bundles became possible, allowing real-time inspection and instrumentation

under visual control. The diameter of these instruments was too large, however, for introduction into the airways.

SHIGETO IKEDA AND THE DEVELOPMENT OF THE FIBERSCOPE

Ikeda, born in 1925, decided to become a specialist in thoracic medicine after recovering from tuberculosis at the age of 23 and started his education in thoracic surgery.[44] In 1962 he joined the National Cancer Center in Tokyo where he also performed rigid bronchoscopy for diagnosis of lung cancer, using, among other instruments, the curette developed by Tsuboi.[45] For better illumination in esophagoscopy he had fiber glass light transmission applied to the rigid optics. With regard to the flexibility of the fibers and the experiences that had been gathered with fiber optics in gastroenterology he considered applying the technique in bronchoscopes. Thus, in 1962 he approached Machida and asked to develop a flexible bronchofiberscope with a diameter of less than 6 mm, containing approximately 15,000 glass fibers of less than 15 mm. In 1964 he obtained the first prototype of this device and, after further improvement in 1966, he was able to present the first useful instrument at a meeting in Copenhagen, a sensation reported in the *New York Times*. After further technical improvements to enhance maneuvering and image quality and including a biopsy channel for taking biopsies, the Machida flexible bronchoscope became commercially available in 1968, considered the year of the second revolution in bronchoscopy.[46] Shortly

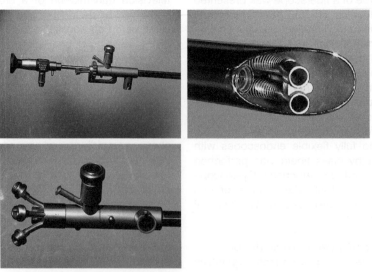

Fig. 6. Modern rigid endoscope (Efer-Dumon) for interventions. The proximal end has various ports for introducing instruments, such as suction catheters and laser probes, and for ventilation and a ring for controlling the bending of the two channels at the distal end.

afterwards, in 1970, the first Olympus model was commercialized with better handling and imaging properties. In 1968 Ikeda demonstrated the new instrument at many international meetings and presented it at the National Institutes of Health and the Mayo Clinic in Rochester, Minnesota, where he also learned about the Mayo mass screening project for early detection of lung cancer in 1970. This was the inspiration for establishing several screening projects in Japan. From 1972 to 1974, the so-called first Ikeda group performed a successful study on early detection of hilar-type lung cancer, including analysis of 3-day pooled sputum and bronchoscopy for localization. After the positive experience with this project, from 1975 to 1978, the second Ikeda group investigated early detection of peripheral nodular lesions by x-ray screening and bronchoscopy. Between the years of 1981 and 1984, a pilot study for mass screening of individuals at risk from smoking was carried out by the third Ikeda group, the results of which led to an even larger mass screening project from 1984 to 1987, supported by the Ministry of Health and Welfare, the results of which were published by Naruke and Kaneko.

Eager to spread the technique of flexible bronchoscopy with the fiberscope, Ikeda organized several investigational groups and many training courses. In 1975 the Anti-Lung Cancer Association was founded in Japan for early detection in smokers over age 40. To enhance understanding and to have a systematic approach, Ikeda developed a new terminology for the bronchial tree and dedicated models for training, correlating in particular with radiographic interpretation. In 1978, the study group for bronchoscopy had its first meeting in Osaka and, with Ideda's enthusiasm and efforts, spread the art of bronchoscopy. The flexible bronchoscope was applied worldwide and the vast majority of bronchoscopies were performed by this technique under local anesthesia. In 1978 Ikeda organized the first World Congress for Bronchology in Tokyo and founded the World Association for Bronchology in 1979, of which he was elected the first chairman. In 1983 the Japan Society for Bronchology was inaugurated.[47]

Ikeda never stopped improving the instrument and developing new techniques in connection with flexible bronchoscopy. His next major achievement was the introduction of video technique, which he began investigating in 1983, which finally was commercialized in 1987. In 1979 Ikeda suffered a cerebral ischemic insult and more followed during the successive years along with several myocardial infarctions, to which he succumbed to in 2001. In Japan, several enthusiastic doctors introduction flexible bronchoscopy to new techniques. Among those pioneers were Arai, performing transbronchial lung biopsies; Kato, treating early lung cancer by photodynamic therapy (PDT)[48–50]; and Watanabe, introducing the spigot for treatment of bronchial fistulae. With the increasing need and popularity of interventional procedures, the necessity for reintroduction of rigid bronchoscopy combined with the flexible bronchoscope became obvious and in 1998 Miyazawa organized the first international conference for this purpose in Hiroshima.

FURTHER DEVELOPMENTS IN FLEXIBLE BRONCHOSCOPY

The ease of application and of access beyond the central airways has led to vast opportunities for introduction of new optical, diagnostic, and therapeutic techniques, starting with transbronchial lung biopsy, performed by Anderson and Zavala after Ikeda's visit to the United States. In 1974 Reynolds published the first experiences with bronchoalveolar lavage. Cortese demonstrated the potential of early lung cancer detection by fluorescence, induced by injection of hematoporphyrine derivates (HPD) in 1978. In the same year Wang had started TBNA of mediastinal lymph nodes via the flexible bronchoscope, which until then was only rarely applied via rigid instruments. The first endobronchial application of the Nd:YAG laser was performed by Toty in the same year and in 1980 Dumon published his results on photoablation of stenoses by Nd:YAG laser treatment, which became the most common therapeutic bronchoscopic procedure in the years to come. In parallel, Hayata and Kato applied PDT after sensitization by HPD for treatment of centrally located early lung cancer. In 1979 Hilaris used radioactive probes for the treatment of central airway cancer for endoscopic high-dose radiation therapy (HDR). With rapid development and miniaturization of electronic imaging by charge-coupled device chips, the first video bronchoscope was developed by Ikeda in cooperation with Pentax in 1987. Two years later, in 1990, the first dedicated stent for the airways was presented by Dumon and in 1991 Lam reported on autofluorescence bronchoscopy without the need for HPD for early detection of lung cancer. The need for local staging of these lesions was met by the introduction of endobronchial ultrasound (EBUS) in 1999 by Becker. This technology was studied with a wide range of applications for diagnosis within the mediastinum and the lung and most recently in connection with transbronchial needle espiration by a dedicated ultrasonic bronchoscope

(2003). This innovation has a potential for replacing mediastinoscopy in staging of lung cancer.

Early detection of lung cancer created further demand for new imaging modalities using high-power magnification video bronchoscopes and narrow band imaging for analysis of subtle vascular structures, headed by the work of Shibuya in 2002. Endoscopic optical coherence tomography, which provides information of the layer structure of the bronchial wall with higher resolution than EBUS (Fujimoto 2002), is currently under investigation for bronchoscopic applications.

Maneuvering smart diagnostic tools inside the airways beyond the visible range has been enhanced by smart electromagnetic navigation (2003), which also supported bronchoscopic treatment of peripheral lesions by insertion of brachytherapy catheters (2005). Recently, the first results of studies for treatment of asthma by thermic destruction of the bronchial muscles and of emphysema by insertion of endobronchial valves have been published (2007).

The rapid growth of Internet communication has opened new ways of communication to enhance consulting, research, and teaching. The first long-distance live transmission on the occasion of the 12th World Congress for Bronchology and 12th World Congress for Bronchoesophagology was performed between Heidelberg, Germany, and Yokohama, Japan, in 2000.

FUTURE DEVELOPMENTS

Current relevant developments are new imaging and image-processing technologies, new devices for interventions and instrument tracking, micro-machines, man-machine interfaces, and navigation technologies for future robots (**Fig. 7**).

Imaging

The gaps in resolution, field of view, and penetration are continuously closing. Chip technology has had a tremendous impact on image quality and miniaturization of the instruments. Miniaturization will enhance incorporation of two lenses, which could provide a 3-D image of the endobronchial tree in the near future. Computerized processing of digital images will enhance endoscopic accuracy in detection and diagnosing diseases and will be a useful addition to 3-D ultrasound imaging. New laser probes will provide accurate measurement of diameter and length of stenoses for objective documentation of results after treatment and as a basis for manufacturing individual stents. Chip endoscopes of up to 100× magnification add zoom technology for endoscopic microscopy and will also be soon available.

Thus, endoscopists will be able to direct diagnostic and therapeutic procedures more accurately. The spatial resolution of endoscopic optical coherence tomography is 10 to 20 mm, with a depth of penetration of up to 2 to 3 mm, and provides visualization of cellular tissue structures beyond the visibility of conventional endoscopes. Microconfocal scanning microscopy (mCosm) allows 800× magnification for visualization of structures within individual cells.

EBUS has been recently introduced and added a new dimension by expanding bronchoscopists' view beyond the airway wall. Resolution of current 20-MHz probes will be further enhanced by probes of 30 MHz. Electrical scanning systems and B-mode Doppler will expand Doppler technology for evaluation of small vessels in tumors and inflammatory lesions. 3-D image reconstruction will improve assessment of tumor volume as basis for dosimetry in PDT or brachytherapy. In particular, the fusion technique with the endoscopic image will dramatically improve orientation in interdisciplinary planning for such treatments. EBUS is the ideal navigation tool for guiding diagnostic biopsy and endotherapy devices. EBUS-controlled transbronchial needle biopsy of lymph nodes is beginning to widely replace mediastinoscopy for staging of lung cancer. It not only will be useful for steering the instruments deeper into organs but also for controlling the effect of therapeutic procedures, such as radiofrequency waves or microwaves by changing the impendence. High-intensity focused ultrasound (HIFU) itself will be an efficient tool for destruction of pathologic tissues. Another new imaging technique will be endoscopic MRI. The reception antenna of the magnetic resonance endoscope will receive signals of extremely high resolution and high signal-to-noise ratio of the mediastinal structures, much superior to conventional technology. New procedures of in vivo imaging of the functional status of the endobronchial tree, such as ciliary beat, local bronchial and pulmonary interstitial inflammation, contraction of the bronchial muscles, bronchial and mediastinal blood flow, and tracheobronchial airflow, will generate new insights into pathomechanisms and new technologies for noninvasive local treatment.

Steering

As new-generation instruments are increasingly steered by remote control, new optical and tactile sensors will assist in guiding endoscopes through the sinuous pathways of the body with minimal discomfort. Force feedback systems will be integrated into "intelligent" instruments, such as

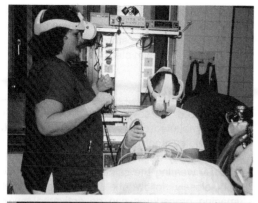
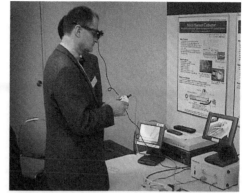
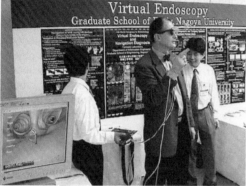
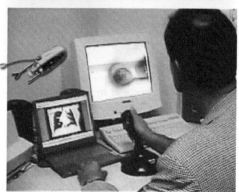

Fig. 7. Prototypes of new instruments. Future technologies might include head-mounted devices with two monitors, providing 3-D images or fusing images from different sources, such as ultrasound and endoscopy (*top left*). Steering of instruments is done via remote control (*top right*). In an advanced system, it could be performed by cybergloves without physical contact with the instruments (*bottom left*). The last example is a vison of remote steering of a capsular endoscope by a joystick via monitor control (*bottom right*).

forceps, needles, snares, baskets, and other probes, that will give an artificial impression of the forces to operators who will no longer maneuver these instruments directly by hand but via telemanipulator or even by joystick on a monitor. Most recent developments integrate chip technology and neuronal structures. In this technology, neurons are directly connected to the computers or computer-driven machines. Thus manipulators will be no longer controlled by hand but by eye trackers and brain-wave sensors. Brainchips and neurochips will be wired directly to the digital world and control devices. This symbiosis between man and machine is a further step towards robotics. True robots will no longer need the interface to a human but will independently perform diagnostic and therapeutic procedures based on computerized feedback data. Humans will only stand by to interfere by trouble shooting.[51]

Energy Transfer

The diameters of instruments are becoming so small that steering by conventional tendon-wire

technology is no longer applicable because of the increasing friction and the lack of rigidity.[52] Currently a miniaturized active bending catheter is in development through which the miniaturized endoscope can be introduced.[53] The bending mechanism is provided by shape memory alloy technology. Recent concepts for future endoscopes abandon the concept of regular hand-guided instruments in favor of remote-controlled capsular endoscopes without connection to the steering unit guided by wireless remote control.[54] As retrieval of these capsules from the lung could be difficult, however, instruments steered by electromagnetic navigation with nanomachines at the tip will be applied (**Fig. 8**).

Navigation

Remote-control instruments need advanced technologies for navigation by magnetic endoscope positioning system. The fields generated by the source coils of endoscopes and probes can be followed on a monitor, thus eliminating the necessity for fluoroscopy.[55] In addition, data provided by

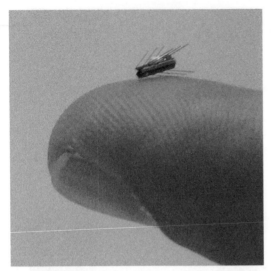

Fig. 8. Prototype of a miniaturized robot that can move along tubular structures by remote control via magnetic control (ViRob, Technion, Haifa, Israel).

3-D CT scanning and ultrasound can be aided by virtual bronchoscopy on a computer screen. The endoscope will be guided down a virtual electronic track to approach the lesion for biopsies and interventional procedures. First experiences proved that this technology can be efficiently applied.

INTERVENTIONAL TECHNOLOGIES

Miniaturized instruments, such as forceps, needles, and suturing devices made from shape memory alloys that currently are applied in neurosurgery, will revolutionize the endoscopic technology. The integration of the hardness sensors to these probes will enhance self-steering of "intelligent instruments." Therapeutic interventions of fine-needle injection of cytotoxic agents or gene therapy will be effectively controlled by these technologies and miniaturized probes, such as those for radio waves, microwaves and HIFU, will be applied with the use of the next-generation endoscopes. The most profound effects on interventional procedures in the future will come from the nanotechnology and bioengineering.[56] With these innovations, surgical procedures will be performed on a cellular or even molecular basis. These devices will be self-organizing micromachines, exactly adapting themselves to the task they have been designed for.[57] In addition, these molecular machines will be the transistors of the next chip generation for new lasers and computers.[58] Biotechnology is applied in seeding grafts and biodegradable devices are under investigation for temporary stenting of the airways. In the future, damaged structures, such as mucosa and cartilage, may be replaced in postintubation stenosis by endoscopic cell seeding or implantation of cultured bioprostheses, eventually cultured from a patient's own stem cells.

Communication

Miniaturized personal operation monitors on a head-mounted device will enhance procedures by providing improved 2-D or 3-D images and ergonomically freeing the hands of interventionists. By wearing the same device, staff personal can closely follow the procedures. Different imaging procedures can be activated by voice command or remote control in picture-in-picture mode, so multiple video sources can be displayed on one monitor. Online tracking of endoscopes and instruments will be supporting a physician's hand in application of man-machine interfaces. Advanced systems will perform the procedures by themselves by steering true robots according to preset programming under a physician's supervision.[59]

System integration will be essential for complete documentation and communication. Heterogeneous devices have to be integrated by complex devices for connection, transformation of images to Moving Picture Experts Group (MPEG) standards, storage on video servers, and steering of complex video networks. Digital systems support documentation and storage of data. They support planning of procedures, rational distribution of resources, manpower, and follow-up of results, all elements of total quality management.

In times of restricted resources, modern communication systems are providing the basis for widespread and evenly distributed patient care on an optimal level. For this purpose, more and more hospitals are connected currently via Integrated Services Digital Network lines by the Internet and even by the electricity net in a high-speed network for communication. Teleconsulting will reduce the need for sending patients to distant specialists for consultation (patient tourism).[60] Also the direct connection of a surgeon with a pathologist via network will reduce time and costs for consultation. The overall result will be an increase in the quality of patient care and reduction of costs. New communication technologies already are used for educational purposes. These can be performed on an individual basis on single monitors or on a large scale in intercontinental live conferences. For teaching new technologies, training groups may be gathered on the Internet, also reducing expenses for travel and accommodation of participants. Telecommunication also will enhance new research strategies by evolution of new self-organizing research teams that without support by conventional hierarchy find themselves in floating teams of varying "chaotic" constellations and goals. This kind of teamwork might prove superior to current systems in generating new ideas and providing rapid results of research work as they are more flexible and independent. Training is available on virtual mannequins in which all diagnostic techniques can be simulated by virtual imaging and procedures can be trained by integration of force feedback systems, providing an impression of real touch and transferring the movements of a surgeon's hand by transformation of its motions into electrical signals. Virtual scenarios will be constructed for the imitation of interventions, such as laser photoresection, stenting, or PDT. Complications can be simulated for training of countermeasures. Even today interventional procedures, such as bypass surgery, can be performed by remote control of instruments from a computer console.[61] With high-speed networks, teleintervention will also be possible over long distance, hospital to hospital, and even continent to continent.

SCENARIOS FOR THE FUTURE

1. A person at risk for developing lung cancer is screened by molecular analysis of his exhalate for suspicious cells. Alterations indicate, by a cluster of oncogenes and suppressor genes, that he has developed early-stage lung cancer. After an overt tumor or peripheral lesions have been excluded by a high-resolution CT, a detached computer-driven endoscope is sent down the airways by navigation according to virtual 3-D bronchoscopy. The endoscope is equipped with imaging devices. By fluorescence imaging, a true early lesion is detected. Closer observation by optical coherence tomography and microcosm are highly suggestive of an early-stage cancer, which is confirmed by a pathologist after transmission of the image to his department. Local staging by 3-D video imaging and high-resolution ultrasound in addition proves that the lesion is localized within the superficial layers of the bronchial wall and lymph node metastasis is excluded. A superfast molecular DNA computer fuses the endoscopic and ultrasonic images and generates a 3-D reconstruction for volume rendering. From the result, a virtual computerized simulation of different treatment modalities is executed. If curative local treatment seems feasible by excision of the tumor, the data are fed to a robot that guides an intelligent molecular nanoknife, which cuts out the lesion exactly

with some safety margin. A local cytotoxic or immunologic sterilizing agent is instilled into the tumor bed before the wound is closed by an intelligent fibrin suture that automatically attaches itself to the rims and closes the gap by traction.

2. In a more advanced localized lesion without lymph node involvement, 3-D reconstruction is generated for planning of treatment by PDT or HDR brachytherapy. According to the reconstruction, exact dosimetry for PDT for deposition of sensitizer, positioning of light source, and duration of illumination is performed. The data are fed to the endoscope and treatment is performed automatically. In cases of brachytherapy, computerized positioning of the radiation source and calculation of radiation time allow exact dosimetry. In addition, a radiosensitizer can be locally instilled.

3. Locally advanced carcinomas are staged and mapped by advanced imaging. After simulation of the most appropriate treatment, exact local instillation of liposomal microcapsulated cytotoxic drugs for inducing controlled apoptosis, immunologic treatment by injection of antibodies, or genetic repair by injection of vectors is performed. High-energy sources are locally applied for controlled tissue destruction, such as lasers, HIFU, microwave, or heat probes, which can be inserted interstitially. The effect is controlled by changes of impedance in the ultrasound image.

4. Small peripheral lesions in the lung tissue detected by high-resolution spiral CT can be approached in a similar way by miniaturized automatic endoscopes on computerized navigation. Removal or destruction is achieved by local excision with intelligent nanoinstruments or by applying destructive energy.

The procedures can be observed by a team of interdisciplinary specialists via a head-mounted display who can step in at crucial moments. Also with advanced computer and communication technologies, these interventions can be performed over long distances, even intercontinentally. Perhaps one day, endoscopic procedures may be possible on a spaceship.[62] The following quotation, dating 1973, might illustrate that we are much closer to seeing these visions become true than we are expecting: "...the two toolholding rods exactly reproduce any movements the surgeon makes outside." He "...can watch the remote operation as closely as if he were bending over the patient, moving the television camera, by a control worked by movements of his head."[63]

A SHORT DISCOURSE ON ETHICAL IMPLICATIONS

There has always been a broader acceptance of developments in "pure" technology, as it is believed that these will improve general health care and life expectancy. So far in this context the only controversial issue is when to limit their application, especially regarding the boundaries of life. With a completely new quality of instruments, this is beginning to change considerably.[64–66] The debate on the necessity of new technologies, such as robotics and nanotechnology, has recently gained worldwide attention and momentum and is currently carried out in international journals. As instruments will be self-controlling, self-repairing, and even identically replicating, especially in connection with gene technology, there is a fear that they might gain uncontrolled artificial life of their own and eventually even endanger mankind and life on earth.[67] According to the alternative position, there will be no choice but to apply these technologies for the survival of the mankind.[68,69] The "National Nanotechnology Initiative: Leading to the Next Industrial Revolution" was a top scientific priority issue of the White House for 2001 and the budget for development of these technologies has been doubled recently.[70] "My budget supports a major new National Nanotechnology Initiative, worth $500 million…Imagine the possibilities: materials with ten times the strength of steel and only a small fraction of the weight…detecting cancerous tumors when they are only few cells in size. Some of our goals may take 20 or more years to achieve, but that is precisely why there is an important role for the federal government." (W. J. Clinton).[71] The specialists who are directly confronted, even involved, in these evolutions will not be able to avoid this confrontation but have to take a position on the basis of a rational analysis. In the author's opinion, direct contact between patient and physician will not be replaced by future technology but computers and related technologies will improve the work. "Generally speaking the basic issue for the future is the ideological question how far mankind decides to propagate the technological acquisition of nature, which has been the recipe for the ascent of mankind from the Savannah of Africa to master and former of the biosphere."[72]

REFERENCES

1. Kollofrath O. Entfernung eines Knochenstücks aus dem rechten Bronchus auf natürlichem Wege und unter Anwendung der directen Laryngoscopie. MMW 1897;38:1038–9.

2. Becker HD, Marsh BR. History of the Rgigid Bronchoscope in: Bolliger CT, Mathur PN (eds): Interventional bronchoscopy. Prog Respir Res Basel (Switzerland), Karger, 2000;30:2–15

3. Becker HD. Gustav Killian—a biographical sketch. J Bronchol 1995;2:77–83.

4. Killian G. Zur Geschichte der Bronchoskopie und Ösophagoskopie. DMW 1911;35:1585–687.

5. Trousseau A, Belloc H. Traité pratique de la phtisie laryngeé. Paris: J.B. Baillière; 1837.

6. Marsh BR. Historic development of bronchoesophagology. Otolaryngol Head Neck Surg 1996; 114:689–716.

7. Elsberg L. Laryngoscopcal medicaton or the local treatment of the diseases of the throat, larynx, and neighboring organs, under sight. New York: William Wood&Co.; 1864.

8. von Eicken C. Zur Geschichte der Endoskopie der oberen Luft- und Speisewege. Giessen (Germany): v. Münchow'sche Universitätsdruckerei; 1921.

9. Richard P. Notice sur l'invention du laryngoscope ou mroirs du larynx (Garcia's Kehlkopfspiegel du Dr. Czermak). Paris: J. Claye; 1861.

10. Garcia M. Beobachtungen über die menschliche Stimme. Wien (Austria): W. Braunmüller; 1878.

11. Czermak J. Physologische Untersuchungen mit Garcia's Kehlkopfspiegel. Wien (Austria): K. Gerold's Sohn; 1858.

12. Türck L. Klinik der Krankheiten des Kehlkopfes und der Luftröhre nebst einer Anleitung zum Gebrauch des Kehlkopfrachenspiegels und zur Localbehandlung der Kehlkopfkrankheiten. Wien (Austria): W. Braunmüller; 1866.

13. Gibb GD. The laryngoscope: llustratons of ist practcal applicaton, and descripton of ts mechanism. London: J. Churchill&Sons; 1863.

14. von Bruns V. Die Larybngoskope und die laryngoskopische Chirurgie. Tübngen (Germany): H. Laupp'-sche Buchhandlung; 1865.

15. Reuter HJ, Reuter MA. Philipp Bozzini und die Endoskopie des 19.Jh. Stuttgart (Germany): Loennicker; 1988.

16. Kluge F. Die Erstanwendung der Ösophago- und Gastroskopie durch A. Kußmaul und seine Assistenten 1868. Fortschr Gastroenerol Endoskope 1986;15:5–9.

17. Mikulicz J. Über Gastroskopie und Ösophagoskopie. Wien (Austria): Urban & Schwarzenberg; 1881.

18. Kirstein A. Autoskopie des larynx und der Trachea (Besichtigung ohne Spegel), Berlin. Kli Wschr 1895;22:476–8.

19. Killian G. Ueber directe bronchoscopie. MMW 1898; 27:844–7.

20. Byck R. Cocain papers by Sigmund Freud. New York: Stonehill; 1974.

21. Killian H. Gustav Killian. Sein Leben. Sein Werk. Remscheid-Lennep (Germany): Dustri Verlag; 1958.
22. Pieniazek. Die Tracheoskopie und die tracheoskopischen Operationen bei Tracheotomierten. Arch Laryng 1896;28:210–30.
23. Killian H. Hinter uns steht nur der Herrgott. Aufzeichnungen eines Chirurgen. Sub umbra dei. München (Germany): Kindler; 1957.
24. Naef HP. The story of thoracic surgery. Toronto: Hogrefe and Huber; 1990.
25. Brünings W, Albrecht W. Direkte Endoskope der Luft- und Speisewege. Neue Deutsche Chirurgie Band 16. Stuttgart (Germany): F. Enke; 1915.
26. Killian G. Über die Behandlung von Fremdkörpern unter Bronchialstenosen. Zschr. Ohrenheilk. 1907; 15:334–70.
27. Killian G. Description abrégée de mon operation radicale sur le sinus frontal. Asnn Mal Oreille Larynx 1902;28:205–9.
28. Killian G. Über den Mund der Speiseröhre. Zschr Ohrenkheilk 1907;55:1–41.
29. Killian G. Die Schwebelaryngoskopie und ihre klinische Verwertung. Berlin: Urban und Schwarzenberg; 1920.
30. Killian G. Zur Geschichte der Endoskopie von den ältesten Zeiten bis Bozzini. Arch Laryngol 1915;29: 247–393.
31. Killian G. A model for Bronchoskopy (sic!). Translation of a paper in Archiv für Laryngologie 13:1, Berlin 1902. Harvard, derby, 1902.
32. Killian G. Bronchoskopie und Lungenchirurgie. Verh Verein Südd Laryngologen. Würzburg (Germany): Stuber's Verlag; 1905.
33. Killian G. Tracheo-bronchoscopy in its diagnostic and therapeutic aspects. Laryngoscope 1906;12: 3–15.
34. Killian G. Die directen Methoden in den jahren 1911 und 1912. Semon's Internat Centralbl Laryngol Rhinol 1913;30:1–28.
35. Killian G. Zwei Fälle von Karzinom. Berlin Klin Wochenschr 1914;7:1–3.
36. Huzly A. Atlas der Bronchoskopie. Stuttgart (Germany): G. Thieme; 1960.
37. Brandt HJ. Endoskopie der Luft- und Speiesewege. Berlin: Springer; 1985.
38. Wiesner B. De Entwicklung der Bronchoskope und der Bronchologie. Ein geschichtlicher Überblick. Atemw Lungenkrankh 1995;21(11):541–7.
39. Jackson: The life of Chevaler Jackson. An autobiography. Macmillan Co., New York, 1938.
40. Cushing H. Boston surgical society: the presentation of the Henry Jacob Bigelow medal. N Engl J Med 1928;199:16.
41. Jackson Ch, Jackson Ch L: Bronchoesophagology. Philadelphia, and London, W.B. Saunders Co., 1950.
42. Ohata M. History and progress of bronchology in Japan. JJSB 1998;20:539–46.
43. Miyazawa T. History of the flexible bronchoscope. In: Bolliger CT, Mathur PN, editors. Interventional bronchoscopy. Prog Respir Res. Basel (Switzerland), Karger, 2000;30:16–21.
44. Shirakawa T. The history of bronchoscopy in Japan. Keynote lecture, the 12th WCB&WCBE, June 18th, 2002, Boston (MA). CD edited by the WAB.
45. Tsuboi E, Ikeda S. Transbronchial biopsy smear for diagnosis of peripheral pulmonary carcinomas. Cancer 1967;20:687–98.
46. Ikeda S, Yanai N. Flexible bronchofiberscope. Kejo J Med 1968;17:1–16.
47. Ikeda S. The development and progress of endoscopes in the field of bronchoesophagology. JJSB 1988;39:85–96.
48. Hayata Y, Kato H, Konaka C, et al. Haematoporphyrine derivate and laser photoradiation in the treatment of lung cancer. Chest 1982;81:269–77.
49. Becker HD. The Impact of current technological development on bronchoscopy. J Japan Bronchoesophagological Soc 2004;55(2):89–91.
50. Becker HD. Bronchoscopy and computer technology. In: Simoff MJ, Sterman DH, Ersnt A, editors. Thoracic endoscopy: advances in interventional pulmonology. Malden (MA): Blackwell Publishers; 2006. p. 88–118.
51. Moravec H. Robot. Mere machine to transcendent mind. New York: Oxford University Press; 2000.
52. Schulz S, Pylatiuk C, Brettauer G. A new class of flexible fluid actuators and their application in medical engineering. Automatisierungstechnik 1999;47(8):390–5.
53. Takizawa H, et al. Development of a microfine active bending catheter equipped with MIF tactile sensors. IEEE MEMS '99, 1999:412–7.
54. Swain P. Pille sendet Videos aus dem Körperinneren Nature. 405, 417, 2000 Available at: http://www.heise.de/newsticker/data/wst-25.05.00-000/. Accessed November 4, 2009.
55. Final report: Steuerbares Flexibles Endoskop für die Minimal Invasive Chirurgie. Forschungszentrum, Karlsruhe, Germany; 2000.
56. Feynman RP. There's plenty of room at the bottom. An invitation to enter a new field of physics. 1960. Available at: http://www.zyvex.com/nanotech/feynman.html. Accessed November 4, 2009.
57. Nanotechnology. Available at: http://www.zyvex.com/nano/. Accessed November 4, 2009.
58. Niemeyer Ch F. Ganz groß im Kleinen. In der DNA liegt die Zukunft der Nanotechnologie. FAZ 2000; 103(52):4.
59. Zylka-Menhorn V. Wenn ein Roboterarm das Skalpell führt. Deutsches Ärzteblatt 2000;97(27):B1580–3.
60. Stein R. Zweite Meinung aus dem Netz. FAZ, 153, 14, 2000 Available at: http://www.uicc-tpcc.charite.de. Accessed November 4, 2009.

61. Virtueller Chirurg. Die Telemedizin holt weit entfernte Experten direkt in den OP. Brennpunkt 4/2000. Information.

62. Norfleet WT. Anesthetic concerns of spaceflight. Anesthesiology 2000;92:1219–22.

63. Thring MW. Man, machines and tomorrow. London: Routledge and Kegan Paul; 1973. Boston, 108–9.

64. Gelernter D. Machine beauty. Elegance and the heart of technology. New York: Basic Books; 1997.

65. Kurzweil R. The age of spiritual machines. New York: Penguin; 1999.

66. Milburn GJ. The Feynman processor. Perseus Books; 1998.

67. Joy B. Warum die Zukunft uns nicht braucht. FAZ 2000;130:49–51.

68. Gelernter D. The second coming – a manifesto. Available at: http://www.edge.org/documents/archive/edge70.html. Accessed November 4, 2009.

69. Kurzweil R. Die Maschinen werden uns davon überzeugen, daß sie Menschen sind. FAZ 2000; 153:51.

70. National nanotechnology initiative. Supplement to the president's FY 2001 Budget. Available at: http://www.nano.gov/nni.pdf. Accessed November 4, 2009.

71. Clinton W.J. National nanotechnology initiative Available at: 2000 California Institute of Technology http://www.nano.gov. Accessed November 4, 2009.

72. Reich J. Erfindung und Entdeckung. FAZ 2000;146:11.

Bronchoscopes of the Twenty-First Century

Lonny Yarmus, DO, FCCP, David Feller-Kopman, MD, FCCP*

KEYWORDS

- Bronchoscopy • Autofluorescence bronchoscopy
- Electromagnetic navigation • Narrow-band imaging
- Confocal fluorescence microendoscopy
- Endobronchial ultrasound–guided transbronchial
  needle aspiration • Endobronchial ultrasound

The bronchoscope has been an invaluable tool for the pulmonologist and surgeon for over a century. In the late 1800s, Dr Gustav Killian performed the first rigid bronchoscopy. The innovative procedure provided physicians with a new glimpse into human anatomy and sparked the growth of pulmonary medicine. Using a metal tube, electric light, and topical cocaine anesthesia, Killian removed a pork bone from a farmer's airway in 1897.

Before the invention of rigid bronchoscopy, over half of the patients who aspirated foreign bodies died, mostly of a postobstructive pneumonia. Rigid bronchoscopy with foreign body removal quickly evolved into the treatment of choice in these patients, with a clinical success rate above 98%.[1] During the early 1900s, Killian published extensively and lectured throughout the world. He further went on to adapt his bronchoscopes, laryngoscopes, and endoscopes, and first described techniques, such as using fluoroscopy and radiographs to define endobronchial anatomy. The design and functionality of the rigid bronchoscope was improved further in 1904 when Chevalier Jackson, the "father of American bronchoesophagology," first equipped his bronchoscope with a suction channel and a small light bulb at the distal tip to provide illumination.

Over the next 150 years, bronchoscopic technology continued to be refined. In 1966, at the 9th International Congress on Diseases of the Chest in Copenhagen, Shigeto Ikeda presented the first prototype flexible fiber-optic bronchoscope. In 1968, the first commercially available flexible bronchoscope was made available by Machita and Olympus.[2] In 1980, Dumon presented his use of the neodymium–yttrium aluminum garnet (Nd:YAG) laser via the fiber-optic bronchoscope. Since then, the flexible bronchoscope has been widely used as both a diagnostic and a therapeutic tool for both diseases of the parenchyma and of the central airways. With the miniaturization of electronic devices, the first video bronchoscope was introduced in 1987. This development enabled endoscopic pictures to be taken and shared for educational purposes. Another major advance in the teaching of bronchoscopy came when physicians no longer needed to look through an eyepiece, but instead could transmit endoscopic images to monitors, enabling an entire bronchoscopy staff to witness procedures.

Although little has changed in the appearance of either the flexible or the rigid bronchoscope since 1968, new technological advances over the past decade have brought improvements to the field of bronchology. This article reviews the current advances in both rigid and flexible bronchoscopy and discusses the diagnostic and therapeutic implications of these tools.

NEW INNOVATIONS IN RIGID BRONCHOSCOPY

Though the design of the rigid bronchoscope has not significantly changed since Jackson first used it in 1897, current designs and accessories have helped make it possible to adapt the

Interventional Pulmonology, Division of Pulmonary and Critical Care, The Johns Hopkins Hospital, 1830 East Monument Street, 5th Floor, Baltimore, MD 21205, USA
* Corresponding author.
E-mail address: dfellerk@jhmi.edu (D. Feller-Kopman).

Clin Chest Med 31 (2010) 19–27
doi:10.1016/j.ccm.2009.11.002

bronchoscope for new technologies. The rigid bronchoscope is made of a hollow cylindrical stainless steel tube with an equal diameter along its entire working length. The adult rigid bronchoscope is usually 40 cm long and has an external diameter ranging from 9 to 14 mm. The distal end has a beveled tip to enable lifting of the epiglottis and safer insertion through the vocal cords. This beveled end can also be used to dilate stenotic lesions and to "core" through tumors, thus achieving rapid airway patency. Fenestrations are present at the distal one third of the broncho-scope to enable contralateral lung ventilation when the bronchoscope is inserted into a mainstem bronchus. In comparison with the bron-choscope, a rigid tracheoscope is shorter—measuring 30 cm—enabling more maneuverability within the trachea to relieve central airway obstruc-tions. Distal fenestrations are absent on the rigid tracheoscope because single lung ventilation is not required while operating within the trachea. The proximal end of the bronchoscope varies by manufacturer as discussed below. Most broncho-scope systems have several ports to enable passage of the telescope, suction catheters, and a variety of instruments for tumor destruction, tumor excision, dilation, and foreign body removal.

Over the past several years, new designs and modifications applied to the standard rigid bron-choscope have made it a more versatile tool for the interventional pulmonologist.

The Bryan-Dumon Series II rigid bronchoscope represents the first major modification to the rigid bronchoscope since the rigid bronchoscope first appeared. The Bryan-Dumon Series II

bronchoscope features an operator head with a universal instrumentation barrel. The operator head (**Fig. 1**) is an interchangeable piece that can be placed on the proximal end of any of the color-coded bronchial and tracheal tubes within the Dumon series. The universal instrumentation barrel is also equipped with three side ports for instruments, ventilation, and anesthesia. In addi-tion, the barrel has a channel for the telescope. The multiple ports of access permit physicians to use various endoscopic tools while maintaining the visualization capabilities of the rigid telescope. The system also has a stent introducer system for the placement of silicone tracheobronchial stents.

Another rigid bronchoscope recently intro-duced is the Texas R.I.B. (Rigid Integrated Bron-choscope) from Wolff. This bronchoscope features separate channels for optics and instru-ments to enable access to a larger working area with uninterrupted visualization. The design combines the operator head with the camera, which limits the loss of working space within the bronchoscope channel taken up by the larger optics. This design may also increase efficiency during procedures because the telescope does not need to be removed before the insertion of accessories. However, the telescope cannot extend distally past the lumen of the broncho-scope and thus vision is limited to only areas at the distal end of the rigid bronchoscope. There is also an irrigation port at the proximal operator end to enable washing of the distal lens for optimal visualization. At the distal tip of the bron-choscope are additional fenestrations to provide 360° viewing.

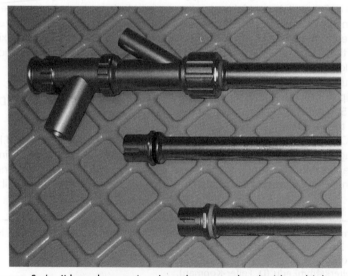

Fig. 1. The Bryan-Dumon Series II bronchoscope's universal operator head with multiple ports, which enable jet or volume ventilation as well as passage of a variety of instruments.

VENTILATION AND MONITORING DURING RIGID BRONCHOSCOPY

Ventilation during rigid bronchoscopy can be achieved in several ways. In 1967, Sanders[3] developed a method of low-frequency jet ventilation to enable effective ventilation and oxygenation while keeping the proximal end of the bronchoscope free for passage of the instruments. In the 1990s, a shift away from this mode followed reports of hypoxemia during spontaneous assisted ventilation with intravenous anesthesia during rigid bronchoscopy in patients with central airway obstruction. Jet Venturi ventilation reemerged as a favored method.[4] Because the system is open to atmosphere, room air is also entrained into the bronchoscope, resulting in a variable fraction of inspired oxygen (FiO_2).[5] Although a safe oxyhemoglobin saturation is usually easily obtained, potential downsides to this system are a limited ability to monitor FiO_2, minute ventilation, and airway pressures. As such, there is a potential increased risk of iatrogenic pneumothorax due to dynamic hyperinflation distal to a stenotic airway.[6]

The Hemer bronchoscope introduced by Wolff is adapted with a measuring port that enables sampling of carbon dioxide and oxygen and monitoring of pressure fluctuations during the procedure. The peak inspiratory pressure of entrained air and jet-pressurized air reaches a plateau within the rigid bronchoscope at a distance of approximately 10 cm from the proximal end of the bronchoscope. By measuring pressure distal to that point, an estimate of mean inspiratory pressure is obtained. The adapted Hemmer bronchoscope has an internal port at 14 cm from the proximal end of the bronchoscope and can be connected to pressure transducers and gas sensors to monitor end-tidal carbon dioxide, enabling real-time monitoring.

NEW INNOVATIONS IN FLEXIBLE BRONCHOSCOPY

Since its first introduction by Ikeda in 1967, the flexible bronchoscope has rapidly emerged as the most adaptable tool for the practicing pulmonologist. Since that time, the field has seen a steady stream of advances. Recently, technological advances have begun to open more doors toward not only improved diagnostic interventions for malignant disease but also for the detection of premalignant lesions. As additional studies are performed and as new data become available, such modalities as endobronchial ultrasound (EBUS), electromagnetic navigation, autofluorescence bronchoscopy, narrow-band imaging, and confocal fluorescence microscopy are emerging as important new technologies for the bronchoscopist.

MODERN VIDEO BRONCHOSCOPES

Despite great advances in the technology within the bronchoscope, the overall appearance of the instrument resembles that of the original fiberoptic design. The external diameter of most working flexible bronchoscopes varies from approximately 4 mm to 6.3 mm. Ultrathin bronchoscopes are also available, with an external diameter of 2.7 mm, and are especially helpful in bypassing obstructing airway lesions to assess distal patency. The diameter of the working channel ranges from 1.2 mm to 3.2 mm. A working channel 2.8 mm or more is recommended for more therapeutic flexible bronchoscopy, as well as EBUS, as it enables better suction and the passage of larger instruments. Most flexible bronchoscopes can flex 180° up and 130° down. Olympus is developing an "endocotoscopy" bronchoscope that provides high-magnification of 450× and a horizontal resolution of 4.2 μm, providing cellular imaging and the possibility of an "optical biopsy."

ENDOBRONCHIAL ULTRASOUND BRONCHOSCOPY AND THE DIAGNOSIS OF LUNG CANCER

Lung cancer remains the leading cause of cancer deaths in the United States and accounted for approximately 161,840 deaths in 2008.[7] It is estimated that 2009 figures will show 219,440 new cases of lung cancer for the year. Meanwhile, the number of lung cancer deaths continues to increase amongst women in the United States.[8] Bronchoscopy has been an invaluable tool in the diagnosis and staging of lung cancer. Transbronchial needle aspiration (TBNA) of mediastinal and hilar lymph nodes has been shown to be an effective means of both diagnosing and staging lung cancer.[9–11] The procedure has consistently been shown to be minimally invasive, safe, and less costly than mediastinoscopy. Also, the procedure can preclude surgery in up to 29% of patients.[12] Despite these facts, the procedure remains underused. A survey performed in 1991 showed that only 12% of pulmonologists routinely use TBNA in evaluating malignant disease. This reluctance to use TBNA is likely due to concerns over lack of training, fear of injuring the bronchial tubes or puncturing a blood vessel, and lack of adequate procedural support.[13] Although traditional TBNA is a safe and effective procedure, the inability to directly visualize mediastinal and hilar lymph nodes as well as surrounding vasculature and lung tissue has been a limitation.

The invention of the integrated EBUS in 2002 used for real-time guidance TBNA solved this issue. The role of EBUS-guided TBNA (EBUS-TBNA) in mediastinal staging and restaging of lung cancer is discussed in detail in the article by Herth and colleagues elsewhere in this issue. The design of the EBUS convex probe flexible bronchoscope differs from that of the standard flexible bronchoscope in widespread use today. The Olympus EBUS bronchoscope is a hybrid bronchoscope incorporating both fiber-optic and video imaging technologies. The bronchoscope incorporates a 7.5-MHz convex transducer, which produces a linear curved array. By making direct contact with the airway wall or by using a water-filled balloon that lies over the tip of the ultrasound transducer, transbronchial ultrasound images of mediastinal and hilar structures can be obtained.

There are currently two Olympus EBUS bronchoscopes available. The Olympus BF-UC160F was the first model widely produced by Olympus. This bronchoscope is larger than standard bronchoscopes. The distal tip has an outer diameter of 6.9 mm and the insertion tube has an outer diameter of 6.2 mm. The working channel is 2.0 mm. The optical vision has a 35° forward oblique view due to the ultrasound transducer at the tip of the bronchoscope and an 80° field of view. This angulation is different from that of standard bronchoscopes and can make the insertion of the bronchoscope into the vocal cords technically more challenging, as discussed below. Recently, Olympus introduced the second-generation EBUS bronchoscope. The BF-UC180F has the same outer dimension as the original model. The working channel is larger at 2.2 mm, enabling better suctioning and accommodating larger-bore needles. The newer bronchoscope is also compatible with the more powerful Olympus Aloka ultrasound system.

Pentax has recently introduced the EB-1970UK EBUS bronchoscope. The Pentax EBUS bronchoscope has a 6.3-mm insertion tube diameter and a 2.0-mm working channel. The angle of view is 100°. The imaging technology on the Pentax bronchoscope uses an all video imaging processor as compared with the hybrid imaging on the Olympus bronchoscopes. This technology allows for a finer visual image at the expense of a slightly larger outer diameter.

Both systems use a dedicated EBUS-TBNA needle. Olympus has produced a 22-gauge needle and recently introduced a 21-gauge TBNA needle. Pentax offers a 22-gauge needle through Medi-Globe.

From a technical standpoint, the EBUS bronchoscope is operated in a slightly different manner than the traditional bronchoscope. This means clinicians must take time to understand the ultrasound anatomy and become familiar with the dedicated needle system.[14] The distal end of the bronchoscope is larger in diameter and the forward view is 30° oblique instead of 0° (straight ahead). As a result, the most distal portion of the bronchoscope cannot be directly visualized, adding an additional challenge when inserting the bronchoscope through the vocal cords.

ENDOBRONCHIAL ULTRASOUND–GUIDED TRANSBRONCHIAL NEEDLE ASPIRATION IN OTHER DISEASES

Initial data examining the yield of EBUS-TBNA primarily concentrated on the diagnosis and staging of lung cancer. As EBUS has become more established, multiple studies have examined its use beyond the scope of lung cancer diagnosis. These applications include those related to sarcoidosis, lymphoma, and pulmonary emboli.[15–17] Several recent studies have shown that EBUS-TBNA may be the preferred diagnostic modality for the investigation of pulmonary sarcoidosis.[15,18,19] One study showed a sensitivity of 85% for the diagnosis of sarcoidosis using EBUS-TBNA as a first-line diagnostic test.[15] A randomized trial by Tremblay and colleagues[18] examined the diagnostic efficacy of EBUS-TBNA versus standard TBNA in sarcoidosis and found an increase in diagnostic yield to 83% from 54% with an increase in sensitivity to 83% from 61% by using EBUS. A recent study by Aumiller and colleagues[17] performed EBUS on patients with computed tomography (CT)–confirmed central pulmonary emboli and reconfirmed the diagnosis in 96% of the cases. Although an interesting finding, the clinical utility of this finding is not yet established.

ENHANCED BRONCHOSCOPIC NAVIGATION

Traditionally, small distal parenchymal lesions less than 2 cm have been difficult to sample bronchoscopically.[20] Often, these lesions must be either followed radiographically or surgically resected.[21] As the large majority of peripheral lung nodules are not malignant, the ability to obtain a minimally invasive diagnosis would significantly reduce the number of unnecessary surgeries.[22] One of the main limitations of bronchoscopy for peripheral lesions is that the size of the bronchoscope precludes direct inspection of distal airways and, as a result, the operator is unable to visualize these lesions. Traditionally, fluoroscopy and, more recently, CT-guided fluoroscopy and radial probe EBUS have been used to attempt localization of peripheral lesion, but these methods were still limited by the bronchoscope's ability to guide a biopsy device successfully to the distal lesion. An electromagnetic guidance system has been adapted to be used with the flexible bronchoscope to assist with peripheral nodule sampling and is discussed in detail in the article by Schwarz and colleagues elsewhere in this issue.

More recently, newer methods of sampling peripheral lesions have emerged. These take advantage of improved CT imaging and complex computer programs, enabling accurate reconstruction of the airways. The distinct advantage of these systems as compared with the electromagnetic guidance systems is that they require no additional guidance equipment during the procedure. A virtual bronchoscopy is created with CT imaging and mapped pathways are determined (**Fig. 2**). Using a flexible ultrathin bronchoscope and the image guidance, the clinician can gain access to small peripheral nodules. In 2006, Asano and colleagues[23] published the first study in the literature using the technology. By using CT virtual bronchoscopy in conjunction with a computer program that generated a pathway to the lesion and an ultrathin bronchoscope, they were able to advance the bronchoscope into the planned route in 36 of 38 cases (94.7%), with a diagnostic rate of 81.6%. A latter study by the same group combined this technology with radial probe EBUS and guide-sheath technology. In this study of 31 patients, 32 peripheral pulmonary lesions were evaluated. The newer program was able to produce virtual images out to a seventh-order bronchi. In all patients, the ultrathin bronchoscope was successfully guided to the lesion. A pathologic diagnosis was obtained in 27 (84.4%) of the samples. With a median total examination time of 22.3 minutes, the procedure time did not appear to be significantly lengthened with the use of the virtual technology.[24]

AUTOFLUORESCENCE BRONCHOSCOPY

For most types of lung neoplasm, surgical resection remains the primary curative modality. Recent efforts have been directed at earlier diagnoses with the hope that such malignancies, caught in earlier stages, could be cured without resection or be surgically removed with a higher likelihood of cure.[25] Early detection of preinvasive lesions within the central airways can be achieved with the autofluorescence.[26] By using blue light (520 nm) instead of white light, dysplasia and carcinoma in situ will appear darker than the surrounding normal tissue because of a loss of normal autofluorescence (**Fig. 3**). There are several autofluorescence devices currently available, including the Laser Induced Fluorescence Endoscope (LIFE) system, the D-Light system, the SAFE-1000 system, and the Autofluorescence Imaging (AFI) system.[27,28] Unfortunately, autofluorescence technology is unable to differentiate between early preinvasive lesions and inflammatory or infectious changes in the epithelium that are benign, thus significantly reducing its specificity.[29] There are several classes of tissue findings in autofluorescence: normal (class I); inflammation and mild dysplasia (class II); and moderate to severe dysplasia, carcinoma in situ, or invasive cancer (class III).[27] To date, this classification does not correlate with degree of invasion or propensity toward a neoplastic process.[30] Because of its poor specificity, and high degree of inter- and intraobserver variability, autofluorescence is not considered an acceptable screening modality, even in high-risk patients, and the utility of this procedure in the lower airway remains in question.[31,32]

NARROW-BAND IMAGING

Narrow-band imaging is a light technology that uses specialized filters to separate wavelengths of white light and select out red, green, and blue

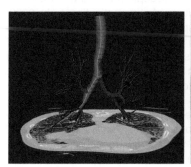 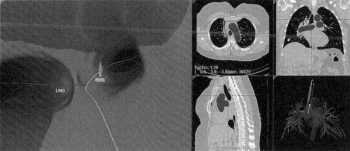

Fig. 2. Virtual bronchoscopic navigation. ([*Left*] *Courtesy of* Vida Diagnostics; with permission. [*Right*] *Courtesy of* Bronchus Technologies; with permission.)

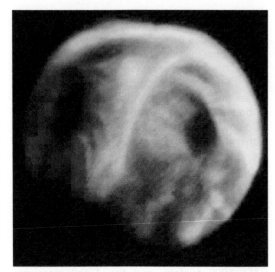

Fig. 3. Carcinoma in situ as seen with autofluorescence bronchoscopy.

bands. Additional filtering technology then intensifies the blue band. By selectively engaging these bands of light, the microvasculature is more clearly visible (**Fig. 4**).[33] This technology has been used to help identify premalignant lesions within the airways.[34] Dysplastic or premalignant lesions have been shown to have abnormal levels of angiogenesis compared with the surrounding normal tissue.[35,36] In a recent pilot study by Vincent and colleagues,[34] narrow-band imaging was compared with white-light bronchoscopy in 22 patients with known or suspected bronchial dysplasia or malignancy. Endobronchial biopsies of lesions suspicious for dysplastic, malignant, and normal (control) areas were then performed. There were four dysplastic and one malignant

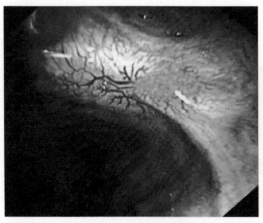

Fig. 4. Neovascularization seen with narrow-band imaging.

lesions in 22 patients detected by narrow-band imaging when findings by white-light imaging were considered normal, which increased the rate of detection of dysplasia and malignancy by 23%. As in the case of autofluorescence, a better understanding of the progression of these lesions and improved specificity is needed before this technology can be recommended for widespread use.

CONFOCAL FLUORESCENCE MICROENDOSCOPY

Alveoloscopy or confocal laser fluorescence microendoscopy (CFM) is a newer technology that enables in vivo microscopic observation of the airways and alveoli. The technology was introduced in 1957 but only in the last decade has the device been adapted for use with bronchoscopy. Similar to autofluorescence, the device uses a blue laser, which has been adapted within a small probe that can be advanced through the working channel of the bronchoscope into the distal airways and alveoli to induce tissue fluorescence. Optical slices of the observed tissue are obtained and in vivo magnified images of the alveoli can be observed.[37]

Although the technology will theoretically enable histologic interpretation of in vivo tissue, several technical issues remain. These need to be resolved before the technology can be put in widespread use. Currently, to adequately fluoresce this live tissue, a contrast dye must be administered within the pulmonary parenchyma and, given the limits of standard bronchoscopy and live imaging, the placement of the confocal probe within the correct area of study cannot yet be accurately controlled. The current data within the pulmonary literature remain limited to studies by Thiberville and colleagues.[37] In 2007, their group performed in vivo CFM bronchoscopically on 29 patients at high risk for lung cancer. The investigators recognized several microscopic patterns that may help in the recognition of dysplastic tissue. In 2009, the same group performed confocal fluorescence microscopy in 41 healthy subjects, including 17 active smokers. In vivo acinar microimaging was obtained from multiple lung segments (**Fig. 5**). The investigators reported that alveolar macrophages were not detectable in nonsmokers, whereas a specific tobacco tar–induced fluorescence was observed in smoking subjects.[38] Although this technology does appear to have promise, given the currently limited data, its accuracy in detecting lung pathology has yet to be defined.

OPTICAL COHERENCE TOMOGRAPHY

Optical coherence tomography (OCT) is an imaging technology similar to ultrasound. Instead of measuring the intensity of back-reflected sound, OCT uses an infrared light to obtain cross-sectional images of tissue. Compared to ultrasound, the resolution of OCT within the airways is significantly higher, which enables a more detailed evaluation of depth of invasion in endobronchial disease (**Fig. 6**).[39] OCT resolution, between 4 and 20 nm in the airway, is approximately 25 times higher than that of other available modalities.[40] It is also an optically based technologically. This means it does not require direct contact with tissue for transmission of a signal and can therefore easily be used within the airways.[41]

OCT's ability to assess the microstructure of the eye has an established role in ophthalmology and has only recently been adapted to the airways.[42] Its potential to produce in vivo images or "optical biopsies" of the microstructure of the lung without the risk of tissue biopsy could be a very useful modality in such fields as interstitial lung disease and lung transplantation.[43,44] As in the other modalities discussed above, further studies are needed to before its true clinical efficacy can be determined.

SUMMARY

Bronchoscopy continues to evolve at a rapid pace and remains an invaluable tool for the practicing pulmonologist. Recent advances have enabled the diagnosis and staging of our patients in a minimally invasive fashion with higher specificity than

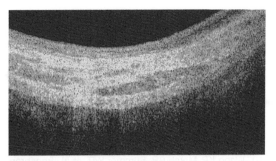

Fig. 6. OCT showing human main bronchus. Scan direction: perpendicular to airway. Image size: 1.5 mm × 4 mm. (*Courtesy of* Tomophase Corp; with permission.)

ever. Further advances and studies in electromagnetic guidance systems, OCT, and CFM may one day allow the bronchoscopist to obtain in vivo diagnoses without tissue destruction. As Chevalier Jackson said:

In the future, as at present, the internist will tap and look and listen on the outside of the chest; the roentgenologist will continue to look through the patient; but in continually increasing proportions of cases, the surgeon, the internist and the roentgenologist will ask the bronchoscopist to look inside the patient.[1]

REFERENCES

1. Becker HD, Marsh BR. History of the rigid bronchoscope. In: Bolliger CT, Mathur PN, editors. Interventional bronchoscopy. Basel (Switzerland): Karger; 2000. p. 2–15.
2. Miyazawa T. History of the flexible bronchoscope. In: Bolliger CT, Mathur PN, editors. Interventional bronchoscopy. Basel (Switzerland): Karger; 2000. p. 16–21.
3. Sanders RD. Two ventilating attachments for bronchoscopes. Del Med J 1967;39:170–92.
4. Perrin G, Colt HG, Martin C, et al. Safety of interventional rigid bronchoscopy using intravenous anesthesia and spontaneous assisted ventilation. A prospective study. Chest 1992;102(5):1526–30.
5. Godden DJ, Willey RF, Fergusson RJ, et al. Rigid bronchoscopy under intravenous general anaesthesia with oxygen Venturi ventilation. Thorax 1982; 37(7):532–4.
6. Fernandez-Bustamante A, Ibanez V, Alfaro JJ, et al. High-frequency jet ventilation in interventional bronchoscopy: factors with predictive value on high-frequency jet ventilation complications. J Clin Anesth 2006;18(5):349–56.

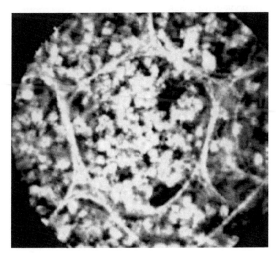

Fig. 5. Confocal microendoscopy showing alveolar septae and alveolar macrophages.

7. American Cancer Society, Inc. Cancer facts and figures 2008. Available at: http://www.cancer.org/downloads/STT/2008CAFFfinalsecured.pdf. Accessed December 8, 2009.

8. National Cancer Institute. SEER cancer statistics review 1975–2005. Available at: http://seer.cancer.gov/statistics/. Accessed December 8, 2009.

9. Dasgupta A, Mehta AC. Transbronchial needle aspiration. An underused diagnostic technique. Clin Chest Med 1999;20(1):39–51.

10. Wang KP, Marsh BR, Summer WR, et al. Transbronchial needle aspiration for diagnosis of lung cancer. Chest 1981;80(1):48–50.

11. Wang KP, Brower R, Haponik EF, et al. Flexible transbronchial needle aspiration for staging of bronchogenic carcinoma. Chest 1983;84(5):571–6.

12. Harrow EM, Abi-Saleh W, Blum J, et al. The utility of transbronchial needle aspiration in the staging of bronchogenic carcinoma. Am J Respir Crit Care Med 2000;161(2 Pt 1):601–7.

13. Prakash UB, Offord KP, Stubbs SE. Bronchoscopy in North America: the ACCP survey. Chest 1991; 100(6):1668–75.

14. Groth SS, Whitson BA, D'Cunha J, et al. Endobronchial ultrasound-guided fine-needle aspiration of mediastinal lymph nodes: a single institution's early learning curve. Ann Thorac Surg 2008; 86(4):1104–10.

15. Garwood S, Judson MA, Silvestri G, et al. Endobronchial ultrasound for the diagnosis of pulmonary sarcoidosis. Chest 2007;132(4):1298–304.

16. Kennedy MP, Jimenez CA, Bruzzi JF, et al. Endobronchial ultrasound-guided transbronchial needle aspiration in the diagnosis of lymphoma. Thorax 2008;63(4):360–5.

17. Aumiller J, Herth FJ, Krasnik M, et al. Endobronchial ultrasound for detecting central pulmonary emboli: a pilot study. Respiration 2009;77(3):298–302.

18. Tremblay A, Stather DR, MacEachern P, et al. A randomized controlled trial of standard vs endobronchial ultrasonography-guided transbronchial needle aspiration in patients with suspected sarcoidosis. Chest 2009;136(2):340–6.

19. Wong M, Yasufuku K, Nakajima T, et al. Endobronchial ultrasound: new insight for the diagnosis of sarcoidosis. Eur Respir J 2007;29(6):1182–6.

20. Savage C, Morrison RJ, Zwischenberger JB. Bronchoscopic diagnosis and staging of lung cancer. Chest Surg Clin N Am 2001;11(4):701–21, vii–viii.

21. Schreiber G, McCrory DC. Performance characteristics of different modalities for diagnosis of suspected lung cancer: summary of published evidence. Chest 2003;123(Suppl 1):115S–28S.

22. MacMahon H, Austin JHM, Gamsu G, et al. Guidelines for management of small pulmonary nodules detected on CT scans: a statement from the Fleischner Society. Radiology 2005;237(2):395–400.

23. Asano F, Matsuno Y, Shinagawa N, et al. A virtual bronchoscopic navigation system for pulmonary peripheral lesions. Chest 2006;130(2):559–66.

24. Asano F, Matsuno Y, Tsuzuku A, et al. Diagnosis of peripheral pulmonary lesions using a bronchoscope insertion guidance system combined with endobronchial ultrasonography with a guide sheath. Lung Cancer 2008;60(3):366–73.

25. Brown WT, Wu X, Amendola B, et al. Treatment of early non-small cell lung cancer, stage IA, by image-guided robotic stereotactic radioablation–CyberKnife. Cancer J 2007;13(2):87–94.

26. Loewen G, Natarajan N, Tan D, et al. Autofluorescence bronchoscopy for lung cancer surveillance based on risk assessment. Thorax 2007;62(4):335–40.

27. Haussinger K, Becker H, Stanzel F, et al. Autofluorescence bronchoscopy with white light bronchoscopy compared with white light bronchoscopy alone for the detection of precancerous lesions: a European randomised controlled multicentre trial. Thorax 2005;60(6):496–503.

28. Lam B, Wong MP, Fung SL, et al. The clinical value of autofluorescence bronchoscopy for the diagnosis of lung cancer. Eur Respir J 2006;28(5):915–9.

29. Kennedy TC, Franklin WA, Prindiville SA, et al. High prevalence of endobronchial malignancy in high-risk patients with moderate dysplasia in sputum. Chest 2004;125(Suppl 5):109S–109a.

30. Hanibuchi M, Yano S, Nishioka Y, et al. Autofluorescence bronchoscopy, a novel modality for the early detection of bronchial premalignant and malignant lesions. J Med Invest 2007;54(3–4):261–6.

31. Feller-Kopman D, Lunn W, Ernst A. Autofluorescence bronchoscopy and endobronchial ultrasound: a practical review. Ann Thorac Surg 2005;80(6):2395–401.

32. Chhajed PN, Shibuya K, Hoshino H, et al. A comparison of video and autofluorescence bronchoscopy in patients at high risk of lung cancer. Eur Respir J 2005;25(6):951–5.

33. Tanaka H, Yamada G, Saikai T, et al. Increased airway vascularity in newly diagnosed asthma using a high-magnification bronchovideoscope. Am J Respir Crit Care Med 2003;168(12):1495–9.

34. Vincent BD, Fraig M, Silvestri GA. A pilot study of narrow band imaging compared to white light bronchoscopy for evaluation of normal airways, pre-malignant and malignant airways disease. Chest 2007; 131(6):1794–9.

35. Keith RL, Miller YE, Gemmill RM, et al. Angiogenic squamous dysplasia in bronchi of individuals at high risk for lung cancer. Clin Cancer Res 2000; 6(5):1616–25.

36. Shibuya K, Fujisawa T, Hoshino H, et al. Fluorescence bronchoscopy in the detection of preinvasive bronchial lesions in patients with sputum cytology suspicious or positive for malignancy. Lung Cancer 2001;32(1):19–25.

37. Thiberville L, Moreno-Swirc S, Vercauteren T, et al. In vivo imaging of the bronchial wall microstructure using fibered confocal fluorescence microscopy. Am J Respir Crit Care Med 2007;175(1):22–31.

38. Thiberville L, Salaun M, Lachkar S, et al. Human in-vivo fluorescence microimaging of the alveolar ducts and sacs during bronchoscopy. Eur Respir J 2009; 33(5):974–85.

39. Whiteman SC, Yang Y, van Pittius DG, et al. Optical coherence tomography: real-time imaging of bronchial airways microstructure and detection of inflammatory/neoplastic morphologic changes. Clin Cancer Res 2006;12(3):813–8.

40. Boppart SA, Bouma BE, Pitris C, et al. In vivo cellular optical coherence tomography imaging. Nat Med 1998;4(7):861–5.

41. Han S, El-Abbadi NH, Hanna N, et al. Evaluation of tracheal imaging by optical coherence tomography. Respiration 2005;72(5):537–41.

42. Hanna N, Saltzman D, Mukai D, et al. Two-dimensional and 3-dimensional optical coherence tomographic imaging of the airway, lung, and pleura. J Thorac Cardiovasc Surg 2005;129(3): 615–22.

43. Bickenbach J, Dembinski R, Czaplik M, et al. Comparison of two in vivo microscopy techniques to visualize alveolar mechanics. J Clin Monit Comput 2009;23(5):323–32.

44. Mertens M, Tabuchi A, Meissner S, et al. Alveolar dynamics in acute lung injury: heterogeneous distension rather than cyclic opening and collapse. Crit Care Med 2009;37(9):2604–11.

Interventional Bronchoscopy from Bench to Bedside: New Techniques for Early Lung Cancer Detection

Henri G. Colt, MD[a,b,]*, Septimiu D. Murgu, MD[a,b]

KEYWORDS

- Autofluorescence bronchoscopy
- High-magnification bronchoscopy • Narrowband imaging
- Multimodality fluorescein imaging
- Endobronchial ultrasonography
- Optical coherence tomography • Confocal endoscopy

RATIONALE FOR EARLY DETECTION

Lung cancer is a leading cause of cancer-related death in the world, and it accounts for more deaths than breast, colon, and prostate cancer combined in the United States.[1] Most patients present with advanced disease, and the overall 5-year survival is approximately 15%.[2] From a historical perspective, the premise behind early lung cancer detection strategy is that if early treatment of lung cancer improves outcome, than early lung cancer detection is justified. Although initially the quest for sputum cytology programs was based on the fact that squamous cell carcinomas represented 70% of all lung cancers, that is no longer the case, as squamous cell cancers now represent only 25% to 30% of all lung cancers. These cancers are thought to be preceded by cellular atypia, reversible preepithelial proliferation, and carcinoma in situ (CIS), as demonstrated in earlier work by Auerbach,[3] and later substantiated in other studies.[4–6]

The incidence of CIS is correlated with the number of cigarette packs smoked. Early-stage squamous cell cancer, defined as a lesion less than 1 cm in diameter and 3 mm in depth, is considered N0 cancer and can be cured using bronchoscopic treatment as an alternative to surgical resection.[3]

The genesis of squamous cell lung cancer seems to require increased genomic instability and cell proliferation early on. Cellular transitions, DNA aneuploidy, and p53 gene overexpression during the transition from bronchial squamous metaplasia to advanced carcinoma, for example, have been identified. These cellular changes may lead to the eventual disruption of basement membrane and extension of intraepithelial carcinoma. The idea of cancer-specific airway-wide injury suggests that cancer-specific alterations in gene expression that occur as a result of smoking might also precede the development of lung cancer, as shown in a study that combined cytopathology of lower airway cells obtained by

Financial disclosures: The authors have no financial disclosures and no conflicts of interest related to the content of this article.

Parts of this article were presented by Dr Colt during the Pasquale Ciaglia Memorial Lecture at CHEST 2008.

[a] Department of Medicine, Pulmonary and Critical Care Medicine, University of California School of Medicine, 101 The City Drive, Irvine, Orange, CA 92868, USA

[b] Department of Medicine, UCI Medical Center, 101 The City Drive South, Building 53, Room 119, Route 81 Orange, CA 92868, USA

* Corresponding author. UCI Medical Center, 101 The City Drive South, Building 53, Room 119, Route 81 Orange, CA 92868.

E-mail address: hcolt@uci.edu (H.G. Colt).

Clin Chest Med 31 (2010) 29–37
doi:10.1016/j.ccm.2009.09.001

bronchoscopy in patients from 5 medical centers, using an 80-gene biomarker, yielding 95% sensitivity and 95% negative predictive value.[7]

The problem is that early morphologic changes occur below the threshold of conventional white-light bronchoscopy (WLB), which has only a 30% sensitivity to detect early-stage cancer in the central airways.[8] Several studies have suggested that a notable percentage of patients with moderate and severe dysplasia subsequently develop invasive carcinoma during a multistep carcinogenesis that might take 3 to 4 years. Approximately 11% of patients with moderate dysplasia and 19% to 46% with severe dysplasia subsequently develop invasive cancer.[5,6] In a recent study, the cumulative risk of developing lung cancer in a patient with a high-grade preoneoplastic lesion, such as severe dysplasia and CIS, was found to be more than 50% at 2 years.[9]

Others have found that capillary loops projecting into a dysplastic bronchial epithelium, referred to as angiogenic squamous dysplasia, might be an additional preneoplastic alteration.[10,11] Breuer and colleagues,[4] however, questioned the idea of progressive cellular alterations by discovering that some of these changes, especially squamous metaplasia, might regress when smokers stop smoking and that other dysplastic cytologic changes can fluctuate over time or progress in a nonstepwise fashion to CIS. Because conventional WLB is not useful for detecting mucosal alterations that might be just a few cells thick, and because it takes an experienced eye indeed to identify the minimal erythema or mucosal swelling that might indicate intraepithelial cancer, new technologies have been and are being developed to better detect these findings. It is possible that the future of bronchoscopic detection will include a multidimensional platform in which each of the following technologies plays a role and is readily available in a single structure, allowing one to change between technologies by the simple flip of a switch.

AUTOFLUORESCENCE BRONCHOSCOPY

Fluorescence bronchoscopy is based on the premise that differences in epithelial thickness, blood flow, and tissue fluorophore concentration cause preinvasive and neoplastic tissues to have diminished red fluorescence and substantially diminished green fluorescence compared with normal tissues when exposed to blue-light excitation of 440 to 480 nm wavelength.[10] Normally, when a surface is illuminated by light, the light can be reflected, backscattered, or absorbed. In addition, light also causes the tissue to fluoresce;

however, this autofluorescence (AF) cannot be seen during conventional WLB because the intensity of fluorescence is very low and is overwhelmed by the reflected and backscattered light. The major chromophores in the airway mucosa are elastin, collagen, flavins, nicotinamide adenine dinucleotide, nicotinamide adenine dinucleotide hydrogen (NADH), and porphyrins. Exposure of the chromophores to light of specific wavelengths excites electrons, and fluorescence is emitted when the electrons return to ground level. Accelerated intracellular metabolism in cancer cells decreases riboflavin and flavin coenzymes and NADH caused by overproduction of lactic acid through glycolysis.[12]

Intraepithelial lesions are only a few cell layers thick, and surface mucosa typically appears normal during conventional WLB. Less than one-third of CIS may be visible, even to the experienced bronchoscopist. In addition, the appearances of CIS may be similar to those produced from chronic bronchitis, which is often present in patients at risk for lung cancer. By the time the mucosa appears distinctly abnormal, the cancer is typically invasive.[10] As mucosal and submucosal disease progresses from normal to metaplasia, dysplasia, and CIS, there is a progressive loss of the green AF, causing a red-brown appearance of the tissue. Areas of abnormal fluorescence are identified as brown regions on a normal green background. Successful localization of a dysplastic lesion is possible using AF, whereas white-light examination is normal. The intensity of green fluorescence is measured, and an abnormally low green fluorescent area is identified as a cold spot on a normal green background.

Optical engineers are working arduously to improve detection of abnormal tissues and discrimination from normal bronchial mucosa. In a study by Gabrecht and colleagues,[13] violet-light excitation at 405 nm was delivered (rather than the 450 nm blue wavelength), and the contrast between preneoplastic and healthy tissue was quantified using off-line image analysis. There was almost 3 times higher contrast when backscattered red light was added to the violet excitation.

AF has been shown to be helpful in high-risk groups, such as in patients with a history of head and neck cancer, chronic obstructive pulmonary disease (COPD), and smokers. Knowing that roentgenographically occult lung cancers are characterized by an incidence of synchronous lesions ranging from 0.7% to 15% and that metachronous lesions might occur in as many as 5% per year,[14,15] it is not surprising that AF bronchoscopy has been advocated as a surveillance tool in these patients, in patients with newly diagnosed early cases before thoracotomy, and in those patients who have undergone curative surgery for non–small cell lung cancer.[16] An increased sensitivity of about 86%, but low specificity of WLB combined with AF has been demonstrated by numerous investigators.[8] Additional concerns are that as a result of the high sensitivity, numerous biopsies are necessary, and even these may alter the natural progression, or lack thereof, of preneoplastic lesions.[17] With this consideration, and for those who accept Breuer's suggestion that each lesion is on an individual time clock and that one cannot predict disease progression based solely on the initial cytopathologic abnormality identified, it becomes clear that a less invasive biopsy method could prove useful.

HIGH-MAGNIFICATION BRONCHOSCOPY

Although the only abnormality of WLB seen in dysplasia is swelling and redness at bronchial bifurcations, histologically there is neovascularization or increased mucosal microvascular growth.[18,19] Furthermore, mucosal blood flow is thought to be influenced by vascular and airway pressures, inspired air conditions, and anatomic neurotransmitters.[18] High-magnification bronchoscopy (HMB) enables observation of vascular networks to identify potential areas of increased vascularity in the bronchial mucosa in patients with respiratory diseases, such as asthma, chronic bronchitis, sarcoidosis, and lung cancer. This system can provide information about the bronchial mucosa with a maximum magnification of 110 times. A dense concentration of subepithelial microvessels mainly observed in the inter cartilage portion, indicating an increase in submucosal circulation, suggests that it may be a useful tool for observing and evaluating subepithelial microvessels in large airways in various pathologies, such as lung cancer or asthma.[18] Areas of increased vessel growth and complex networks of tortuous vessels in the bronchial mucosa that are detected using HMB at sites of abnormal fluorescence may enable discrimination between bronchitis and dysplasia. At sites of abnormal fluorescence established by fluorescence bronchoscopy, HMB detects bronchial dysplasia more accurately than fluorescence bronchoscopy alone, the sensitivity and specificity being 70% and 90%, respectively.[18] Measurements of subepithelial vessels showed that vessel area density and vessel length density are significantly increased in subjects with asthma compared with control subjects and patients with COPD.[20] On the other hand, subepithelial microvessels of

smokers are notably decreased and narrow, which suggests a decrease in microcirculation in the subepithelial layer of the large airway.[21] One shortcoming of HMB, however, is that a significant number of subepithelial vessels have a diameter of less than 20 μm, which is below the limits of HMB detection. Furthermore, HMB cannot distinguish new vessels from vascular engorgement or vasodilation.[20]

NARROWBAND IMAGING

Microvascular structures are further observed if a new narrowband filter is used instead of the conventional red/green/blue broadband filter. This narrowband imaging (NBI) technique uses a 415-nm blue light, which is absorbed by hemoglobin contained in the capillary network on the mucosal surface and a 540-nm green light that is absorbed by blood vessels located a bit deeper below the capillary layer.[11] Compared with WLB, NBI was shown to increase the rate of detection of dysplasia or malignancy by 23%.[22] In a recent study, investigators found that NBI has a higher specificity than AF imaging, without significantly compromising sensitivity. Combining AF imaging and NBI did not increase diagnostic yield significantly. NBI might thus become an alternative to AF imaging in the detection of early lung cancers.[23]

MULTIMODALITY FLUORESCEIN IMAGING

Researchers are investigating a multimodality technique whereby fluorescein imaging, analogous to that used in ophthalmology, in conjunction with high-resolution computed tomography (CT) scanning, bronchoscopy, and four-dimensional spatial reconstructions allow detailed examination of the bronchial microcirculatory system.[24–26] The idea is to develop a macro-optical technique that would allow large field visibility of alterations in blood flow to identify focused regions of interest for micro-optical techniques, such as optical coherence tomography (OCT).

Fluorescein is a highly fluorescent compound that fluoresces yellow-green after excitation with a blue light. Although a large portion binds to serum protein in the blood stream, much of it remains unbound, and it is this unbound portion that is responsible for the observed yellow-green light emission. Fluorescein stays in the body for about 36 hours before being metabolized by the kidneys. In one study, changes in rabbit trachea fluorescence were noted after the injection of potent vasodilators and vasoconstricting agents, such as bradykinin and cocaine.[24] In another study, texture mapping and identification of distal airway tumor infiltration beyond an area of initial endobronchial obstruction was possible using simultaneous application of 4 different imaging modalities, including white light and color bronchoscopy after fluorescein injection and three-dimensional multi-detector CT.[26]

ENDOBRONCHIAL ULTRASONOGRAPHY

Ultrasound and Doppler ultrasound image tissue structure and blood flow, but are limited in spatial resolution to approximately 50 to 200 µm because of their relatively long acoustic wavelengths (**Fig. 1**A, B). Endobronchial ultrasound (EBUS), however, has been used to accurately measure the depth of tumor invasion beyond the cartilaginous layer and to identify the structural layers of the airway wall that are important in defining and

understanding various central airway disorders, such as relapsing polychondritis, tuberculosis, tracheomalacia, and lung cancer.[27–32]

It is known that lymph node invasion in radio-occult cancers changes staging and subsequently the treatment and prognosis in non–small cell lung cancer. The general probability is about 5% but very rare in CIS (1%) and not seen in lesions that are less than 3 mm thick, 10 mm in surface area, or those with an invasion index less than 20 mm in the large central bronchi.[33,34] However, significant rates of lymph node invasion have been reported (10%–30%) in case of invasion of the cartilage.[35–37] Furthermore, 70% of patients presenting with radiographically occult lung cancer were shown to have more advanced cancer using a combination of autofluorescence bronchoscopy and high-resolution CT rather than a conventional initial evaluation.[38] An accurate assessment of

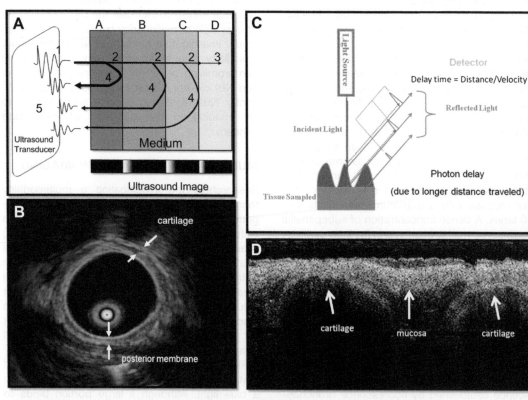

Fig. 1. (*A*) Ultrasound image formation. The transducer sends out a brief pulse of high-frequency sound (**1**) that penetrates and propagates (**2**) through various substances (referred to as medium). Ultrasound waves attenuate (**3**) as they propagate through a medium and get reflected (**4**) from tissue boundaries and interfaces back to the transducer, which serves as the sensor and the source of signal (**5**). (*B*) Endobronchial ultrasound image obtained with radial scanning using a 20 MHz probe for a normal airway (left main bronchus). The cartilaginous rings and the posterior membrane layers are visualized. (*C*) OCT image formation. Light is emitted from the source, shined into tissues, and reflected off internal structures. The longer the distance traveled, the longer the delay in returning to a detector. The delay in the returning light from deeper structures compared with shallow structures is used to reconstruct images. (*D*) OCT image of the trachea using a longitudinal scanning direction showing the mucosa and the upper part of the cartilaginous rings.

cartilaginous and peribronchial tumor invasions are likely to be important before selecting or proposing endoscopic treatment modalities.

For this purpose, the radial EBUS probe has been proved to be useful.[31] The standard frequency for radial probe EBUS is 20 MHz, which allows for a resolution of less than 1 mm and a depth of penetration of approximately 4 to 5 cm (**Fig. 2**). This frequency allows for delineation of the layers of the airway wall and peribronchial structures.[30] Using this technique, Herth and colleagues[31] showed that EBUS clearly defines bronchial wall layers and adjacent anatomic structures and is an excellent tool for distinguishing airway tumor invasion from external compression and for determining the depth of endobronchial tumor invasion.

Hayata and colleagues[39] found that photodynamic therapy (PDT) is less effective in achieving a complete response when tumor is extended beyond the cartilaginous layer. Using this principle of extracartilaginous extension, Miyazu and colleagues[40] further demonstrated the role of EBUS in selecting patients for endobronchial therapies. If the tumor invades beyond the cartilaginous layer, PDT should not be applied, and surgery should be proposed, if possible. More recently, it was shown that in 28% of patients referred for presumed CIS or early cancer, EBUS established disease extent that would have made

endoscopic curative treatment impossible.[31] Thus, EBUS might guide clinicians in deciding on bronchoscopic treatments or open resection in patients with early lung cancer and might be an important component of future multimodality diagnostic bronchoscopy platforms in patients with airway abnormalities.

OCT

The search for a rapid acquisition, high-spatial resolution, and noninvasive technique for endoscopic imaging of in vivo tissue structure and function has resulted in the development of OCT systems. OCT resembles ultrasound but uses light rather than acoustic waves. In ultrasound, the imaging is obtained by measuring the delay time (echo delay) for an incident ultrasonic pulse to be reflected back from structures within tissues (**Fig. 1C, D**). Because the velocity of sound is relatively slow, this delay time can be measured electronically. However, ultrasound and Doppler ultrasound, used clinically to image tissue structure and blood flow, are limited in spatial resolution to approximately 50 to 200 μm because of their relatively long acoustic wavelengths.

For optical diagnostic technologies, the velocity of light is 200,000 times greater than the velocity of sound, such that measurements

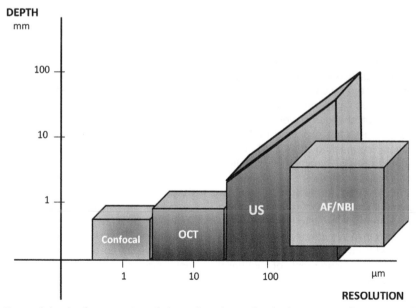

Fig. 2. Resolution and depth of penetration of airway imaging technologies. In general, systems with good depth of penetration have low resolution and cover large areas, whereas systems with shallow depth of penetration have high resolution and cover small areas. Confocal, confocal microscopy; OCT, optical coherence tomography; US, ultrasound; AF, autofluorescence; NBI, narrowband imaging.

of delay cannot be performed directly by electronic techniques. Therefore, a technique known as low-coherence interferometry is used. Latest ultrahigh-resolution OCT systems are capable of up to 2 orders of magnitude greater resolution (1–2 μm) than ultrasound at depths of up to 2 mm in optically scattering tissues (see **Fig. 2**).[41] The depth range of OCT is thus sufficient to penetrate through the upper layers of exposed tissues on airway surfaces (maximal depth average 2–3 mm), where many endobronchial and bronchogenic carcinomas originate or spread, and is equivalent to the depth that standard endobronchial forceps can sample.[42] OCT uses a noncontact probe, which does not influence the special resolution. The procedure is straightforward and adds less than 5 minutes to a standard WLB procedure under local anesthesia and moderate sedation. Rigid probes can of course be used during rigid bronchoscopy, but technology using fiberoptic probes provides miniaturization to enable imaging of airways down to the terminal bronchiole beyond the range of a standard flexible video bronchoscope. Although some images obtained show potentially characteristic architectural changes in malignancy, and exact OCT-surgical pathology correlations are promising, further study is warranted in cancer and many other disorders.[43]

Whiteman and colleagues[44] examined freshly excised lung specimens and showed the ability to differentiate tissue structural characteristics of normal airway and airway malignancy using a 10 μm resolution time-domain OCT benchtop prototype. However, they were unable to define individual cellular profiles. In a study by Brenner and colleagues,[45] statistically and clinically significant increases were detected by OCT in the thickness of the lower trachea and bronchial airways, whereas only modest changes developed in the higher trachea 6 hours after exposing rabbits to smoke inhalation, suggesting that OCT might also be a means to study dynamic in vivo alterations of airway wall architecture.

Studies were designed to determine whether OCT could characterize preneoplastic changes in the bronchial epithelium identified by AF bronchoscopy. CIS and invasive carcinoma were able to be distinguished from normal bronchial epithelium.[46] Quantitative measurement of epithelial thickness showed that invasive carcinoma was significantly different from CIS and that dysplasia was significantly different from metaplasia or hyperplasia.[47]

Other applications of OCT systems include measuring lower and upper airway calibers.

Coxson and colleagues[48] analyzed third and fourth generation airways and found excellent correlation between OCT- and CT-based estimates of airway luminal area. OCT might be a more sensitive method than CT for discriminating changes in the more distal airways of subjects with a range of expiratory flow limitations. Therefore, this tool may become useful in detecting airway remodeling in asthma or COPD or in evaluating disease progression over time. In other studies, OCT measurements during quantitative real-time imaging of human upper airways were found to correlate with CT-derived measurements.[49] Thus, OCT has a potential application in determining the site and length of the collapsing airway, which might be important in patients with obstructive sleep apnea and expiratory central airway collapse.

OCT technology is evolving rapidly. Time-based OCT is limited because it is time consuming. On the other hand, ultrafast frequency-domain OCT is limited only by the speed at which the mirrors used need to move and by the lasers used to bounce light off those mirrors because light penetration itself is measured rather than the time it takes for the light to travel. Current challenges include the need to access the tissues using small probes, and therefore necessitating further miniaturization, the need to acquire data quickly and process the data in real time, and the need to improve the overall resolution of the images obtained. The ability to deliver this technology to the region of interest, therefore, is also critical, and requires development of specialized probes and, most importantly, the ability to miniaturize the technology onto probes or needle-based systems that are capable of penetrating deeply into regions that would otherwise be inaccessible using surface technologies.

Three-dimensional OCT imaging is another area of major advancement. Three-dimensional imaging allows organized image acquisition from volume-based regions. This information is potentially invaluable for three-dimensional reconstructions, reconstructions of vascular and functional tissue information, and more thorough and complete investigations of tissue alterations, such as malignant transformations.[50] Three-dimensional imaging, however, requires rapidly responsive three-dimensional probes and very fast acquisitional OCT technologies. By using three-dimensional hysteresis, mechanical movement is avoided, and real-time OCT scanning is possible.

Improvements in OCT resolution are necessary for image analysis. This increasingly involves the use of broadband lasers. Current laser systems can deliver images with 1-μm resolution, such as those obtained using a prototype system where the structural elements of onion skin and in vivo tadpole cells are readily visible. Methods for reducing the acquisition time are needed to obtain rapid three-dimensional in vivo imaging. A major advance in acquisition time is obtained by using spectral domain technologies. In spectral domain technologies, a moving mirror is not required to perform depth scanning. Instead, depth information is obtained from the frequency-dependent differences in the interference signal reflections. Thus the speed of acquisition can be improved more than 100-fold over time-domain systems.[51]

CONFOCAL ENDOSCOPY

Another major area of optical technology advances for endoscopic imaging is confocal endoscopy/endomicroscopy. Confocal endoscopy/endomicroscopy has the capabilities for submicrometer-level resolution imaging but has even further limitations in depth of penetration (approximately 0.5 mm compared with approximately 2–3 mm with OCT) (see **Fig. 2**). Confocal endoscopy uses principles that are analogous to confocal microscopy, where the source light is focused through a pinhole to localize the specific point in space from which the signal is obtained from tissues. Three-dimensional imaging can be reconstructed with very high resolution by moving the endoscopic source beam.[52] Fluorescein sodium can be used to produce tissue contrast, and in the future, biomarkers common to precancerous states or declared lung cancers might become detectable because of specific fluorescent staining patterns. Dynamic changes in respiratory epithelial structure, primarily at the level of the microvasculature, and enhanced visualization of angiogenesis might also help in the study of the pathophysiology of airway disease involving central or peripheral airways.

SUMMARY

Studies increasingly demonstrate the importance of structural wall changes, angiogenesis, cellular proliferation, and genetic alterations in the pathogenesis of benign and malignant airway abnormalities. Angiogenesis in malignancy, airway remodeling in asthma, and destruction of the airway cartilage by cancer or in malacia can already be explored in vivo using bronchoscopic optical technologies.

New optical technologies such as those presented in this article allow dynamic study of these processes at the cellular level, and it is hoped that opportunities for targeted therapy will be provided in the future. The authors thus envision a future where these optical technologies provide a window to intracellular structures in vivo, replacing traditional in vitro analyses of cellular components using conventional tissue biopsy specimens. Indeed, we are on the verge of discovering a multidimensional bronchoscopic platform that can be used to narrow in on airway structures, explore vascular flow and angiogenesis, and discover new features of bronchogenic carcinogenesis.

REFERENCES

1. Horner MJ, Ries LAG, Krapcho M, et al, editors. SEER cancer statistics review, 1975–2006. Bethesda (MD): National Cancer Institute. Available at: http://seer.cancer.gov/csr/1975_2006/. based on November 2008 SEER data submission, posted to the SEER web site, 2009. Accessed August 1, 2009.
2. Ries L, Eisner M, Kosary C, editors. Cancer statistics review, 1975–2002. Bethesda (MD): National Cancer Institute; 2005.
3. Auerbach O, Stout AP, Hammond EC, et al. Changes in bronchial epithelium in relation to cigarette smoking and in relation to lung cancer. N Engl J Med 1961;265:253–68.
4. Breuer RH, Pasic A, Smit EF, et al. The natural course of preneoplastic lesions in bronchial epithelium. Clin Cancer Res 2005;11:537–43.
5. Band PR, Feldstein M, Saccomanno G. Reversibility of bronchial marked atypia: implication for chemoprevention. Cancer Detect Prev 1986;9:157–60.
6. Venmans BJ, van Boxem TJ, Smit EF, et al. Outcome of bronchial carcinoma in situ. Chest 2000;117:1572–6.
7. Spira A, Beane JE, Shah V, et al. Airway epithelial gene expression in the diagnostic evaluation of smokers with suspect lung cancer. Nat Med 2007;13:361–6.
8. Ikeda N, Hayashi A, Iwasaki K, et al. Comprehensive diagnostic bronchoscopy of central type early stage lung cancer. Lung Cancer 2007;56:295–302.
9. Jeremy GP, Banerjee AK, Read CA, et al. Surveillance for the detection of early lung cancer in patients with bronchial dysplasia. Thorax 2007;62:43–50.
10. Keith RL, Miller YE, Gemmill RM, et al. Angiogenic squamous dysplasia in bronchi of individuals at high risk for lung cancer. Clin Cancer Res 2000;6:1616–25.
11. Shibuya K, Hoshino H, Chiyo M, et al. High magnification bronchovideoscopy combined with narrow band imaging could detect capillary loops of angiogenic squamous dysplasia in heavy smokers at high risk for lung cancer. Thorax 2003;58:989–95.

12. Interventional bronchoscopy. Progress in respiratory research, vol. 30. Switzerland: Springer Kaarger; 2000. p. 243.

13. Gabrecht T, Glanzmann T, Freitag L, et al. Optimized autofluorescence bronchoscopy using additional backscattered red light. J Biomed Opt 2007;12: 064016.

14. Furukawa K, Ikeda N, Miura T, et al. Is autofluorescence bronchoscopy needed to diagnose early bronchogenic carcinoma? Pro: autofluorescence bronchoscopy. J Bronchol 2003;10:64–9.

15. Pierard P, Vermylen P, Bosschaerts T, et al. Synchronous roentgenographically occult lung carcinoma in patients with resectable primary lung cancer. Chest 2000;117:779–85.

16. Weigel TL, Yousem S, Dacic S, et al. Fluorescence bronchoscopic surveillance after curative surgical resection for non-small-cell lung cancer. Ann Surg Oncol 2000;7:176–80.

17. Bota S, Auliac JB, Paris C, et al. Follow-up of bronchial precancerous lesions and carcinoma in situ using fluorescence endoscopy. Am J Respir Crit Care Med 2001;164:1688–93.

18. Shibuya K, Hoshino H, Chiyo M, et al. Subepithelial vascular patterns in bronchial dysplasias using a high magnification bronchovideoscope. Thorax 2002;57:902–7.

19. Yamada G, Takahashi H, Shijubo N, et al. Subepithelial microvasculature in large airways observed by high-magnification bronchovideoscope. Chest 2005;128:876–80.

20. Tanaka H, Yamada G, Saikai T, et al. Increased airway vascularity in newly diagnosed asthma using a high-magnification bronchovideoscope. Am J Respir Crit Care Med 2003;168:1495–9.

21. Yamada G, Shijubo N, Kitada J, et al. Decreased subepithelial microvasculature observed by high magnification bronchovideoscope in the large airways of smokers. Intern Med 2008;47:1579–83.

22. Vincent BD, Fraig M, Silvestri GA. A pilot study of narrow-band imaging compared to white light bronchoscopy for evaluation of normal airways and premalignant and malignant airways disease. Chest 2007;131:1794–9.

23. Herth FJ, Eberhardt R, Anantham D, et al. Narrow-band imaging bronchoscopy increases the specificity of bronchoscopic early lung cancer detection. J Thorac Oncol 2009;4:1060–5.

24. Suter M, Reinhardt J, Montague P, et al. Bronchoscopic imaging of pulmonary mucosal vasculature responses to inflammatory mediators. J Biomed Opt 2005;10:034013.

25. Suter M, McLennan G, Reinhardt JM, et al. Macro-optical color assessment of the pulmonary airways with subsequent three-dimensional multidetector-x-ray-computed-tomography assisted display. J Biomed Opt 2005;10:051703.

26. Suter MJ, Reinhardt JM, McLennan G. Integrated CT/bronchoscopy in the central airways: preliminary results. Acad Radiol 2008;15:786–98.

27. Iwamoto Y, Miyazawa T, Kurimoto N, et al. Interventional bronchoscopy in the management of airway stenosis due to tracheobronchial tuberculosis. Chest 2004;126:1344–52.

28. Lee P, Low S, Liew H, et al. Endobronchial ultrasound for detection of tracheomalacia from chronic compression by vascular ring. Respirology 2007; 12:299–301.

29. Miyazu Y, Miyazawa T, Kurimoto N, et al. Endobronchial ultrasonography in the diagnosis and treatment of relapsing polychondritis with tracheobronchial malacia. Chest 2003;124:2393–5.

30. Kurimoto N, Murayama M, Yoshioka S, et al. Assessment of usefulness of endobronchial ultrasonography in determination of depth of tracheobronchial tumor invasion. Chest 1999;115:1500–6.

31. Herth F, Ernst A, Schulz M, et al. Endobronchial ultrasound reliably differentiates between airway infiltration and compression by tumor. Chest 2003; 123:458–62.

32. Murgu S, Kuromoto N, Colt H. Endobronchial ultrasound morphology of expiratory central airway collapse. Respirology 2008;13:315–9.

33. Nagamoto N, Saito Y, Ohta S, et al. Relationship of lymph node metastasis to primary tumor size and microscopic appearance of roentgenographically occult lung cancer. Am J Surg Pathol 1989;13:1009–13.

34. Nagamoto N, Saito Y, Sato M, et al. Clinicopathological analysis of 19 cases of isolated carcinoma in situ of the bronchus. Am J Surg Pathol 1993;17:1234–43.

35. Akaogi E, Ogawa I, Mitsui K, et al. Endoscopic criteria of early squamous cell carcinoma of the bronchus. Cancer 1994;74:3113–7.

36. Woolner LB, Fontana RS, Cortese DA, et al. Roentgenographically occult lung cancer: pathologic findings and frequency of multicentricity during a 10-year period. Mayo Clin Proc 1984; 59:453–66.

37. Saito Y, Nagamoto N, Ota S, et al. Results of surgical treatment for roentgenographically occult bronchogenic squamous cell carcinoma. J Thorac Cardiovasc Surg 1992;104:401–7.

38. Sutedja TG, Codrington H, Risse EK, et al. Autofluorescence bronchoscopy improves staging of radiographically occult lung cancer and has an impact on therapeutic strategy. Chest 2001;120: 1327–32.

39. Hayata Y, Kato H, Furuse K, et al. Photodynamic therapy of 168 early stage cancers of the lung and esophagus: a Japanese multi-centre study. Lasers Med Sci 1996;11:255–9.

40. Miyazu Y, Miyazawa T, Kurimoto N, et al. Endobronchial ultrasonography in the assessment of centrally located early-stage lung cancer before

photodynamic therapy. Am J Respir Crit Care Med 2002;165:832–7.

41. Drexler W, Morgner U, Kärtner FX, et al. In vivo ultra-high-resolution optical coherence tomography. Opt Lett 1999;24:1221–3.

42. Fujimoto JG, Brezinski ME, Tearney GJ, et al. Optical biopsy and imaging using optical coherence tomography. Nat Med 1995;1:970–2.

43. Colt H, Murgu SD, Ahn YC, et al. Multimodality bronchoscopic imaging of tracheopathica osteochondroplastica. J Biomed Opt 2009;14: 034035.

44. Whiteman SC, Yang Y, Gey van Pittius D, et al. Optical coherence tomography: real-time imaging of bronchial airways microstructure and detection of inflammatory/neoplastic morphologic changes. Clin Cancer Res 2006;12:813–8.

45. Brenner M, Kreuter K, Ju J, et al. In vivo optical coherence tomography detection of differences in regional large airway smoke inhalation induced injury in a rabbit model. J Biomed Opt 2008;13: 034001.

46. Tsuboi M, Hayashi A, Ikeda N, et al. Optical coherence tomography in the diagnosis of bronchial lesions. Lung Cancer 2005;49:387–94.

47. Lam S, Standish B, Baldwin C, et al. In vivo optical coherence tomography imaging of preinvasive bronchial lesions. Clin Cancer Res 2008;14: 2006–11.

48. Coxson HO, Quiney B, Sin DD, et al. Airway wall thickness assessed using computed tomography and optical coherence tomography. Am J Respir Crit Care Med 2008;177:1201–6.

49. Armstrong JJ, Leigh MS, Sampson DD, et al. Quantitative upper airway imaging with anatomic optical coherence tomography. Am J Respir Crit Care Med 2006;173:226–33.

50. Jung W, McCormick DT, Ahn YC, et al. In vivo three-dimensional spectral domain endoscopic optical coherence tomography using a microelectromechanical system mirror. Opt Lett 2007;32:3239–41.

51. Su J, Zhang J, Yu L, et al. Real-time swept source optical coherence tomography imaging of the human airway using a microelectromechanical system endoscope and digital signal processor. J Biomed Opt 2008;13:030506.

52. Thiberville L, Moreno-Swirc S, Vercauteren T, et al. In vivo imaging of the bronchial wall microstructure using fibered confocal fluorescence microscopy. Am J Respir Crit Care Med 2007;175:22–31.

Early Diagnosis of Lung Cancer

Kazuhiro Yasufuku, MD, PhD

KEYWORDS

- Lung cancer • Early detection
- Autofluorescence bronchoscopy
- Endobronchial ultrasound

Early detection and surgical resection is essential for the treatment of lung cancer. Although the introduction of low-dose spiral computed tomography (CT) is considered to be one of the most promising clinical research developments, CT screening is used for detecting small peripheral lesions. However, tumors arising in the central airways require other techniques for early detection. Centrally arising squamous cell carcinoma of the airway, especially in heavy smokers, is thought to develop through multiple stages from squamous metaplasia to dysplasia, followed by carcinoma in situ (CIS), progressing to invasive cancer.[1,2] It would be ideal to be able to detect and treat preinvasive bronchial lesions, defined as dysplasia and carcinoma in situ, before they progress to invasive cancer.[3,4] Hence, great efforts have been made to develop new bronchoscopic imaging techniques capable of detecting these lesions. Bronchoscopic imaging techniques capable of detecting preinvasive lesions and currently available in clinical practice include autofluorescence bronchoscopy (AFB), high magnification bronchovideoscope, and narrow band imaging (NBI). For a more precise evaluation of newly detected preinvasive lesions, endobronchial ultrasound (EBUS) and optical coherence tomography (OCT) can be used.

AFB improves the sensitivity for detection of preinvasive lesions in the central airway[3–5] and increases the diagnostic accuracy for squamous dysplasia, CIS, and early lung carcinoma when used simultaneously with conventional white light bronchoscopy (WLB).[5–16] In addition to single center studies, 3 multicenter and 2 randomized clinical trials have documented the usefulness of AFB as an adjunct to WLB for detecting intraepithelial neoplasia and CIS.[5,13–16] However, the specificity of AFB for diagnosing preinvasive lesions is low.[13] Distinguishing between preinvasive lesions and other benign epithelial changes such as bronchitis is problematic. To increase the specificity, a new autofluorescence imaging (AFI) bronchovideoscope system has been developed where preinvasive lesions and benign changes may be differentiated by color.[17]

AFB displays areas of epithelial thickness and hypervascularity as abnormal fluorescence, which suggests a role for neovascularization or increased mucosal microvascular growth in bronchial dysplasia.[12,13] To focus on the mucosal microvascular structure, the high magnification bronchovideoscope was developed.[18] The high magnification bronchovideoscope is a combination of 2 systems: a video observation system for high magnification observation and a fiber observation system for orientation of the bronchoscope tip. The magnification is 110 times or 4-fold that of a conventional bronchovideoscope. This enables visualization of the vascular networks of the bronchial mucosa.[18] High magnification can detect increased vessel growth and complex networks of tortuous vessels of various sizes in the bronchial mucosa.[18]

Focusing on the visualization of the vascular network in the bronchial mucosa, a new imaging technology, NBI, was developed after high magnification.[19,20] NBI is an optical image technology that enhances vessels in the surface mucosa by using the light absorption characteristics of hemoglobin at a specific wavelength. NBI enhances the clinical value of magnification bronchoscopy by

Division of Thoracic Surgery, Department of Surgery, Toronto General Hospital, University Health Network, University of Toronto, 200 Elizabeth Street, 9N-957, Toronto, Ontario M5G2C4, Canada
E-mail address: kazuhiro.yasufuku@uhn.on.ca

Clin Chest Med 31 (2010) 39–47
doi:10.1016/j.ccm.2009.08.004

allowing the visualization of abnormal distribution and dilatation of blood vessels.[19,20]

This article reviews new bronchoscopic imaging techniques, including AFI, NBI, and EBUS and describes their roles in the early diagnosis and treatment of lung cancer.

AFI VIDEOSCOPE SYSTEM

AFI is a video-endoscopic system that exploits the fact that different wavelengths of light can be used to highlight the distinction between tumorous lesions and normal tissues.[17] AFI produces diagnostic images using light that is affected by blood constituents and autofluorescence. The system has a high resolution imaging charge-coupled device (CCD) at the distal end of the bronchovideoscope (BF-F260, Olympus Medical Systems Corp, Tokyo, Japan). By combining autofluorescence and a high resolution bronchovideoscope, subtle differences in mucosal structures that would be difficult to detect in normal observation can be visualized. In addition to fluorescence light observation with high image quality, this system also provides the detailed normal light images required for observation of the vascular structures

in the mucosa. With one touch of a button, one can easily switch back and forth between normal images and fluorescence images.

Attenuation of autofluorescence is caused by (1) absorption and scattering of light because of hyperplasia of the mucosal epithelium and (2) absorption of light by hemoglobin in the blood. The limitation of conventional AFB was that it displayed inflammatory lesions in the same way as neoplastic lesions, which resulted in low specificity for detection of preinvasive lesions. The new AFI can easily distinguish between neoplastic lesions and normal tissue by changes in color.

AFI exploits the characteristics of 2 different wavelengths: (1) autofluorescence (460–690 nm) is attenuated when a neoplastic lesion is irradiated with blue excitation light (390–440 nm), and (2) components absorbed by the blood are reflected when irradiated with green light (540–560 nm). Both types of light are emitted from the AFI-dedicated rotary filter installed in front of the light source bulb. These 2 types of light are captured by the CCD at the distal end of the scope and converted into electrical signals. The barrier filter installed in front of the CCD cuts excessive blue excitation light to detect weak autofluorescence.

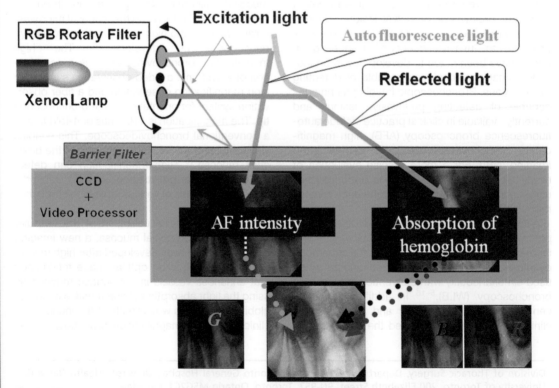

Fig. 1. AFI system configuration. AFI exploits the characteristics of 2 different wavelengths: (1) autofluorescence (460–690 nm) is attenuated when a neoplastic lesion is irradiated with blue excitation light (390–440 nm) , and (2) components absorbed by the blood are reflected when irradiated with green light (540–560 nm).

In the video processor, the autofluorescence light signal is converted into green data and the green reflected light is converted into red and blue data. The data are then synthesized into the AFI color image data that is displayed on the monitor (**Fig. 1**). As a result, AFI displays normal areas in light green, areas with abundant blood flow and blood vessels in darker green, and neoplastic lesions in magenta (**Fig. 2**).

REPRESENTATIVE CASES OF AFI

Representative cases of bronchitis, squamous dysplasia, and squamous cell carcinoma are shown. Arrows indicate abnormal areas of bronchial epithelium. **Fig. 3A** shows a case of bronchitis affecting the bifurcation of the right B4 and 5. Lung imaging fluorescence endoscopy (LIFE) demonstrated abnormal autofluorescence and the AFI image was green. **Fig. 3B** shows a case of squamous dysplasia at the bifurcation of the left B3a and B3bc. Although WLB demonstrated normal bifurcation, LIFE demonstrated abnormal autofluorescence, and the AFI image was magenta. **Fig. 3C** shows a case of squamous cell carcinoma. Irregular mucosa and protruding nodules are identified at the bifurcation of the right middle and lower lobe bronchi by WLB, LIFE, and AFI. The AFI image clearly is magenta at the abnormal area.

APPLICATIONS OF AFI

Besides the detection of preinvasive bronchial and malignant lesions, AFI is useful for the confirmation of the extent of tumor invasion in central type lung cancer.

This case was referred for abnormal chest radiograph. On the chest CT scan, the left upper lobe bronchus was seen to be completely occluded by the tumor. On bronchoscopic examination, a tumor obstructing the left upper lobe bronchus was seen under white light examination. On the AFI image, the extent of the tumor margins was clearly identified as magenta. Left upper lobectomy, bronchoplasty, and pulmonary artery angioplasty were performed on this patient and the margins had negative results for malignancy (**Fig. 4**).

COMPARISON OF WLB, LIFE, AND AFI

The first prospective study on the effectiveness of AFI in the evaluation of preinvasive lesions and inflammation was based on the hypothesis that color analyses of the different wave lengths would improve the ability to differentiate between inflammation and preinvasive lesions.[17] To prove this hypothesis, a total of 32 patients with suspected or known lung cancer were entered into this study. Conventional WLB and LIFE were performed before using AFI.

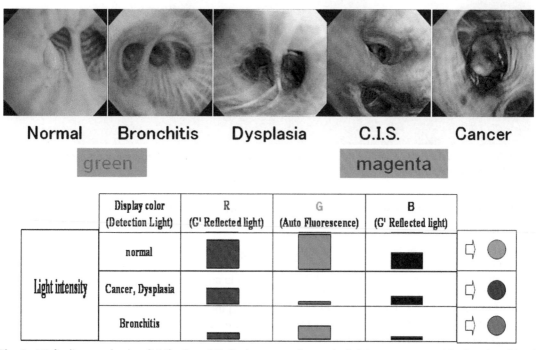

	Display color (Detection Light)	R (G' Reflected light)	G (Auto Fluorescence)	B (G' Reflected light)	
Light intensity	normal				
	Cancer, Dysplasia				
	Bronchitis				

Fig. 2. AFI findings and color distribution. AFI displays normal areas in light green, areas with abundant blood flow and blood vessels in darker green, and neoplastic lesions in magenta.

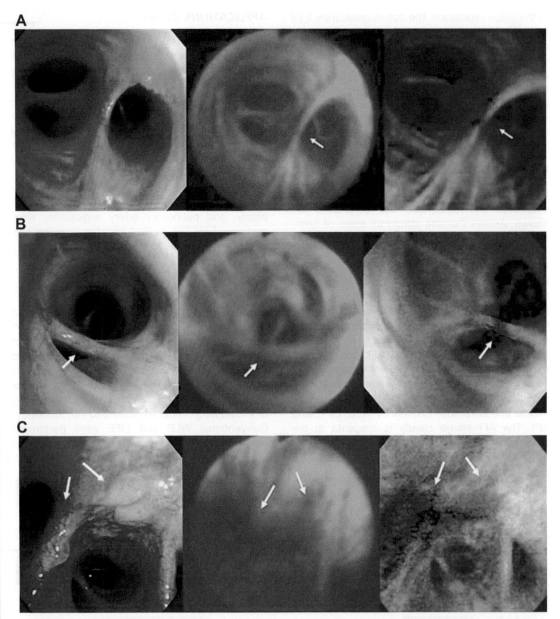

Fig. 3. Images of WLB, lung imaging fluorescence endoscopy (LIFE), and AFI. Representative cases of (A) bronchitis, (B) squamous dysplasia, and (C) squamous cell carcinoma.

WLB and LIFE detected 62 lesions, including lung cancers (n = 2), squamous dysplasias (n = 30), and bronchitis (n = 30). By using AFI, 24 dysplasias and 2 cancer lesions were displayed in magenta and 25 bronchitis lesions, blue. The sensitivities of detecting dysplasia by LIFE and AFI were 96.7% and 80%, respectively. The specificity of AFI (83.3%) was significantly higher than that of LIFE (36.6%) (P = .0005). The conclusion of this prospective study was that AFI seems to represent a significant advance in distinguishing preinvasive and malignant lesions from bronchitis

or hyperplasia under circumstances where LIFE would identify all these as abnormal lesions.

NBI

NBI is an optical image enhancement technology that enhances vessels in the surface mucosa by using the light absorption characteristic of hemoglobin at a specific wavelength (BF-6C260, Olympus Medical Systems Corp, Tokyo, Japan). In a normal WLB observation, an endoscopic light source radiates wide spectrum light to ensure that

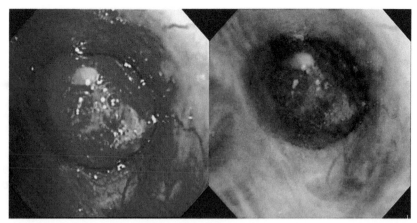

Fig. 4. Images of WLB and AFI in invasive lung cancer. WLB and AFI images of a tumor occluding the left upper lobe bronchus.

the colors in the reproduced images of the mucosal tissues look as natural as possible. However, this eliminates the contrast generated by blood vessels in the submucosa. NBI, in contrast, uses narrow spectrum light (narrow band light) specifically suited to the optical characteristics of mucosal tissues and hemoglobin in blood. This results in the improvement of contrast of the image relevant to diagnosis and delivers images with excellent visualization capability. NBI enhances the clinical value of magnification bronchoscopy by allowing the visualization of

abnormal distribution and dilatation of blood vessels (**Fig. 5**).

By optimizing the light wavelength at 415 nm (blue light) and 540 nm (green light) and keeping the spectral width narrow (narrow band), NBI enhances the contrast to ensure that blood vessels in the mucosa stand out clearly (see **Fig. 5**). The 415 nm blue light is absorbed by capillary vessels in the surface layer of the mucosa, whereas the 540 nm is strongly absorbed by blood vessels located below the capillary vessels in the surface layer of the mucosa. Finer blood vessels near the surface are

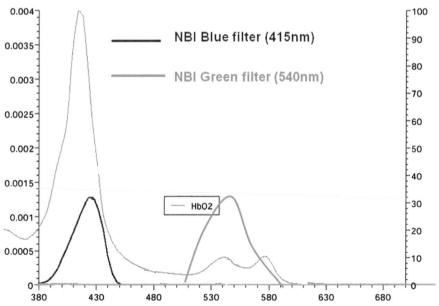

Fig. 5. Hemoglobin absorption characteristics. The peak of wavelength of hemoglobin O_2 absorption is the same as the peak of the NBI blue filter (415 nm). NBI enhances the contrast to ensure that blood vessels in the mucosa stand out clearly.

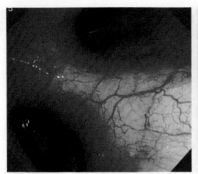
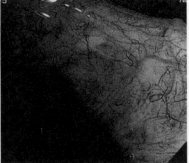

Fig. 6. Normal mucosa. Finer blood vessels near the surface are displayed in brown, whereas thicker vessels in deeper layers are displayed in cyan.

displayed in brown, whereas thicker vessels in deeper layers are shown in cyan (**Fig. 6**).

NBI FINDINGS

Various types of vascular networks can be visualized in the bronchial membrane using NBI. Because centrally arising squamous cell carcinoma is thought to develop through multiple stages from squamous metaplasia to dysplasia and CIS, detection of these lesions is important. In addition, differential diagnosis of these lesions without the need for biopsies would be ideal. NBI images may have potential for these purposes.

As shown in **Fig. 7**, complex networks of tortuous vessels appear in squamous dysplasia. In angiogenic squamous dysplasia, dotted vessels along with the tortuous vessels become evident. When preinvasive lesions develop into squamous cell carcinoma, scattered dotted vessels and capillary loops of tortuous vessels of various sizes are seen (**Figs. 8** and **9**).

NBI FOR DETECTION OF PRECANCEROUS LESIONS

In lung cancer, promising results have been shown for the detection of malignant precursors

and early cancers using the new NBI system.[20] The first report was on the efficacy of high magnification bronchovideoscopy combined with NBI for the detection of capillary blood vessels in angiogenic squamous dysplasia (ASD). In 48 patients with sputum cytology specimens suspicious or positive for malignancy, conventional white light and fluorescence bronchoscopy was first performed, followed by observations of abnormal fluorescence with high magnification NBI. The microvessels, vascular networks of various grades, and dotted vessels in ASD tissues were observed in NBI-B1 images. The diameters of the dotted vessels visible on NBI-B1 images corresponded with diameters of ASD capillary blood vessels diagnosed by pathologic examination. Capillary blood vessels were also clearly visualized by green fluorescence using confocal laser scanning microscopy. There was a significant association between the frequency of dotted vessels by NBI-B1 imaging and tissues confirmed as ASD pathologically ($P = .002$). This study showed the possibility of distinguishing between ASD and other preinvasive bronchial lesions.

Although there are growing numbers of reports on the effectiveness of NBI for detailed observation of the superficial mucosal and vascular patterns in

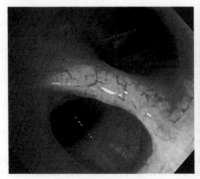
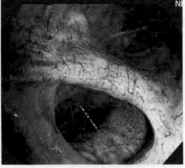

Fig. 7. Squamous dysplasia. Complex networks of tortuous vessels are clearly identified by NBI.

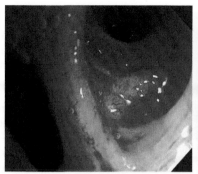
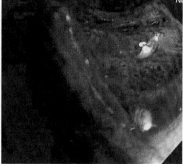

Fig. 8. CIS. Dotted vessels and tortuous vessels are clearly identified by NBI.

the gastrointestinal tract,[21–25] there are only a few studies on NBI in the evaluation of the airway. The high potential for NBI in the detection of preinvasive lesions in the tracheobronchial tree raises the importance of a single internationally accepted classification of the mucosal and vascular patterns by NBI. The author and fellow investigators have created their own classification of the different mucosal and vascular patterns, and preliminary data show a high correlation with histologic features.[26]

EBUS

Two types of EBUS are currently available for clinical use. The radial probe EBUS was first described in 1992[27] and is used for the evaluation of the bronchial wall structure,[28,29] visualization of detailed images of the surrounding structures for assisting transbronchial needle aspiration (TBNA),[30,31] and detection of peripheral intrapulmonary nodules.[32,33] In contrast, the convex-probe EBUS, first described in 2004, has a built-in ultrasound probe on a flexible bronchoscope that enables bronchoscopists to perform real-time TBNA of mediastinal and hilar lesions.[34–36]

For optimal imaging, the miniaturized 20 MHz radial probes (UM-BS20-26R, Olympus Medical Systems) are fitted with a catheter that carries a water-inflatable balloon at the tip. The balloon optimizes the contact between the probe and the bronchial wall and allows visualization of detailed images of the surrounding structures and the bronchial wall structure.[28,29] The structure of the cartilaginous portion of the central bronchial wall has been described as a 5- or 7-layer structure by different investigators.[28,29] This enables the evaluation of tumor infiltration into the airway.

EBUS IN EARLY LUNG CANCER

Premalignant lesions or small intrabronchial radiologically invisible tumors are being detected more frequently because of evolving mucosal imaging technologies. The decision to use endoscopic therapeutic intervention depends on the extent of tumor within the different layers of the bronchial wall. Conventional radiological imaging alone is not capable of distinguishing the tumor extent. In contrast, the radial probe EBUS is a sensitive method for detection of alterations of the multilayered structure of the bronchial wall, even in small

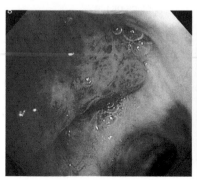
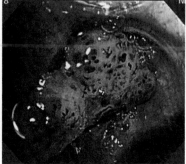

Fig. 9. Squamous cell carcinoma (invasive). Capillary loops of tortuous vessels of various sizes are identified by NBI.

tumors. After performing a needle-puncture experiment in 45 normal tissue specimens, a comparison between the ultrasonograms and the histologic findings in 24 lung cancer cases revealed that the depth diagnosis was the same in 23 lesions (95.8%).[28] Another study in a series of 15 patients showed a high diagnostic yield of 93% for predicting tumor invasion into the tracheobronchial wall.[37] EBUS also improves the specificity (from 50% to 90%) for predicting malignancy in small AF-positive lesions that were negative in white light bronchoscopy.[38]

Other than surgical resection, photodynamic therapy (PDT) is an alternative treatment for selected patients with early-stage lung cancer. In 18 biopsy-proven early-stage squamous cell carcinomas, including 3 CIS, EBUS was performed to evaluate tumor extent.[39] Nine lesions were diagnosed as intracartilaginous by EBUS, and PDT was subsequently performed. The other 9 patients had extracartilaginous tumors undetected by CT scanning; they were considered candidates for other therapies, such as surgical resection, chemotherapy, and radiotherapy, although 2 were invisible to high-resolution CT, 3 were superficial, and 5 were less than 1 cm in diameter. Using EBUS, 100% complete remission rate was achieved in the endoluminal-treated group. At a mean follow-up of 32 months, none of the patients had recurrence.

SUMMARY

The attraction of the AFI and NBI bronchovideoscope is easy handling, requiring only a single touch of a button. For a bronchoscopist, it is just the same as performing a routine WLB without any complicated procedures necessary. Interpretation of the results seems to be fairly straightforward. AFB and NBI are complimentary. The high sensitivity of autofluorescence is its strength, allowing it to pick up potentially neoplastic lesions, whereas its moderate specificity is a potential limitation. On the other hand, NBI enhances the mucosal and vascular patterns, which is best suited for detailed inspection of the mucosa. In the future, a combination of autofluorescence and NBI into a single bronchovideoscope system would decrease the time for the procedure and the number of unnecessary biopsies.

EBUS is an excellent tool for the evaluation of the airway structure, which is useful for the determination of the depth of tumor invasion. Minimally invasive treatment may be suitable for selected patients with early-stage lung cancer.

REFERENCES

1. Niklinski J, Niklinski W, Chyczewski L, et al. Molecular genetic abnormalities in premalignant lung lesions: biological and clinical implications. Eur J Cancer Prev 2001;10:213–26.
2. Thiberville L, Payne P, Vielkinds J, et al. Evidence of cumulative gene losses with progression of premalignant epithelial lesions to carcinoma of the bronchus. Cancer Res 1995;155:5133–9.
3. Lam S, MacAulay C. Endoscopic localization of preneoplastic lung lesions. In: Martinet Y, Hirsch FR, Martinet N, et al, editors. Clinical and biological basis of lung cancer prevention. Basel: Birkhauser Verlag; 1997. p. 231–8.
4. George PJ. Fluorescence bronchoscopy for the early detection of lung cancer. Thorax 1999;54: 180–3.
5. Lam S, Kennedy T, Unger M, et al. Localization of bronchial intraepithelial neoplastic lesions by fluorescence bronchoscopy. Chest 1998;113: 696–702.
6. van Rens MT, Schramel FM, Elbers JR, et al. The clinical value of lung imaging fluorescence endoscope for detecting synchronous lung cancer. Lung Cancer 2001;32:13–8.
7. Kusunoki Y, Imamura F, Uda H, et al. Early detection of lung cancer with laser-induced fluorescence endoscopy and spectrofluorometry. Chest 2000; 118:1776–82.
8. Sato M, Sakurada A, Sagawa M, et al. Diagnostic results before and after introduction of autofluorescence bronchoscopic in patients suspected of having lung cancer detected by sputum cytology in lung cancer mass screening. Lung Cancer 2001;32:247–53.
9. Pierard P, Martin B, Verdebout JM, et al. Fluorescence bronchsocpy in high-risk patients – a comparison of LIFE and Pentax systems. J Bronchol 2001;8: 254–9.
10. Chhajed PN, Shibuya K, Hoshino H, et al. A comparison of video and autofluorescence bronchoscopy in patients at high risk of lung cancer. Eur Respir J 2005;25:951–5.
11. Weigel TL, Kosco PJ, Dacic S, et al. Postoperative fluorescence bronchoscopic surveillance in non-small cell lung cancer patients. Ann Thorac Surg 2001;71:967–70.
12. Shibuya K, Fujisawa T, Hoshino H, et al. Fluorescence bronchoscopy in the detection of preinvasive bronchial lesions in patients with sputum cytology suspicious or positive for malignancy. Lung Cancer 2001;32:19–25.
13. Haussinger K, Becker H, Stanzel F, et al. Autofluorescence bronchoscopy with white light bronchoscopy compared with white light bronchoscopy alone for the detection of precancerous lesions: a European

randomised controlled multicentre trial. Thorax 2005; 60:496–503.

14. Hirsch FR, Prindiville SA, Miller YE, et al. Fluorescence versus white light bronchoscopy for detection of preneoplastic lesions: a randomized study. J Natl Cancer Inst 2001;93:1385–91.

15. Ernst A, Simoff MJ, Mathur PN, et al. D-light autofluorescence in the detection of premalignant airway changes: a multicenter trial. J Bronchol 2005;12:133–8.

16. Edell E, Lam S, Pass H, et al. Detection and localization of intraepithelial neoplasia and invasive carcinoma using fluorescence-reflectance bronchoscopy – an international, multicenter clinical trial. J Thorac Oncol 2009;4:49–54.

17. Chiyo M, Shibuya K, Hoshino H, et al. Effective detection of bronchial preinvasive lesions by a new autofluorescence imaging bronchovideoscope system. Lung Cancer 2005;48(3):307–13.

18. Shibuya K, Hoshino H, Chiyo M, et al. Subepithelial vascular patterns in bronchial dysplasias using a high magnification bronchovideoscope. Thorax 2002;57:902–7.

19. Yamada G, Shijubo N, Kitada J, et al. Decreased subepithelial microvasculature observed by high magnification bronchovideoscope in the large airways of smokers. Intern Med 2008;47(18):1579–83.

20. Shibuya K, Hoshino H, Chiyo M, et al. High magnification bronchovideoscopy combined with narrow band imaging could detect capillary loops of angiogenic squamous dysplasia in heavy smokers at high risk for lung cancer. Thorax 2003;58:989–95.

21. Gono K, Obi T, Yamaguchi M, et al. Appearance of enhanced tissue features in narrow-band endoscopic imaging. J Biomed Opt 2004;9:568–77.

22. Muto M, Katada C, Sano Y, et al. Narrow band imaging: a new diagnostic approach to visualize angiogenesis in superficial neoplasia. Clin Gastroenterol Hepatol 2005;3:S16–20.

23. Sharma P. Narrow band imaging in Barrett's esophagus. Clin Gastroenterol Hepatol 2005;3:S21–2.

24. Kuznetsov K, Lambert R, Rey JF. Narrow-band imaging: potential and limitations. Endoscopy 2006;38:76–81.

25. Kara MA, Ennahachi M, Fockens P, et al. Detection and classification of the mucosal and vascular patterns in Barrett's esophagus by using narrow band imaging. Gastrointest Endosc 2006;64:155–66.

26. Shibuya K, Nakajima T, Yasufuku K, et al. Narrow band imaging with high resolution bronchovideoscopy: a new approach to visualize angiogenesis in squamous cell carcinoma of the lung. Eur Respir J 2006;28(Suppl 50):601s.

27. Hurter T, Hanrath P. Endobronchial sonography: feasibility and preliminary results. Thorax 1992;47: 565–7.

28. Kurimoto N, Murayama M, Yoshioka S, et al. Assessment of usefulness of endobronchial ultrasonography in determination of depth of tracheobronchial tumor invasion. Chest 1999;115: 1500–6.

29. Baba M, Sekine Y, Suzuki M, et al. Correlation between endobronchial ultrasonography (EBUS) images and histologic findings in normal and tumor-invaded bronchial wall. Lung Cancer 2002; 35:65–71.

30. Herth FJ, Becker HD, Ernst A. Ultrasound-guided transbronchial needle aspiration: an experience in 242 patients. Chest 2003;123:604–7.

31. Herth FJ, Becker HD, Ernst A. Conventional vs endobronchial ultrasound-guided transbronchial needle aspiration: a randomized trial. Chest 2004;125: 322–5.

32. Kurimoto N, Murayama M, Yoshioka S, et al. Analysis of the internal structure of peripheral pulmonary lesions using endobronchial ultrasonography. Chest 2002;122:1887–94.

33. Kurimoto N, Miyazawa T, Okimasa S, et al. Endobronchial ultrasonography using a guide sheath increases the ability to diagnose peripheral pulmonary lesions endoscopically. Chest 2004;126: 959–65.

34. Yasufuku K, Chhajed PN, Sekine Y, et al. Endobronchial ultrasound using a new convex probe: a preliminary study on surgically resected specimens. Oncol Rep 2004;11:293–6.

35. Yasufuku K, Chiyo M, Sekine Y, et al. Real-time endobronchial ultrasound guided transbronchial needle aspiration of mediastinal and hilar lymph nodes. Chest 2004;126:122–8.

36. Yasufuku K, Chiyo M, Koh E, et al. Endobronchial ultrasound guided transbronchial needle aspiration for staging of lung cancer. Lung Cancer 2005;50: 347–54.

37. Tanaka F, Muro K, Yamasaki S, et al. Evaluation of tracheo-bronchial wall invasion using transbronchial ultrasonography (TBUS). Eur J Cardiothorac Surg 2000;17:570–4.

38. Herth FJ, Becker HD. EBUS for early lung cancer detection. J Bronchol 2003;10:249.

39. Miyazu Y, Miyazawa T, Kurimoto N, et al. Endobronchial ultrasonography in the assessment of centrally located early-stage lung cancer before photodynamic therapy. Am J Respir Crit Care Med 2002; 165:832–7.

Role of Bronchoscopy in the Evaluation of Solitary Pulmonary Nodules

Christopher A. Hergott, MD, FRCPC,
Alain Tremblay, MDCM, FRCPC, FCCP*

KEYWORDS

- Solitary pulmonary nodule • Peripheral pulmonary lesion
- Flexible bronchoscopy • Ultrathin bronchoscopy
- Endobronchial ultrasound
- Electromagnetic navigational bronchoscopy

Since the first rigid bronchoscopy by Gustav Killian in 1897, the bronchoscope has evolved to play a central role in the diagnosis and treatment of patients with pulmonary diseases. The development of the flexible bronchoscope revolutionized the approach to pulmonary lesions and spawned the development of many technologies designed to effectively and efficiently diagnose a wide range of pulmonary diseases.

Solitary pulmonary nodules (SPNs) are usually defined as lesions less than 3 cm in size and surrounded by normal lung tissue. These lesions present special difficulties for flexible bronchoscopists, as they usually cannot be visualized through a standard bronchoscope, resulting in unsatisfactory diagnostic results.

The past decade has witnessed several attempts at increasing the reach of the flexible bronchoscope in order to improve diagnostic accuracy in the setting of SPNs. Ultrathin bronchoscopes have been developed in the hopes that they might improve visualization of more proximal SPNs and guide biopsy tools in the correct subsegments for the more peripheral lesions. Patients have undergone bronchoscopy under CT fluoroscopy to allow more accurate visualization and sampling. Real-time confirmation of lesions has been made possible by small peripheral endobronchial ultrasound (pEBUS) probes, and accurate navigation of the complex branches of the tracheobronchial tree has been achieved with the use of virtual bronchoscopic (VB) mapping and electromagnetic navigational bronchoscopy (ENB) techniques.

Given the high diagnostic yield of CT-guided transthoracic needle aspiration (CT-TTNA)[1,2] in addition to its low procedural costs, the question of why seemingly more complicated and expensive bronchoscopic techniques need to be developed might be asked. One reason is the frequent occurrence of pneumothorax, approximately 20%, as a complication of CT-guided biopsy with approximately 7% of patients requiring chest tube drainage. Another is that certain lesions remain difficult to access via CT-guided biopsy, because of their location, distance from the pleura, or presence of bullous lung disease. Increased distance from the pleura, presence of obstructive airways disease or emphysema, and biopsy of smaller nodules all are associated with increased risk of pneumothorax.[1,3] Distance from the pleura also affects diagnostic accuracy, which drops to 60% or less when the needle path length exceeds 40 mm.[4] Another concern is that the diagnostic accuracy for benign lesions, critical to avoid thoracotomy, has been highly variable with CT-guided biopsy (16% to 68%) and the ability to obtain more tissue from bronchoscopy instruments could improve these results. Finally, bronchoscopic approaches may also allow the sampling of

Division of Respiratory Medicine, University of Calgary, 3330 Hospital Drive NW, Calgary, Alberta T2N 4N1, Canada
* Corresponding author.
E-mail address: alain.tremblay@ucalgary.ca (A. Tremblay).

Clin Chest Med 31 (2010) 49–63
doi:10.1016/j.ccm.2009.08.003
0272-5231/10/$ – see front matter © 2010 Elsevier Inc. All rights reserved.

multiple lesions and mediastinal nodes during the same procedure, adding to the diagnostic and staging capacity of the test.

The following sections endeavor to describe and present the most pertinent evidence surrounding the use of advanced bronchoscopic techniques for diagnosis of SPNs.

ASSESSMENT OF THE LITERATURE ON DIAGNOSTIC TESTS

The majority of the literature surrounding the bronchoscopic approach to SPN is comprised of case series data, retrospectively or prospectively collected, without comparison to a gold standard technique. As such, comparisons of different techniques usually can only be inferred from examination of separate studies, performed on variable patient populations and using different primary outcome measures and gold standards. The reader is referred to the *JAMA*'s "Users' Guides to the Medical Literature" regarding interpretation of articles on diagnostic tests for further assistance in interpreting individual studies.[5,6]

The literature on bronchoscopic approach to peripheral lung lesions often does not limit inclusion criteria to the SPN (<3 cm). As lesion size is highly likely to influence the performance characteristics of the various approaches, results must always be interpreted accordingly. This article, when possible, reports the results of studies based on analysis of lesions 3 cm or less, which the authors believe is the population most likely to benefit from advanced bronchoscopic techniques. Conversely, nodules less that 1 cm are rarely included in such trials and many of these lesions are probably best investigated by serial radiologic examinations.[7]

Another frequent difficulty in the studies of interest is the absence of an independent reference standard with regards to final diagnosis, which ideally should be pathologic analysis after surgical resection of the nodule. As such, in most trials, calculations of sensitivity and negative predicted values (NPV) are impossible to perform or are based on the assumption of benignity by clinical follow-up of variable duration. Because of this difficulty, diagnostic yield (the number of positive tests/the total number of tests performed) has been a popular primary outcome measure, as a final diagnosis after negative results is not required for its calculation. Although practical, this assumes the absence of false-positive results and varies significantly with the patient population studied (for example, with nodule size or prevalence of malignancy), making comparison

between trials problematic. In addition, the definition of a positive test can be variable between studies, with some investigators including findings, such as nonspecific inflammation, in the definition of a positive diagnostic test. Although diagnostic yield can be an important test characteristic, others, such as NPV, could be as, or even more, important according to the clinical setting. For example, consider patients with an SPN assessed at intermediate risk for malignancy. In this setting, a test with a high NPV value for malignancy may be most useful in avoiding a thoracotomy for benign disease, whereas a test with high diagnostic yield or sensitivity for malignancy may not prevent this. If these techniques are to become entrenched in the approach to patients with SPN beyond a role of confirming disease in patients with advanced or inoperable disease, these issues will require additional consideration.

STANDARD FLEXIBLE BRONCHOSCOPY

Standard flexible bronchoscopy can offer an overall diagnostic sensitivity for malignant peripheral lesions of 36% to 88% (average 78%),[2] but this includes lesions of all sizes and relatively central lesions, with the definition of peripheral lesion usually inclusive of any lesion with no proximal visualized endobronchial component. Lesion size is often missing altogether from some publications,[8–10] making direct comparisons between trials difficult.

The yield of standard bronchoscopy for a true SPN is likely lower, and the relationship of lesion size to diagnostic yield or sensitivity has been noted by several investigators.[11–13] A summary of publications performed as part of the American College of Chest Physicians lung cancer guidelines suggests that for lesions of less than 2 cm, sensitivity of bronchoscopy is only 34%.[2] Other factors that may influence these results include distance from the hilum,[11,12,14] presence of a CT-bronchus sign,[15,16] and the lobe or subsegment of the lesion of interest (lower lobes and apical segment of upper lobes having lower yield),[17] although it is not clear if all of these factors are independent predictors of diagnostic yield.

Several sampling techniques can be used through the working channel of the flexible bronchoscope and with the more advanced techniques (described later). Transbronchial biopsy, transbronchial needle aspiration (TBNA), cytology brush, and bronchoalveolar lavage can all be of use in the diagnosis of peripheral lesions, with sensitivities of 57%, 65%, 54%, and 43%, respectively.[2] Several studies attest to the additive value of combining these various methods, with a substantial number of cases diagnosed solely by one of each instrument.[8,9,11,12,18,19]

Fluoroscopy was used in the majority of publications investigating bronchoscopic approaches for peripheral lung lesions. This involves radiation exposure to patients and the bronchoscopy team,[20] and equipment can be expensive even if commonly available in most hospitals. Although fluoroscopy is often thought to improve the diagnostic yield of bronchoscopy,[2,14] no comparative trials have been published, and similar diagnostic yields have been described without its use.[21]

Although bronchoscopy can be useful for peripheral lesions as a whole, its role in the true SPN seems limited. This has led to recommendations that in cases where a preoperative diagnosis is warranted, a CT-guided approach should be preferred and "that bronchoscopy (only) be performed when an air bronchogram is present or in centers with expertise in newer guided techniques."[7] This article examines these newer techniques.

ULTRATHIN BRONCHOSCOPY

The quest to improve diagnostic yield for peripheral pulmonary lesions led to the development of smaller, ultrathin bronchoscopes designed to be driven further into the airways to identify and biopsy peripheral lesions. Initial devices were designed to fit inside the working channel of standard flexible scopes but did not themselves have a working channel through which lesions could be sampled.[22,23] Nevertheless, these early prototypes confirmed that small peripheral airways could be navigated and visualized and that peripheral lesions could be identified. This lead to the development of an ultrathin bronchoscope with a 2.7-mm outer diameter and a small 0.8-mm working channel allowing the passage of a 0.7-mm cytology brush.[24] Seventeen patients with a variety of respiratory conditions underwent bronchoscopy with this device; their airways were examined and collection of epithelial cells was performed. In five patients with known peripheral lung cancer not seen with conventional bronchoscopy, the ultrathin bronchoscope, introduced through a standard bronchoscope working channel and assisted by fluoroscopy down to the ninth-generation bronchi, successfully allowed the collection of malignant cells from each lesion.[24]

In an attempt to overcome the limitations of the small working channels of the ultrathin devices, an alternative approach has been investigated. The ultrathin scope is used to navigate towards a peripheral lesion under fluoroscopic imaging in order to determine the most appropriate path, followed by an attempt to sample the lesion along the same path with a standard endoscope and forceps. This approach was applied to 17 consecutive patients with peripheral lung lesion seen on CT scan.[25] A diagnostic yield of 64.7% was achieved for lesions between 1.5 and 7.0 cm (mean 3.2 cm), even though the lesion was visualized in only four cases. The investigators credit ultrathin bronchoscopy for allowing them to establish a correct path to the lesion, essentially ensuring that the correct subsegment was accessed with the biopsy forceps.

More recently, thin bronchoscopes with larger working channels (1.2–1.7 mm) have been developed, allowing insertion of small biopsy forceps. The first study performed with a 1.2-mm channel targeted 35 peripheral lesions of mean diameter of 21.7 mm (range 10–40 mm).[26] The investigators performed sampling of the lesions through a standard bronchoscope and with the thin scope. Although an overall diagnostic yield of 60% was achieved with the thin bronchoscope, in only three cases was the diagnosis made exclusively via this method, suggesting an incremental yield over standard bronchoscopy of only 8.6%. In a second phase of this study, 13 of 32 (40.6%) patients with lesions 12 to 55 mm (mean 24.4 mm) in size and negative on-site rapid cytology after standard bronchoscopy had a diagnosis confirmed by ultrathin bronchoscopy.[26]

In the most recent and largest case series, 102 patients with peripheral lung lesions underwent bronchoscopy with a 3.5-mm thin bronchoscope with a 1.7-mm working channel.[27] The ultrathin bronchoscope was wedged into the corresponding bronchus and transbronchial biopsies (1.5-mm forceps) and bronchial washings with 10 to 20 mL of saline were performed under fluoroscopic guidance. An overall diagnostic yield of 69% was attained in lesions between 1.1 and 7.6 cm (mean 3.4 cm) with the peripheral lesion visualized in only 14 patients (13.7%).[27]

No randomized trial has yet confirmed that ultrathin bronchoscopy in isolation can increase the diagnostic yield of standard bronchoscopy, making it difficult to comment on any incremental yield afforded by this technique. It is conceivable that the ultrathin bronchoscope placed into more distal airways allows for a more direct path for the transbronchial biopsy forceps and lessens the likelihood of the biopsy forceps entering the wrong segmental bronchus. Only a small percentage of peripheral lesions, however, are visualized with this technique,[25,27] likely accounting for the modest yields achieved. Given that this instrument can navigate all the way to the pleura,[28] difficult visualization with advancement into smaller airways and the sheer complexity of the tracheobronchial tree are likely the main impediments to finding these lesions. It is likely that the future of ultrathin bronchoscopy lies not in isolation but in combination with additional techniques (discussed later).

CT FLUOROSCOPY

In an attempt to improve localization of pulmonary lesions often poorly visualized on standard fluoroscopy, several groups have attempted to use CT fluoroscopy as a more precise localization tool. This approach is performed in the CT scan suite with intermittent CT scanning of the region of interest to confirm appropriate location of the bronchoscope and biopsy forceps in relationship to the airway and lesion of interest. As CT fluoroscopy can help localize the position of the instruments and the lesion but cannot help guide or navigate towards the lesion, several investigators also make use of preprocedure VB mapping and ultrathin bronchoscope to advance it as distal as possible (fifth- to eighth-generation bronchi) towards the lesion before deploying sampling instruments.[29–31] This may be an important consideration during CT fluoroscopy and other techniques as diagnostic yield seems to improve according to the depth which the bronchoscope can be inserted from the third- to sixth-generation bronchus.[29]

An impressive diagnostic yield of 66.6% from an initial small pilot study[32] has been replicated by two other centers in larger case series despite small mean nodule size (1.3 and 1.7 cm).[29,31] Nevertheless, a recent randomized trial of CT fluoroscopy versus standard fluoroscopy for the diagnosis of suspected lung cancer did not demonstrate any significant differences in sensitivity for malignancy between the two groups.[33] This result may be explained by the larger size of the nodules/masses (mean 3.7 cm) as compared to the prior studies and resulting high sensitivity of bronchoscopy with standard fluoroscopy in the control arm, as smaller nodules are probably the ones most likely to demonstrate improved results with advanced bronchoscopic techniques. Another difference was the absence of VB planning and use of a standard-size bronchoscope, which may have limited the ability to navigate towards a lesion, even if identified on CT. As pointed out by Ost and colleagues, "often we could see that we were missing the lesion, but we could not do much about it."[33] **Table 1** lists a summary of studies using CT fluoroscopy.

A disadvantage of this technique is the radiation exposure to patients and operators. Unlike the practice for percutaneous CT-guided biopsy techniques, an operator cannot leave the room during acquisition of the CT images. Mean CT fluoroscopy exposure time has been measured at 228 to 240 seconds per procedure.[32,33] Displacing the bronchoscopy suite to the CT suite may also bring up logistic, time, and cost issues.

FLEXIBLE BRONCHOSCOPY WITH PERIPHERAL ENDOBRONCHIAL ULTRASOUND GUIDANCE

Endobronchial ultrasound allows the visualization of central structures beyond the airway wall and also can be used to image the peripheral compartments of the lung in real time during bronchoscopy[34] and applied in the diagnosis of peripheral lesions. Twenty-MHz, radial-type, ultrasound probes have been developed with outer diameters of 1.4 mm and 1.8 mm coupled with corresponding guide sheaths (GSs), which can fit in 2.0-mm and 2.8-mm working channels, respectively. Before the procedure, sampling instruments (biopsy forceps, cytology brush, and TBNA needles) are introduced into the GS until the tip of the instrument protrudes out of the distal end of the sheath. The location at which the proximal end of the instrument and the GS meet is then marked with indelible marker, tape, or a rubber stopper, allowing a bronchoscopist to eventually place the instrument in the correct position to obtain the cytopathologic specimens.

The bronchoscope is advanced into the segment or subsegment of interest after careful interpretation of the location of the peripheral lesion on CT images. Use of smaller pEBUS probes and GS, which can be inserted in smaller bronchoscope, allows more distal navigation towards the lesion before the pEBUS is deployed. The radial ultrasound probe is then inserted into the GS such that the ultrasound probe is protruding approximately 1 cm from the distal end of the GS. The pEBUS-GS is then inserted through the working channel (**Fig. 1**A) and fed into the suspected bronchus until the lesion is detected by the ultrasound image. The lesion is identified when the ultrasound image turns from the normal snowstorm appearance to the darker more homogeneous appearance often associated with a bright border (see **Fig. 1**D; **Fig. 2**B). Once the lesion is identified, the pEBUS radial probe is turned off and removed from the GS, which remains in position in or near the lesion. The biopsy forceps, cytologic brush, or TBNA needles can then be advanced into the GS to the appropriate depth and samples obtained. It is the

Table 1
Published results of CT fluoroscopy for peripheral lung lesions

Author and Year, Study Design	Method	Number of Nodules (Mean Size)	Prevalence of Malignancy	Overall Diagnostic Yield	Diagnostic Yield for Lesions ≤2 cm	Diagnostic Yield for Lesions ≤3 cm
White 2000, case series[32]	TBNA	12 (2.2 cm)	42%	66.6%	50%	66.6%
Tsushima 2006, case series[31]	VB, UT	82 (1.7 cm)	69%	62%	56%	NA
Shinagawa 2007,[a] case series[29]	VB, UT	85 (1.3 cm)	52%	66%	66%	All ≤2 cm
Ost 2008, RCT versus fluoroscopy[33]	TBNA, TBBX, Brush	21 (3.7 cm)	72%	71%	NA	NA

Abbreviations: NA, data not available; RCT, randomized controlled trial; UT, ultrathin bronchoscopy.
[a] Patients from report, Shinagawa N, Yamazaki K, Onodera Y, et al. CT-guided transbronchial biopsy using an ultrathin bronchoscope with virtual bronchoscopic navigation. Chest 2004;125(3):1138–43, also included in this publication.

authors' practice to obtain approximately five to six transbronchial biopsies and one cytologic brush sample per peripheral lesion in addition to a standard bronchoalveolar lavage in the segment of interest. Peripheral TBNA can also be performed through the GS (discussed later).

The technique has also been described without the use of a GS.[35–37] With this approach, a measurement of the distance to which the pEBUS probe is introduced beyond the tip of the bronchoscope to reach the lesion is taken, followed by insertion of biopsy instruments to the same depth. Although the diagnostic yields in these studies are similar to those using GS (**Table 2**), the use of a GS affords two major benefits over simply using the pEBUS radial probe. The most appealing reason to use GS is that, given the number of branch points within the peripheral bronchial tree, there is a risk that the biopsy instrument may follow an alternate route when reinserted without a GS even if the lesion was identified by pEBUS. The use of a GS ensures that the diagnostic implement is guided directly to the lesion. In addition, the presence of the GS may help tamponade any bleeding that may have occurred during the biopsy procedure.

A summary of the results from several studies using pEBUS in the diagnosis of peripheral pulmonary lesions is in **Table 2**. Diagnostic yields in all studies range from 34% to 84.4%. Overall, diagnostic yields for smaller lesions are lower, although this is not a consistent finding in all studies. Results range from 58% to 79% for lesions less than or equal to 3 cm and from 18% to 73% for lesions less than or equal to 2 cm. In a large single-center trial, one group did not find any statistically significant decrease in diagnostic yield with smaller lesion size of less than 10 mm.[38]

The results of these studies suggest improved diagnostic rates over historical reports of standard bronchoscopy for pulmonary lesions, especially considering lesions less than 3 cm. This has been confirmed by a prospective randomized trial in which 206 patients with peripheral pulmonary lesions were randomized to pEBUS (without GS) or conventional transbronchial biopsies (without fluoroscopy).[37] Overall sensitivity for malignancy was significantly improved (79% vs 55%) for the pEBUS group. When results were stratified based on size of the lesion, no difference in sensitivity was found for lesions greater than 3.0 cm (82.8% vs 77.3%). In lesions less than or equal to 3 cm and less than or equal to 2 cm, however, pEBUS had significantly improved sensitivity (75% vs 31% and 71% vs 23%, respectively) over standard bronchoscopy.[37] These data suggest that the localization of peripheral

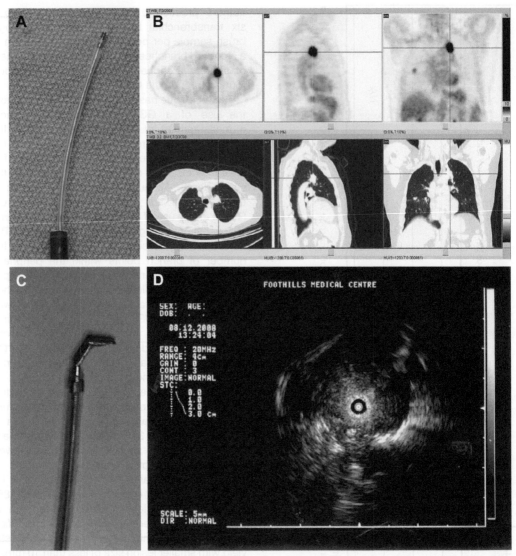

Fig. 1. pEBUS of a left upper-lobe tumor. (*A*) View of tip of bronchoscope with GS and ultrasound probe advanced out of working channel. (*B*) PET-CT demonstrating centrally located, left upper-lobe lesion. (*C*) Bihinged curette used to guide the GS in a medial direction after failing to identify mass with pEBUS/GS alone. (*D*) Ultrasound image of the left upper-lobe lesion. Transbronchial biopsy performed through the GS confirmed an adenocarcinoma.

pulmonary lesions with pEBUS improves the diagnostic yield of transbronchial biopsies, particularly in the setting of the SPN.

One of the inherent difficulties in the diagnosis of peripheral pulmonary lesions is correctly directing the biopsy implement to the lesion. The use of pEBUS-GS allows for visual confirmation that the probe is within the lesion but does not guarantee that the lesion will be found. Bihinged curettes (see **Fig. 1C**)[38–43] and fluoroscopy[38–42,44] have been used in several studies to help guide the pEBUS probe to the lesion. In one particular study, pEBUS-GS was unable to identify the lesion in 10

cases. In those 10 lesions, fluoroscopy was used to direct the angulated curette into the correct bronchus. This procedure allowed for diagnosis in 3 of 10 of these lesions,[38] suggesting that these additional tools may improve diagnostic yield in selected cases (see **Fig. 1**). The routine use of fluoroscopy may not be essential with this technique. In one trial, fluoroscopy was unable to identify that the forceps were in the lesion in 54 of 81 lesions less than or equal to 20 mm (67%),[38] suggesting fluoroscopy is unlikely to be helpful in guiding the pEBUS probe to these smaller lesions. Even though fluoroscopy was unable to confirm

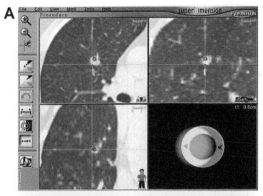

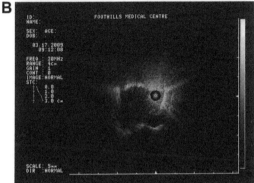

Fig. 2. Combination of electromagnetic navigation bronchoscopy (*A*) and pEBUS (*B*) for localization of a 1.5-cm, PET-positive, right upper-lobe lesion in a 65-year-old nonsmoking woman.

that the biopsy forceps were in the lesion, the diagnostic yield was similar whether or not fluoroscopy identified the lesion.[38]

The ability to place the instruments within the lesion using pEBUS is a key to obtaining diagnostic specimen. Diagnostic yield has been shown in two studies to be significantly higher if the pEBUS probe is seen within the lesion (see **Figs. 1**D and **2**B) than if it is seen adjacent to the lesion (**Fig. 3**): 87% versus 42% (P<.0001)[38] and 78.3% versus 47.2% (P<.001), respectively.[35] It is likely that in cases where an adjacent position is achieved, the lesion remains extrabronchial and out of reach of the instruments. The use of a TBNA needle to penetrate the airways in this situation intuitively is useful. In a prospective randomized trial of pEBUS using bronchial wash and transbronchial biopsies with or without TBNA biopsies, the yield in the pEBUS-TBNA group was significantly higher than the pEBUS without TBNA group (78.4% vs 60.6%; P = .015).[35] Although overall diagnostic yield was again highest if the pEBUS probe was within the lesion, the diagnostic yield of pEBUS-TBNA alone was not affected by this factor (63.6% vs 59.1%).[35] This suggests that the addition of

peripheral TBNA coupled with pEBUS improves the diagnostic yield of the procedure over and above transbronchial biopsy and cytology brush and that the use of TBNA is most important when the pEBUS probe is located adjacent to the lesion.

Given the importance of positioning the pEBUS probe and GS in the center of the lesions, further work has gone into methods of navigating towards these lesions. The use of VB through the reformatting of CT images has emerged as a new and helpful technique in directing pEBUS biopsies. VB images that allowed the creation of a map to the lesion have been used to guide a pediatric bronchoscope to the target bronchus, reaching a median of the fifth-order bronchi.[45] A smaller 1.4-mm pEBUS probe and GS were then used to find the lesion and transbronchial biopsies performed. In this study, a high proportion (30 of the 32) of the lesions were visualized with pEBUS (93.8%) despite a median nodule size of only 2.1 cm, resulting in a diagnostic yield of 84.4%—the best results described with pEBUS to date.[45]

In an effort to define the relative indications of pEBUS and CT-TTNA, investigators have compared 140 prospective pEBUS-GS bronchoscopies to a retrospective analysis of 121 CT-TTNA performed in the same institution during the same time period. Although lesion size was slightly smaller in the pEBUS group (2.9 cm vs 3.7 cm), the overall diagnostic sensitivity was similar (pEBUS 66% and CT-TTNA 64%).[44] pEBUS-GS had higher sensitivity for lesions not touching the visceral pleura compared with lesions touching the visceral pleura (74% vs 35%; P<.01) but the yield of CT-TTNA was not affected by this factor. Complications occurred more frequently in the CT-TTNA group with 9.1% of patients experiencing hemoptysis compared with no patients in the PEBUS-GS group. Rates of pneumothorax and tube thoracostomy were significantly greater in the CT-TTNA group compared to the EBUS-GS group (28% vs 1% for pneumothorax; 6% vs 0% for tube thoracostomy; P<.001) with fewer pneumothoraces for the CT-TTNA group when the lesions were pleural based (2.6% vs 31.7%). These results suggest that pleural-based lesions are still better suited to CT-TTNA given the low risk of pneumothorax and poor yield of pEBUS in this setting. Alternatively, in patients with lesions not adjacent to the visceral pleura and higher risk of pneumothorax, pEBUS-GS biopsies may be associated with fewer complications and an equal chance at achieving a diagnosis.

Some investigators have attempted to extract diagnostic information from the pEBUS image of

Table 2
Published results of peripheral endobronchial ultrasonography for peripheral lung lesions

Author and Year, Study Design	Method	Number of Nodules (Mean Size)	Prevalence of Malignancy	Overall Diagnostic Yield	Diagnostic Yield for Lesions ≤2 cm	Diagnostic Yield for Lesions ≤3 cm
Herth 2002, prospective crossover study[36]	pEBUS, fluoroscopy, no GS	50 (3.3 cm)	90%	80%	NA	NA
Shirakawa 2004, case series[41]	pEBUS, fluoroscopy, some GS, curette	50 (NA)	48%	34%	NA	NA
Kikuchi 2004, case series[40]	pEBUS-GS, fluoroscopy, curette	24 (1.8 cm)	92%	58.3	53%	58.3%
Kurimoto, 2004, case series[38]	pEBUS-GS ± curette/fluoroscopy	150 (NA)	67%	77%	72%	73%
Paone 2005 RTC TBBx[37]	pEBUS no GS	87 (NA)	70%	76%[a]	71%[a]	75%[a]
Asahina 2005, case series[39]	pEBUS-GS, VB, curette, fluoroscopy	30 (1.9 cm)	76%	63.3%	44%	63%
Chung 2007, RCT[69]	pEBUS no GS	158 (2.5 cm)	NA	49%	NA	NA
Eberhardt 2007, RTC ENB[58]	pEBUS-GS	39 (2.6 cm)	78%	69%	78%	72%
Dooms 2007, case series[70]	pEBUS no GS	50 (3.7 cm)	≥74%	68%	18%	NA
Yoshikawa 2007, case series[43]	pEBUS-GS, curette	123 (3.1 cm)	87%	62%	30%	44%
Yamada 2007, case series[42]	pEBUS-GS ± curette/fluoroscopy	158 (2.1 cm)	70%	67%	49%	67%
Fielding 2008, case series[44]	pEBUS-GS, fluoroscopy	140 (2.9 cm)	53%	66%	NA	NA
Asano 2008, case series[45]	pEBUS-GS virtual guidance	32 (2.1 cm median)	88%	84.4%	73%	79%
Chao 2008, RCT[35]	EBUS, no GS, TBNA	182 (3.5 cm)	77%	78%	NA	NA

Abbreviations: NA, not available; RCT, randomized controlled trial; TBBX, transbronchial biopsy.
[a] Value represents sensitivity, not diagnostic yield.

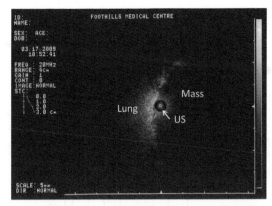

Fig. 3. pEBUS of a right middle-lobe mass. The ultrasound probe (US) is seen at the periphery of the lesion (Mass). The typical snowstorm appearance of normal lung parenchyma is noted (Lung).

peripheral lesions beyond simply using it to confirm GS position.[46–48] An initial report created three specific classes and six subclasses of lesion based on the internal structure of the lesion on the pEBUS image. The defining features of the internal structure of the lesion included internal echoes, vascular and bronchial patency, and the morphology of the hyperechoic areas. In type I lesions, 23 of 25 lesions were benign (92%) whereas 98 of 99 type II and III lesions were malignant (99%).[48] In a more recent study, a simplified classification was created from previous publications and a training set of 20 lesions defining three specific ultrasound characteristics favoring malignancy: the presence of a continuous margin; nonlinear, dotted, or mottled air bronchograms; and heterogeneous echogenicity.[47] These characteristics were then applied to a set of 131 lesions. The NPV for malignancy of a lesion with none of the three ultrasound features was 93.7% and the positive predictive value for malignancy of a lesion with any two of the three ultrasound internal features was 89.2%.[47] The most useful application of these results may be in cases where cytopathologic samples are nondiagnostic to aid in the decision to proceed to resection versus after a watch and wait approach. Nevertheless, the interpretation of such images remains challenging, and further validation of these findings is required.

In summary, pEBUS-guided biopsies of peripheral pulmonary lesions show improved accuracy and sensitivity compared to conventional transbronchial biopsies, its improved sensitivity most apparent in smaller peripheral lesions. The use of TBNA through the GS seems important, especially in cases where the probe is seen adjacent to the lesion of interest. This technique is safe and efficacious and offers benefits over conventional

fluoroscopic transbronchial and CT-TTNA biopsies. As with most bronchoscopic procedures, however, the NPV for pEBUS-GS biopsies of peripheral nodules is not sufficiently high enough to rule out a diagnosis of lung cancer. Additional refinements to increase the ability to reach lesions with the probe and GS likely will improve results obtained with this technique.

VIRTUAL BRONCHOSCOPY–ASSISTED BRONCHOSCOPY

VB reconstruction of chest CT data has been used to noninvasively assess airway lesions and even guide TBNA of mediastinal lymph nodes. The use of VB techniques for assistance in bronchoscopic diagnosis of peripheral lesions (see the article by Asano elsewhere in this issue) has more recently been made possible by two technologic advancements. The first is the development of thin-slice CT, which now allows higher resolution imaging of peripheral airways. The second is the availability of ultrathin bronchoscopes with large enough working channels to navigate these same airways and guide sampling instrument further into the tracheobronchial tree. With this approach, analysis of VB images are used to guide bronchoscopists towards a peripheral lesion without having to examine a large number of bifurcations in the tracheobronchial tree, hopefully shortening the length of the examination and increasing the chance that a lesion can be accessed.

After a first case report of this approach was published in 2002,[49] a case series was published in 2004 in which VB, ultrathin bronchoscopy, and CT fluoroscopy were used to access 26 small (mean 1.3-cm) peripheral lesions. A diagnostic rate of 65% was obtained, which is impressive given the small size of the lesions. After these early successes, there have significant refinements in the VB systems beyond having a bronchoscopist simply review the CT images prior to the procedure. A system capable of rotating the VB image and advancing from one bifurcation to another during the procedure with the use of a foot pedal in order to maintain location and orientation of VB and bronchoscopic images in sync was tested in 38 peripheral nodules (≤3 cm, median 1.85 cm).[50] Again, an impressive diagnostic yield of 81.6% was obtained and the planned route could be followed by the bronchoscope in 95% of cases. A similar study in which standard rather than CT fluoroscopy was used obtained less favorable results (63.5 diagnostic yield, lesions ≤3 cm, mean 1.67 cm).[51] This suggests that the combination of technologies used may be as important as the primary technique of interest in a particular study.

Newer VB systems are being developed that will help navigate towards peripheral lesions by coordinating,[52] or even fusing,[53,54] VB images to those generated in real time by the bronchoscope and adding computer-generated graphics to the VB image.[55]

It has recently been documented that physician selection of the appropriate endobronchial path towards lung lesions is a source of error and that VB techniques may improve accuracy.[56] Undoubtedly, in order for bronchoscopists to successfully access small peripheral lung lesions, they will need some form of guidance to ensure that the correct path is taken.

ELECTROMAGNETIC NAVIGATIONAL BRONCHOSCOPY

One of the most recent techniques introduced for bronchoscopic sampling of peripheral lung lesions is electromagnetic navigational bronchoscopy (ENB). These systems use an electromagnetic field to track a locatable guide in real time, correlating its position in the tracheobronchial tree to a patient's CT scan. A path to a peripheral lung lesion can be planned and the locatable guide advanced towards it with use of a steerable probe through the working channel of a regular bronchoscope. Once the guide has reached the lesion, it is removed, leaving a GS in place through which forceps, brushes, or needles can be advanced. The most widely used system to date has been the inReach system (superDimension, Hertzliya, Israel),[57–63] although experience with other devices has been published.[64,65] This technique is reviewed in detail in the article by Schwarz elsewhere this issue.

Several studies have been published with the inReach system on a total of 285 patients, with diagnostic yields between 59% and 77% overall and 54% to 75% in nodules less than or equal to 3 cm (**Table 3**).[57–63] The actual yields may be slightly lower given concerns with study designs, such as exclusion of patients in which the procedure was attempted in the calculation of diagnostic yield,[57,60,63] and inclusion of nonspecific benign features, such as inflammation[57] and atypical cell,[63] that were confirmed only by clinical follow-up[59,60] but included in the definition of positive results. The technique can be performed with or without additional fluoroscopy guidance, but it is unclear if this has an impact on results, as these approaches have not been formerly compared. The results between series using both approaches seem similar. No study has been published comparing ENB to standard bronchoscopy techniques to date.

Table 3
Published results of electromagnetic navigation bronchoscopy for peripheral lung lesions

Author and Year, Study Design	Method	Number of Nodules (Mean Size)	Prevalence of Malignancy	Overall Diagnostic Yield	Diagnostic Yield for Lesions ≤2 cm	Diagnostic Yield for Lesions ≤3 cm
Becker 2005, case series[57]	Fluoroscopy, pEBUS, GA	30—1 excluded (2.9 cm)	83%	69%	NA	NA
Schwarz 2006, case series[63]	CS, fluoroscopy	15—2 excluded (3.4 cm)	92%	69%	50% (2 lesions)	60% (5 lesions)
Gildea 2006, case series[60]	CS, fluoroscopy	56 (2.3 cm)	77%	74%	74.1%	72.1%
Makris 2007, case series[62]	GA, no fluoroscopy	40 (2.4 cm)	83%	63%	50%	56%
Eberhardt 2007, case series[59]	GA/CS, no fluoroscopy	92 (2.4 cm)	76%	67%	63%	67%
Eberhardt 2007, RCT (ENB arm)[58]	GA/CS, no fluoroscopy	39 (2.8 cm)	74%	59%	75% (4 lesions)	54%
Lamprecht 2009, case series[61]	GA, ROSE, no fluoroscopy	13 (3.0 cm)	69%	77%	75% (4 lesions)	75%

Abbreviations: CS, conscious sedation; GA, general anesthesia; NA, not available; RCT, randomized controlled trial; ROSE, rapid on-site cytopathologic evaluation.

It has long been recognized that lung lesions can move significantly with respiration, especially in lower lobes.[66] The main drawback of the technique is that there is no real-time confirmation that a lesion has been reached but only that the probe is in the location of the lesion based on a CT scan done on a different day, at a different lung volume. Another issue is the cost of the disposables associated with this equipment, which significantly exceeds those associated with other techniques discussed.

COMBINED APPROACHES

The diagnostic capabilities of the bronchoscope for SPNs have improved significantly over the past few years. Unfortunately, diagnostic yield remains below 70% for the most part, resulting in unacceptably low NPVs for malignancy. As such, patients without a diagnosis after bronchoscopy still require additional testing or surgery.

These techniques have various strengths and weaknesses and the combination of more than one technique can exploit the advantages of each tool. Advanced bronchoscopic techniques for diagnosis of pulmonary nodules can be subdivided into three main categories (**Table 4**).

The first category of procedures aims to improve the maneuverability of instruments, allowing specific bifurcations to be accessed as opposed to the straight-line path of a standard bronchoscopy forceps. These techniques include ultrathin bronchoscopy, which, as discussed previously, can help advance the bronchoscope from the third- or fourth-generation airways to the seventh or ninth generation. The bihinged curette inserted through a GS can also be used to maneuver into specific airways towards lung lesions. Also, the steerable navigation catheter of the inReach system can be bent and rotated in an effort to guide it in the correct direction.

The second category of procedures is those that offer bronchoscopists specific knowledge about the optimal path between the central airway to the target lesion. In its most basic form, this information can be gathered from careful examination of a patient's chest CT but is facilitated by VB reconstruction of the images and even further by formal VB guidance systems with or without electromagnetic localization.

Finally, the third category of procedures confirms that the lesion of interest has been reached by the GS or biopsy forceps. Standard fluoroscopy can be useful for this, but CT fluoroscopy and pEBUS can confirm with near certainty that a lesion has been reached.

The authors believe that an optimal approach to bronchoscopy for sampling of peripheral lung nodules needs to incorporate systems that achieve the goals of all three categories. Bronchoscopists' tools need to inform them of the best path to take, offer the ability to take that path, and confirm that the destination has been reached. Several combined approaches have been discussed previously, such as the combination of VB and pEBUS,[45] but in this case, the ability to maneuver toward a lesion is still limited by the depth to which the bronchoscope can be advanced, so that not all three criteria are met. The combination of pEBUS with thinner scopes and VB guidance may continue to improve this approach as the size of the ultrasound probes get smaller and smaller, but current probes cannot be used with ultrathin bronchoscopes.

Another combination, discussed previously, includes the integration of ultrathin bronchoscopes (maneuverability), VB (path), and CT fluoroscopy (destination), bringing all three necessary components in the bronchoscopic diagnosis of SPNs together.[31,50] One such study showed particularly impressive results, with a diagnostic yield of 81.6% in patients with nodules less than or equal to 3 cm (median 1.85 cm).[50]

Perhaps the most interesting multimodality strategy to date, and one of few subjected to a randomized trial, is the combination of ENB (maneuverability and path) and pEBUS (destination). The ENB system can be applied as described previously, but prior to performing sampling procedures through the GS, the pEBUS

Table 4		
Components of a combined approach to the peripheral lung nodule		
		Confirmation of Destination
ManeuverabilityTechniques	Path/RoadmapTechniques	Techniques
Ultrathin bronchoscopy	VB	Fluoroscopy
Electromagnetic navigation (steerable probe component)	Electromagnetic navigation	CT fluoroscopy pEBUS
Bihinged curette		

probe is inserted to confirm that the lesion of interest has been reached. If the lesion is not seen on pEBUS, the locator probe is reinserted and repeated navigation attempted until confirmation is documented by pEBUS. Once the GS position is confirmed to be in the lesion of interest via pEBUS, the ultrasound probe is removed and biopsy forceps advanced to the correct location. In a three-way randomization design, 118 patients with peripheral lung lesions (mean 2.6 cm, ±6 mm) underwent ENB, pEBUS, or the combination of techniques with diagnostic yield as the primary outcome measure.[58] Statistically significant differences between the three groups were reported, with diagnostic yields for ENB, pEBUS, and the combination of 59%, 69%, and 88%, respectively.[58] The NPV for combined ENB and pEBUS was 75%, which is similar to CT-TTNA.[2]

The authors anticipate that combination approaches will be critical for bronchoscopic techniques, offering a viable alternative to CT-guided and surgical diagnostic sampling procedures. The challenge is to find the most effective combination without increasing complications while maintaining costs competitive with other techniques.

DIAGNOSTIC APPROACH

There are several different technologies available for the diagnosis of peripheral pulmonary lesions. The choice of one particular technology over another depends on several different factors. In addition to those discussed previously, observation, PET scanning, CT-TTNA. and surgical resection can all be considered according to the clinical scenario, patient preference, availability of each technology, bronchoscopist expertise, and cost factors.

Given the poor NPV of most of the bronchoscopic modalities for SPN, the authors believe that they should not routinely be applied to patients with a high clinical likelihood of early-stage, surgically resectable lung malignancy. In such cases, a negative result would still require surgical resection, and alternative (benign) diagnoses are rare. Bronchoscopic tests may be best applied to confirm the diagnosis of lung cancer in patients when an extensive resection is required, in high-risk patients prior to surgery, in medically inoperable patients with early-stage disease but who are candidates for high-dose radiation treatments, and in patients with advanced disease but without alternatives for safer, less-invasive biopsy (eg, those with solitary lung mass with brain metastasis). In such cases, a CT-guided approach may be more cost effective if the lesion is accessible (pleural based) and the risk of pneumothorax is not considered increased.

Other situations that may be suited to a bronchoscopic approach include diagnosis of multiple lung lesions; diagnosis of suspected benign lesions, in cases when a lesion is not accessible or thought high risk for CT-guided biopsy; possibility of staging of bronchogenic carcinoma; or after a negative result from this TTNA.

SUMMARY

The past decade has witnessed the application of many advanced bronchoscopic modalities to improve access to the SPN. Although many of the techniques are being applied on a regular basis by bronchoscopists, which technique—or more likely which combination of techniques—will offer the best performance and cost-effectiveness remains to be determined. The authors anticipate that bronchoscopic approaches to the SPN will continue to proliferate as technologic advances are implemented and clinical data accumulate. Research should focus on combinations of techniques, cost-effectiveness, and incorporation of these tools in diagnostic algorithms for lung nodules/masses. Perhaps even more interesting are early reports of using such technologies not only for diagnosis but also for treatment of lung malignancies.[67,68]

REFERENCES

1. Klein JS, Zarka MA. Transthoracic needle biopsy. Radiol Clin North Am 2000;38(2):235–66.
2. Rivera MP, Mehta AC. Initial diagnosis of lung cancer: ACCP evidence-based clinical practice guidelines (2nd edition). Chest 2007;132(Suppl 3): 131S–48S.
3. Heyer CM, Reichelt S, Peters SA, et al. Computed tomography-navigated transthoracic core biopsy of pulmonary lesions: which factors affect diagnostic yield and complication rates? Acad Radiol 2008; 15(8):1017–26.
4. Ohno Y, Hatabu H, Takenaka D, et al. CT-guided transthoracic needle aspiration biopsy of small (<= 20 mm) solitary pulmonary nodules. Am J Roentgenol 2003;180(6):1665–9.
5. Jaeschke R, Guyatt G, Sackett DL. Users' guides to the medical literature. III. How to use an article about a diagnostic test. A. Are the results of the study valid? Evidence-Based Medicine Working Group. JAMA 1994;271(5):389–91.
6. Jaeschke R, Guyatt GH, Sackett DL. Users' guides to the medical literature. III. How to use an article about a diagnostic test. B. What are the results and will they help me in caring for my patients?

The Evidence-Based Medicine Working Group. JAMA 1994;271(9):703–7.

7. Gould MK, Fletcher J, Iannettoni MD, et al. Evaluation of patients with pulmonary nodules: when is it lung cancer?: ACCP evidence-based clinical practice guidelines (2nd edition). Chest 2007;132(Suppl 3):108S–30S.

8. Buccheri G, Barberis P, Delfino MS. Diagnostic, morphologic, and histopathologic correlates in bronchogenic carcinoma. A review of 1,045 bronchoscopic examinations. Chest 1991;99(4):809–14.

9. Kawaraya M, Gemba K, Ueoka H, et al. Evaluation of various cytological examinations by bronchoscopy in the diagnosis of peripheral lung cancer. Br J Cancer 2003;89(10):1885–8.

10. Zavala DC. Diagnostic fiberoptic bronchoscopy: techniques and results of biopsy in 600 patients. Chest 1975;68(1):12–9.

11. Baaklini WA, Reinoso MA, Gorin AB, et al. Diagnostic yield of fiberoptic bronchoscopy in evaluating solitary pulmonary nodules. Chest 2000;117(4):1049–54.

12. Stringfield JT, Markowitz DJ, Bentz RR, et al. The effect of tumor size and location on diagnosis by fiberoptic bronchoscopy. Chest 1977;72(4):474–6.

13. Wallace JM, Deutsch AL. Flexible fiberoptic bronchoscopy and percutaneous needle lung aspiration for evaluating the solitary pulmonary nodule. Chest 1982;81(6):665–71.

14. Cox ID, Bagg LR, Russell NJ, et al. Relationship of radiologic position to the diagnostic yield of fiberoptic bronchoscopy in bronchial carcinoma. Chest 1984;85(4):519–22.

15. Gaeta M, Pandolfo I, Volta S, et al. Bronchus sign on CT in peripheral carcinoma of the lung: value in predicting results of transbronchial biopsy. Am J Roentgenol 1991;157(6):1181–5.

16. Naidich DP, Sussman R, Kutcher WL, et al. Solitary pulmonary nodules. CT-bronchoscopic correlation. Chest 1988;93(3):595–8.

17. Chechani V. Bronchoscopic diagnosis of solitary pulmonary nodules and lung masses in the absence of endobronchial abnormality. Chest 1996;109(3):620–5.

18. Baba M, Iyoda A, Yasufuku K, et al. Preoperative cytodiagnosis of very small-sized peripheral-type primary lung cancer. Lung Cancer 2002;37(3):277–80.

19. Popp W, Rauscher H, Ritschka L, et al. Diagnostic sensitivity of different techniques in the diagnosis of lung tumors with the flexible fiberoptic bronchoscope. Comparison of brush biopsy, imprint cytology of forceps biopsy, and histology of forceps biopsy. Cancer 1991;67(1):72–5.

20. Jain P, Fleming P, Mehta AC. Radiation safety for health care workers in the bronchoscopy suite. Clin Chest Med 1999;20(1):33–8, x.

21. Lee CH, Wang CH, Lin MC, et al. Multiple brushings with immediate Riu's stain via flexible fibreoptic bronchoscopy without fluoroscopic guidance in the diagnosis of peripheral pulmonary tumours. Thorax 1995;50(1):18–21.

22. Tanaka M, Kawanami O, Satoh M, et al. Endoscopic observation of peripheral airway lesions. Chest 1988;93(2):228–33.

23. Tanaka M, Kohda E, Satoh M, et al. Diagnosis of peripheral lung cancer using a new type of endoscope. Chest 1990;97(5):1231–4.

24. Tanaka M, Takizawa H, Satoh M, et al. Assessment of an ultrathin bronchoscope that allows cytodiagnosis of small airways. Chest 1994;106(5):1443–7.

25. Rooney CP, Wolf K, McLennan G. Ultrathin bronchoscopy as an adjunct to standard bronchoscopy in the diagnosis of peripheral lung lesions. Respiration 2002;69(1):63–8.

26. Yamamoto S, Ueno K, Imamura F, et al. Usefulness of ultrathin bronchoscopy in diagnosis of lung cancer. Lung Cancer 2004;46(1):43–8.

27. Oki M, Saka H, Kitagawa C, et al. Novel thin bronchoscope with a 1.7-mm working channel for peripheral pulmonary lesions. Eur Respir J 2008;32(2):465–71.

28. Oki M, Saka H, Kitagawa C, et al. Visceral pleural perforation in two cases of ultrathin bronchoscopy. Chest 2005;127(6):2271–3.

29. Shinagawa N, Yamazaki K, Onodera Y, et al. Factors related to diagnostic sensitivity using an ultrathin bronchoscope under CT guidance. Chest 2007;131(2):549–53.

30. Shinagawa N, Yamazaki K, Onodera Y, et al. CT-guided transbronchial biopsy using an ultrathin bronchoscope with virtual bronchoscopic navigation. Chest 2004;125(3):1138–43.

31. Tsushima K, Sone S, Hanaoka T, et al. Comparison of bronchoscopic diagnosis for peripheral pulmonary nodule under fluoroscopic guidance with CT guidance. Respir Med 2006;100(4):737–45.

32. White CS, Weiner EA, Patel P, et al. Transbronchial needle aspiration: guidance with CT fluoroscopy. Chest 2000;118(6):1630–8.

33. Ost D, Shah R, Anasco E, et al. A randomized trial of CT fluoroscopic-guided bronchoscopy vs conventional bronchoscopy in patients with suspected lung cancer. Chest 2008;134(3):507–13.

34. Tremblay A. Endobronchial ultrasonography: bronchoscopy beyond the airway wall. Can Respir J 2008;15(Suppl):17C–8C.

35. Chao TY, Chien MT, Lie CH, et al. Endobronchial ultrasonography-guided transbronchial needle aspiration increases the diagnostic yield of peripheral pulmonary lesions: a randomized trial. Chest 2009;136(1):229–36.

36. Herth FJ, Ernst A, Becker HD. Endobronchial ultrasound-guided transbronchial lung biopsy in solitary pulmonary nodules and peripheral lesions. Eur Respir J 2002;20(4):972–4.

37. Paone G, Nicastri E, Lucantoni G, et al. Endobronchial ultrasound-driven biopsy in the diagnosis of peripheral lung lesions. Chest 2005;128(5):3551–7.

38. Kurimoto N, Miyazawa T, Okimasa S, et al. Endobronchial ultrasonography using a guide sheath increases the ability to diagnose peripheral pulmonary lesions endoscopically. Chest 2004;126(3):959–65.

39. Asahina H, Yamazaki K, Onodera Y, et al. Transbronchial biopsy using endobronchial ultrasonography with a guide sheath and virtual bronchoscopic navigation. Chest 2005;128(3):1761–5.

40. Kikuchi E, Yamazaki K, Sukoh N, et al. Endobronchial ultrasonography with guide-sheath for peripheral pulmonary lesions. Eur Respir J 2004;24(4):533–7.

41. Shirakawa T, Imamura F, Hamamoto J, et al. Usefulness of endobronchial ultrasonography for transbronchial lung biopsies of peripheral lung lesions. Respiration 2004;71(3):260–8.

42. Yamada N, Yamazaki K, Kurimoto N, et al. Factors related to diagnostic yield of transbronchial biopsy using endobronchial ultrasonography with a guide sheath in small peripheral pulmonary lesions. Chest 2007;132(2):603–8.

43. Yoshikawa M, Sukoh N, Yamazaki K, et al. Diagnostic value of endobronchial ultrasonography with a guide sheath for peripheral pulmonary lesions without X-ray fluoroscopy. Chest 2007;131(6):1788–93.

44. Fielding DI, Robinson PJ, Kurimoto N. Biopsy site selection for endobronchial ultrasound guide-sheath transbronchial biopsy of peripheral lung lesions. Intern Med J 2008;38(2):77–84.

45. Asano F, Matsuno Y, Tsuzuku A, et al. Diagnosis of peripheral pulmonary lesions using a bronchoscope insertion guidance system combined with endobronchial ultrasonography with a guide sheath. Lung Cancer 2008;60(3):366–73.

46. Chao TY, Lie CH, Chung YH, et al. Differentiating peripheral pulmonary lesions based on images of endobronchial ultrasonography. Chest 2006;130(4):1191–7.

47. Kuo CH, Lin SM, Chen HC, et al. Diagnosis of peripheral lung cancer with three echoic features via endobronchial ultrasound. Chest 2007;132(3):922–9.

48. Kurimoto N, Murayama M, Yoshioka S, et al. Analysis of the internal structure of peripheral pulmonary lesions using endobronchial ultrasonography. Chest 2002;122(6):1887–94.

49. Asano FMD, Matsuno YMD, Matsushita TMD, et al. Transbronchial diagnosis of a pulmonary peripheral small lesion using an ultrathin bronchoscope with virtual bronchoscopic navigation [report]. Journal of Bronchology 2002;9(2):108–11.

50. Asano F, Matsuno Y, Shinagawa N, et al. A virtual bronchoscopic navigation system for pulmonary peripheral lesions. Chest 2006;130(2):559–66.

51. Tachihara M, Ishida T, Kanazawa K, et al. A virtual bronchoscopic navigation system under X-ray fluoroscopy for transbronchial diagnosis of small peripheral pulmonary lesions. Lung Cancer 2007;57(3):322–7.

52. Bricault I, Ferretti G, Cinquin P. Registration of real and CT-derived virtual bronchoscopic images to assist transbronchial biopsy. IEEE Trans Med Imaging 1998;17(5):703–14.

53. Gibbs JD, Graham MW, Higgins WE. 3D MDCT-based system for planning peripheral bronchoscopic procedures. Comput Biol Med 2009;39(3):266–79.

54. Higgins WE, Helferty JP, Lu K, et al. 3D CT-video fusion for image-guided bronchoscopy. Comput Med Imaging Graph 2008;32(3):159–73.

55. Helferty JP, Sherbondy AJ, Kiraly AP, et al. Computer-based system for the virtual-endoscopic guidance of bronchoscopy. Comput Vis Image Underst 2007;108(1–2):171–87.

56. Dolina MY, Cornish DC, Merritt SA, et al. Interbronchoscopist variability in endobronchial path selection: a Simulation Study. Chest 2008;133(4):897–905.

57. Becker HDM, Herth FM, Ernst AM, et al. Bronchoscopic biopsy of peripheral lung lesions under electromagnetic guidance: a Pilot Study. Journal of Bronchology Dedicated to Bronchoscopy and Interventional Pulmonology 2005;12(1):9–13.

58. Eberhardt R, Anantham D, Ernst A, et al. Multimodality bronchoscopic diagnosis of peripheral lung lesions: a randomized controlled trial. Am J Respir Crit Care Med 2007;176(1):36–41.

59. Eberhardt R, Anantham D, Herth F, et al. Electromagnetic navigation diagnostic bronchoscopy in peripheral lung lesions. Chest 2007;131(6):1800–5.

60. Gildea TR, Mazzone PJ, Karnak D, et al. Electromagnetic navigation diagnostic bronchoscopy: a Prospective Study. Am J Respir Crit Care Med 2006;174(9):982–9.

61. Lamprecht B, Porsch P, Pirich C, et al. Electromagnetic navigation bronchoscopy in combination with PET-CT and rapid on-site cytopathologic examination for diagnosis of peripheral lung lesions. Lung 2009;187(1):55–9.

62. Makris D, Scherpereel A, Leroy S, et al. Electromagnetic navigation diagnostic bronchoscopy for small peripheral lung lesions. Eur Respir J 2007;29(6):1187–92.

63. Schwarz Y, Greif J, Becker HD, et al. Real-time electromagnetic navigation bronchoscopy to peripheral lung lesions using overlaid CT images: the First Human Study. Chest 2006;129(4):988–94.

64. Chen W, Chen L, Yang S, et al. A novel technique for localization of small pulmonary nodules. Chest 2007;131(5):1526–31.

65. Hautmann H, Schneider A, Pinkau T, et al. Electromagnetic catheter navigation during bronchoscopy: validation of a novel method by conventional fluoroscopy. Chest 2005;128(1):382–7.

66. Stevens CW, Munden RF, Forster KM, et al. Respiratory-driven lung tumor motion is independent of tumor size, tumor location, and pulmonary function. Int J Radiat Oncol Biol Phys 2001; 51(1):62–8.
67. Anantham D, Feller-Kopman D, Shanmugham LN, et al. Electromagnetic navigation bronchoscopy-guided fiducial placement for robotic stereotactic radiosurgery of lung tumors: a feasibility study. Chest 2007;132(3):930–5.
68. Harms W, Krempien R, Grehn C, et al. Electromagnetically navigated brachytherapy as a new treatment option for peripheral pulmonary tumors. Strahlenther Onkol 2006;182(2):108–11.
69. Chung YH, Lie CH, Chao TY, et al. Endobronchial ultrasonography with distance for peripheral pulmonary lesions. Respir Med 2007;101(4):738–45.
70. Dooms CA, Verbeken EK, Becker HD, et al. Endobronchial ultrasonography in bronchoscopic occult pulmonary lesions. J Thorac Oncol 2007;2(2):121–4.

Electromagnetic Navigation

Yehuda Schwarz, MD, FCCP[a,b,*]

KEYWORDS

- Electromagnetic navigation bronchoscopy
- Peripheral lung lesion • Transbronchial needle aspiration
- Fiducial markers • Stereotactic radiosurgery

The first bronchoscopic procedure was performed in 1897 by Gustav Killian using a laryngoscope and a rigid esophageal tube to remove a foreign body from the trachea.[1] During the next century, bronchoscopy evolved from being a rigid technique to one that uses a flexible bronchoscope developed by Ikeda and colleagues[2] in 1968, opening new horizons in the diagnosis and treatment of pulmonary diseases. Flexible bronchoscopy is a minimally invasive procedure, obviating general anesthesia and eliminating potential associated complications. New technological developments emerged in the 80s to improve the yield in diagnosis; these innovations included videobronchoscopy, endobronchial ultrasonography (EBUS), autofluorescence bronchoscopy, and lately, narrow-band imaging.[3,4] Endoscopic therapeutic procedures have also kept pace with these developments, with the introduction of laser photoresection, cryotherapy, electrocautery, and stent technology.[5] The field of imaging also underwent technological transformation at the same time.

The incidence of peripheral non-small–cell lung cancer (NSCL, adenocarcinoma subgroup) has also increased significantly during the last 30 years; probably because of the introduction and use of filtered cigarettes and the subsequent distal delivery of smaller cigarettes particles.

Patients with pulmonary nodules and masses are routinely referred to pulmonologists, radiologists, and thoracic surgeons for evaluation and tissue diagnosis. The rapidly increasing use of chest computed tomography (CT) for screening and ruling out pulmonary embolism and various other indications has led to a significant increase in the detection of lung nodules.[6] More than 6.5 million CT scans of the chest were performed in the United States alone in 2001, highlighting the gravity of this clinical scenario.[7]

Choosing the invasive diagnostic procedures to perform a biopsy for tissue diagnosis in cases of small peripheral nodules or opacities remains a clinical challenge. The main options are bronchoscopy, percutaneous needle aspiration, and thoracoscopic lung biopsy. Percutaneous needle aspiration biopsy still plays an important role in the diagnosis of peripheral lung cancers, yet the associated pneumothorax (20%–34%) and hemoptysis are unacceptable.[8–11] The high incidence of pneumothorax in percutaneous techniques can be partially explained by the fact that most patients diagnosed with a peripheral lung lesion also may have some degree of emphysematous changes and poor pulmonary function from smoking. Thoracoscopic and open surgical biopsy have the obvious disadvantages of the procedures being invasive, the patients having to undergo general anesthesia, and the need to tolerate single-lung ventilation during the procedure. The rate of mortality for this procedure can be 0.5% to 5.3%.[12]

In patients with a high probability of lung cancer and good lung function, it is often not necessary to obtain tissue diagnosis. For all others, however, there is a need for an approach with a low complication rate, especially in those with multiple nodules and compromised lung function. Cohort studies have demonstrated that most nodules so detected are benign.[13] As such, surgery, with its associated morbidity and mortality, is not

a Department of Pulmonology, Tel-Aviv Sourasky Medical Center, 6 Weisman Street, Tel-Aviv, 64239, Israel
b Sackler Faculty of Medicine, Tel Aviv University, Ramat Aviv 69978, Israel
* Department of Pulmonology, Tel-Aviv Sourasky Medical Center, 6 Weisman Street, Tel-Aviv, 64239, Israel.
E-mail address: schwarz@tasmc.health.gov.il

Clin Chest Med 31 (2010) 65–73
doi:10.1016/j.ccm.2009.08.005
0272-5231/10/$ – see front matter © 2010 Published by Elsevier Inc.

indicated for most patients who present with incidentally discovered pulmonary nodules. Tissue diagnosis, on the other hand, is frequently essential.[12]

The conventional flexible bronchoscopy procedure is of limited diagnostic value in peripheral lung nodules, that is, those located at the peripheral third of the lung. Biopsy success is further compromised if the lesion is smaller than 2 cm in diameter.[14] The main limitation of the bronchoscopic approach is the difficulty in reaching peripheral lesions with the biopsy tools. The tools used to obtain biopsy tissue are difficult to steer to the desired location. Once extended beyond the tip of the bronchoscope, the physician performing the bronchoscopy is faced with the difficulty of precisely localizing the lesion under fluoroscopy, whereas the alternatives of CT-guided bronchoscopy and EBUS are more technically demanding and require special training. EBUS enables the operator to "see" the lesion but it cannot provide guidelines to the bronchoscopist for choosing the correct airway to reach a given peripheral lesion.

Moderate sedation is the current practice in standard bronchoscopy and the procedure is safe in the hands of trained personnel. Because the mortality for bronchoscopy is low (1 in 4000) and the complication rate for pneumothorax with transbronchial biopsy is also much lower than all the other available approaches (<2%), it would be worthwhile to use it as the procedure of choice if the yield could be improved.

The recently introduced electromagnetic navigation bronchoscopy (EMB) system (inReach system, superDimension Ltd, Herzliya, Israel) is a new technology that includes the use of virtual bronchoscopy (VB) and real-time 3-dimensional CT images, allowing the bronchoscopist to localize peripheral lung lesions and to introduce endobronchial accessories for performing biopsies of peripheral lesions. The technology uses a processor, an amplifier, and a location board. By means of low-frequency electromagnetic waves emitted from a board placed under the head of the bronchoscopy table, the monitor picks up the signal emitted by the sensor. Electromagnetic waves preclude the use of the system on patients with devices such as pacemakers and automatic cardioverter-defibrillators. The sensor is 1 mm in diameter and 8 mm in length at the tip of a flexible metal cable (the "locatable guide" [LG]) (**Fig. 1**A). Once the sensor is placed within the electromagnetic field generated by the board placed under the mattress of the bronchoscopic bed (see **Fig. 1**B), its position in the X, Y, and Z planes and its orientation (roll, pitch, and yaw

movements) are visualized on the monitor in real-time (see **Fig. 1**C). The guide is mounted on a tool that allows its distal section to be steered in 8 directions, translating into 360° of steerability. The fully retractable sensor is integrated into a flexible catheter that serves as an extended working channel (EWC) of the bronchoscope (see **Fig. 1**D). The LG has a built-in bending mechanism for active steering that allows bending of the tip toward the selected target (see **Fig. 1**A). The catheter is left in place once it reaches the desired location, enabling easy access for bronchoscopic accessories. The computer software and monitor allow the bronchoscopist to view the reconstructed 3-dimensional CT scans of the patient's anatomy in coronal, sagittal, and axial views, with superimposed graphic information depicting the position of the sensor probe (**Fig. 2**). Information on location, orientation, and movement is then superimposed on a previously acquired CT scan and displayed on a monitor in real time.

Navigation bronchoscopy is performed in several steps. The first step is the planning of the procedure, which is performed by importing the CT data into the software. The software presents the CT images in axial, sagittal and coronal cuts and also provides VB images (**Fig. 3**A). The planner marks the main carina and major bronchial bifurcations as reference points on the VB images (see **Fig. 3**B) and the targeted lesions (mediastinal lymph nodes and lung nodules) on the CT images. The physician can track a lesion by following the CT images and "flying" though the VB images. The quality of the virtual environment is dependent on the quality of the CT scan; so it is essential to plan the procedure in great detail. To perform a transbronchial needle aspiration (TBNA), the tracheal wall on the VB images can be made transparent to place a marker as reference to a site for needle insertion (**Fig. 4**). The next step is the alignment of the VB images at preselected points of the carina and major bronchial bifurcations. These easily recognizable points act as anatomic landmarks during the bronchoscopy and are aligned with the VB images for the purpose of "registration" (**Fig. 5**). The software then aligns both environments (VB and endoscopy), thus enabling the sequential presentation of the CT cuts while the sensor (LG) is advanced through the patient's airways. Registration errors could then be reduced by either repositioning a misplaced registration point or by eliminating the registration points with the greatest deviation. Navigation is performed by steering the LG probe with its extending working channel (EWC) to the lesion, by following the multiplanar CT images and the "tip-view." The latter also provides information on the

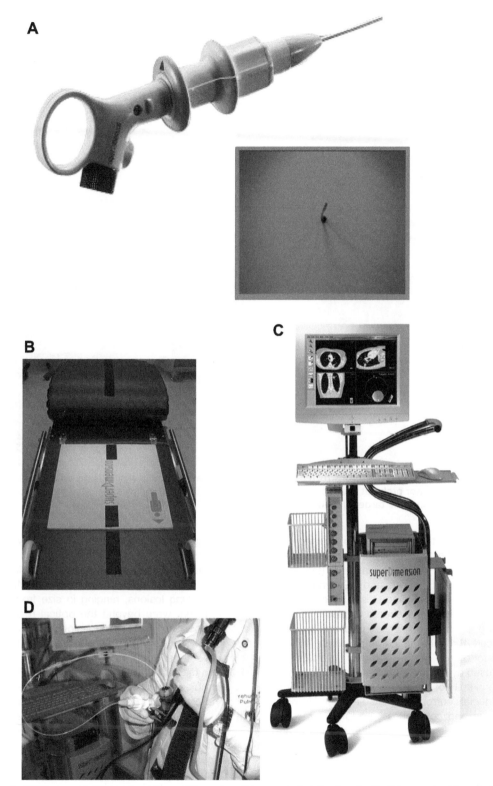

Fig. 1. (*A*) The sensor (1 mm diameter and 8 mm length) mounted at the tip of a flexible metal cable—the LG. The LG has a built-in bending mechanism for active steering in 8 directions that allows bending of the tip. *Courtesy of* superDimension, Inc., Minneapolis, MN; with permission. (*B*) The LG with the sensor is integrated into the extended working channel (EWC). The EWC is left at the desired location once it has been reached with the aid of the sensor, enabling easy access for bronchoscopic accessories. (*C*) The monitor and computer are placed on a trolley to receive input and visualization of the sensor's position on the monitor in all orientations (X, Y, and Z planes and roll, pitch, and yaw movements) in real time. *Courtesy of* superDimension, Inc., Minneapolis, MN; with permission. (*D*) Magnetic board placed under the mattress of the bronchoscopy bed.

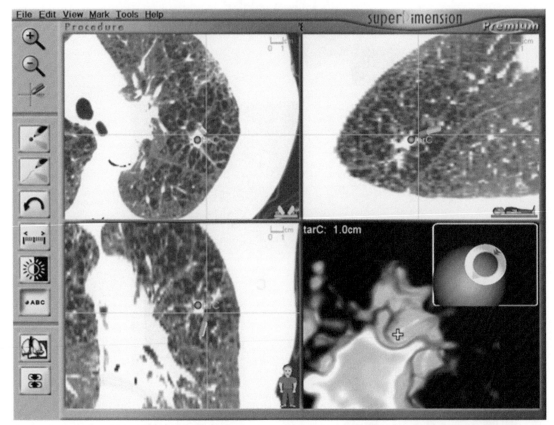

Fig. 2. The monitor depicting the reconstructed 3-dimensional CT scans (coronal, sagittal, and axial views), with the position of the sensor probe at the "tip-view" showing a ring with an arrow giving an accurate direction to bend the LG for reaching the targeted lesion and 3-dimensional CT images of the focal sensor's area.

direction in which to bend the LG to move toward the lesion (see **Fig. 2**). The fully retractable probe is incorporated into a flexible catheter (the EWC sheath) that is 130 cm long and 1.9 mm in diameter. Once the area of interest is reached, the LG is removed leaving the sheath in place. Various tools and endoscopic accessories can now be introduced through the catheter: these include forceps for biopsy, needle, brush or curette, radial EBUS (used by some researchers for confirmation of the proximity of the sensor to the nodule), or to place fiducials surrounding the diagnosed tumors.

Schwarz and colleagues[15] performed the first trial to determine the practicality, accuracy, and safety of real-time EMB in locating artificial peripheral lung lesions in a swine model. The study showed a registration accuracy of 4.5 mm on average. No adverse effects, such as pneumothorax or internal bleeding, were encountered in any animal. The authors concluded that real-time electromagnetic positioning with previously acquired CT scans is an accurate technology that can augment standard bronchoscopy to assist in reaching peripheral lung lesions and in

performing biopsies. The first human study was a prospective controlled clinical investigation that was opened in June 2003; its result was published in 2006.[16] Of 15 subjects, 13 underwent EMB for peripheral lung lesions, ranging in size from 1.5 to 5 cm, that were beyond the optical reach of a bronchoscope. Four of the lesions were in the left upper lobe, 3 in the right upper lobe; 5 in the right lower lobe, and 1 in the right middle lobe. A definitive diagnosis was established in 9 (69%) of the 13 subjects. No device-related adverse events were reported during or up to 48 hours after the study. A parallel study[17] was performed in Germany from July to December, 2003, which also attained diagnostic yield of 69%. There were no serious complications. Both studies concluded that real-time EMB with CT images is a feasible and safe method for obtaining biopsies of peripheral lung lesions.

At the end of the 2006, a larger prospective study involving 60 patients was performed by Gildea and colleagues[18]; the results showed an improved yield of 74%, although 57% of lesions were smaller than 20 mm in size. Their study

A

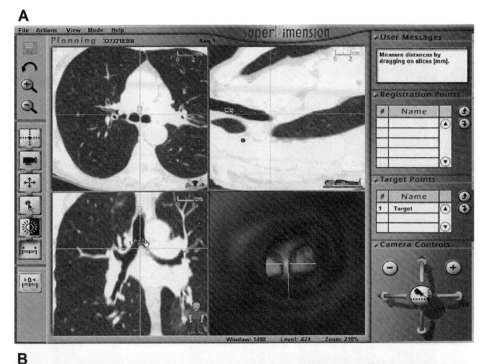

B

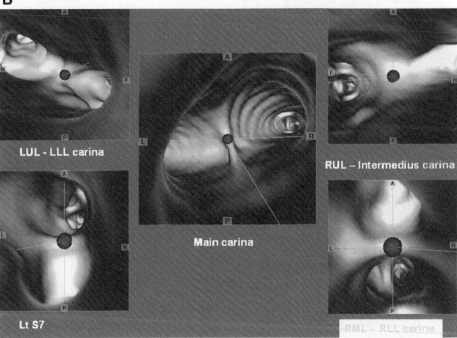

Fig. 3. (*A*) CT data represented by the system software in axial, sagittal, and coronal cuts and VB images. (*B*) Carina and major bronchial bifurcations on the VB images marked as reference points for the registration phase.

was the first to demonstrate another application of the navigation system, that is, the diagnosis of mediastinal lymph nodes. By adding lymph node sampling, they improved the overall patient diagnosis accuracy to 80.3%. Complications were limited to pneumothorax, which occurred in 3.5% of the patients. By giving the bronchoscopist access to the peripheral lung area, it became apparent that there are cases in which the steerable probe cannot be advanced to all the lesions, as the bronchus leading to the lesion may not exist.

A

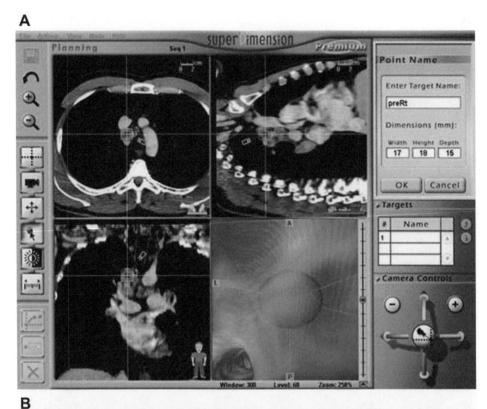

B

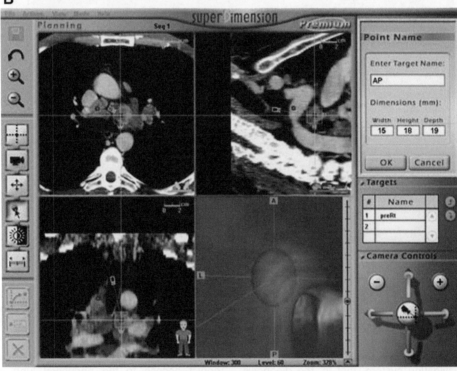

Fig. 4. Targeting the mediastinal lymph nodes for TBNA. The software "on-demand" shows a transparent VB image of the tracheal wall, thus allowing a view of the previously marked mediastinal lymph node for aspiration. (*A*) R4 lymph node and (*B*) lymph node at the aortopulmonary window.

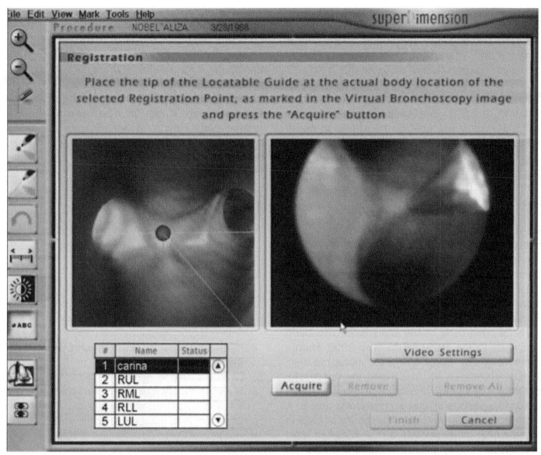

Fig. 5. Registration step: during the bronchoscopy the carina and the major bronchial bifurcations are marked on the VB images at the planning step in the same position using the sensor applied lightly on the carina mucosa.

Makris and colleagues[19] described their experience using the same EMB system in 40 patients with lesions between 17 to 39 mm in size. They emphasized that the average of CT-to-body divergence, which represents the radius of the expected difference in location between the tip of the sensor probe in the actual patient and where the tip is expected to be was 4.6015 mm, whereas the distance between sensor probe and the center of the lesion was 8.7608 mm. The yield they reached was 62.5% in 25 out of the 40 cases, improving if the CT-to-body divergence was less than 4 mm. The sensitivity and negative predictive value of EMB for malignancy were 57 and 25%, respectively.

Eberhardt and colleagues[20] reported their experience with EMB in 89 subjects in whom they reached a diagnostic yield of 67%, (independent of lesion size). They had a CT-to-body divergence of 4.6 ± 1.8 mm (range, 1 to 31). There was no occurrence of pneumothorax. The mean navigation error was 9 ± 6 mm. These investigators also found that size of the lesion was not

a determinant in diagnostic yield, and noted that the time needed for the electromagnetic navigation method is around 30 minutes or less. This is similar to the time for performing bronchoscopy on patients with interstitial lung diseases and for obtaining a transbronchial biopsy.

The same group[21] compared the added value of using the US probe to verify and correct the position of the sensor once it had reached the lesion, as indicated by the software. By doing so, they were able to correct the position of the sensor and thereby improved their yield. They concluded that combined EBUS and EMB enhance the diagnostic yield of flexible bronchoscopy in peripheral lung lesions without compromising patient safety. Specifically, combined EBUS/EMB had a significantly higher diagnostic yield (88%) compared with EBUS (69%) or EMB alone (59%; P = .02), with an overall pneumothorax rate of 6%.

Several explanations were given by the users of the EMB for the failure to reach near 100% success, one being the absence of an airway leading to the targeted nodule, another being the lesion extrinsic to an airway making adequate tissue sampling difficult.

Wilson and Bartlett[22] performed a larger EMB retrospective consecutive study in a community bronchoscopic unit using rapid on-site cytologic evaluation (ROSE) on 248 patients referred for diagnosis of peripheral lesions or mediastinal lymph nodes (71). Pneumothorax was reported in 1.2%, mainly because of the efforts to reach a diagnosis, which occurred in 70%. Mean size of targeted peripheral lung lesion (PLL) and lymph nodes was 2.1 ± 1.4 (SD) cm and 1.8 ± 0.9 (SD) cm, respectively. The mean follow-up period was 6 ± 5 (SD) months. Fifty-one percent of PLLs were in the upper lobes; EMB + ROSE success was 96% for PLL (3–4 samples per patient with forceps and needle). Lymph nodes success was 94.3% (5–6 samples with needle biopsy). Overall diagnosis was made in 173 patients of the 248 (70%). The investigators used fluoroscopy to verify the location of the LG and biopsy forceps.

Therapeutic uses of the EMB have also been described in the literature. In year 2006, Harms and colleagues[23] applied EMB technology to therapeutic objectives and described the successful placement of a brachytherapy catheter after navigation to a peripheral, unresectable lung cancer. A second article showing the applicability of EMB in therapeutics was published by Kupelian and colleagues.[24] They placed metallic markers for radiation therapy for a small early-stage lung cancer using the EMB system transbronchially. They concluded that the markers placed using this less invasive method remained stable within the tumors throughout the treatment duration without any incidence of pneumothorax as compared with the 8 out of 15 in whom the transthoracic route was used and who developed the complication.

Anantham and colleagues[25] reported their experience with placement of 39 fiducial markers in 9 patients. The success rate was 89% (8 of 9 patients). The mean number of fiducial markers placed in each patient was 4.9 + 1.0 (range, 4 to 6). No migration was encountered in 90% of the patients.

Weiser and colleagues[26] published their experience in diagnosis and in placing fiducial markers in and around the lesions to enable stereotactic radiosurgery. They used ROSE and in case of a negative result, they continued surgically for additional biopsies. Krimsky and colleagues[27] used the EMB system to tattoo the subpleural area of the lung nodules after malignant diagnosis and to perform a therapeutic video-assisted thoracoscopic surgery.

Electromagnetic navigation bronchoscopy using overlaid CT images is a safe procedure. It improves the diagnostic yield of the flexible bronchoscopy for peripheral lesions and also allows sampling of the mediastinal lymph nodes. Also, the system affords several other advantages: there is no additional radiation, and it has a short learning curve. It can also be used for fiducial marker placement for brachytherapy or stereotactic radiosurgery. It plays a complementary role to other modalities such as an ultrathin bronchoscopy or an EBUS.

REFERENCES

1. Killian G. Meeting of the Society of Physicians of Freiburg. December 17, 1897. Munchen Med Wschr 1989;45:378.
2. Ikeda S, Yanai N, Ishikawa S. Flexible bronchofiberscope. Keio J Med 1968;17:1–16.
3. Lam S, Kennedy T, Unger M, et al. Localization of bronchial intraepithelial neoplastic lesions by fluorescence bronchoscopy. Chest 1998;113:696–702.
4. Herth FJF, Becker HD. Endobronchial ultrasound of the airways and the mediastinum. Monaldi Arch Chest Dis 2000;55:36–45.
5. Baram D. Palliation of endobronchial disease: flexible and rigid bronchoscopic options. Respir Care Clin N Am 2003;9:237–58.
6. Healthcare Cost and Utilization Project. Rockville (MD): Agency for Healthcare Research and Quality; 2001.
7. Sharma SK, Pande JN, Dey AB, et al. The use of diagnostic bronchoscopy in lung cancer. Natl Med J India 1992;5:162–6.
8. Laurent F, Michel P, Latrabe V, et al. Pneumothoraces and chest tube placement after CT-guided transthoracic lung biopsy using a coaxial technique. Am J Roentgenol 1999;172(4):1049–53.
9. Mullan CP, Kelly BE, Ellis PK, et al. CT-guided fine-needle aspiration of lung nodules: effect on outcome of using coaxial technique and immediate cytological evaluation. Ulster Med J 2004;73(1):32–6.
10. Baaklini WA, Reinoso MA, Gorin AB, et al. Diagnostic yield of fiberoptic bronchoscopy in evaluating solitary pulmonary nodules. Chest 2000;117: 1049–54.
11. Santambrogio L, Nosotti M, Bellaviti N, et al. CT-Guided fine-needle aspiration cytology of solitary pulmonary nodules. Chest 1997;112(2):423–5.
12. Gould MK, Sanders GD, Barnett PG, et al. Cost-effectiveness of alternative management strategies for patients with solitary pulmonary nodules. Ann Intern Med 2003;138:724–35.
13. Swensen SJ, Jett JR, Hartman TE, et al. Lung cancer screening with CT: Mayo Clinic experience. Radiology 2003;226:756–61.

14. Schreiber G, McCrory DC. Performance characteristics of different modalities for diagnosis of suspected lung cancer. Summary of published evidence. Chest 2003;123:115S–28S.

15. Schwarz Y, Mehta AC, Ernst A, et al. Electromagnetic navigation during flexible bronchoscopy. Respiration 2003;70(5):516–22.

16. Schwarz Y, Greif Y, Becker H, et al. Real-time electromagnetic navigation bronchoscopy to peripheral lung lesions using overlaid ct images: the first human study. Chest 2006;129(4):988–94.

17. Heinrich D, Becker HD, Herth F, et al. Bronchoscopic biopsy of peripheral lung lesions under electromagnetic guidance. A pilot study. J Bronchol 2005;12:9–13.

18. Gildea TR, Mazzone PJ, Karnak D, et al. Electromagnetic navigation diagnostic bronchoscopy: a prospective study. Am J Respir Crit Care Med 2006;174(9):982–9.

19. Makris D, Scherpereel A, Leroy S, et al. Electromagnetic navigation diagnostic bronchoscopy for small peripheral lung lesions. Eur Respir J 2007;29(6):1187–92.

20. Eberhardt R, Anantham D, Herth F, et al. Electromagnetic navigation diagnostic bronchoscopy in peripheral lung lesions. Chest 2007;131(6):1800–5.

21. Eberhardt R, Anantham D, Ernst A, et al. Multimodality bronchoscopic diagnosis of peripheral lung lesions: a randomized controlled trial. Am J Respir Crit Care Med 2007;176(1):36–41.

22. Wilson DS, Bartlett RJ. Improved diagnostic yield of bronchoscopy in a community practice: combination of electromagnetic navigation system and rapid on-site evaluation. J Bronchol 2007;14:227–32.

23. Harms W, Krempien R, Grehn C, et al. Electromagnetically navigated brachytherapy as a new treatment option for peripheral pulmonary tumors. Strahlenther Onkol 2006;182:108–11.

24. Kupelian PA, Forbes A, Willoughby TR, et al. Implantation and stability of metallic fiducials within pulmonary lesions. Int J Radiat Oncol Biol Phys 2007;69:777–85.

25. Anantham D, Feller-Kopman D, Shanmugham LN, et al. Electromagnetic navigation bronchoscopy guided fiducial placement for robotic stereotactic radiosurgery of lung tumors—a feasibility study. Chest 2007;132:930–5.

26. Weiser TS, Hyman K, Yun J, et al. Electromagnetic navigational bronchoscopy: a surgeon's perspective. Ann Thorac Surg 2008;85:S797–801.

27. Krimsky W, Sethi S, Cicenia JC. Tattooing of pulmonary nodules for localization prior to vats. Chicago, IL: ACCP meeting, October 22, 2007, Volume 132, Issue 4.

Virtual Bronchoscopic Navigation

Fumihiro Asano, MD, FCCP

KEYWORDS

- Virtual bronchoscopy
- Lung neoplasms and solitary pulmonary nodule/diagnosis
- Transbronchial biopsy • Three-dimensional imaging
- Endobronchial ultrasonography • User-computer interface

In recent years, solitary peripheral pulmonary lesions are being encountered more frequently because of the widespread use of CT scanning.[1] For the diagnosis of these lesions, bronchoscopy is routinely considered because it is safe and minimally invasive. However, its overall diagnostic yield is inadequate. The guidelines of the American College of Chest Physicians (ACCP) in 2007 showed a diagnostic yield of 57% for all lesions and 34% for lesions less than 2 cm in diameter.[2] The lesion-associated factors affecting the transbronchial diagnosis of solitary peripheral pulmonary lesions includes the lesion size,[3,4] its location,[3] the presence/absence of bronchial involvement,[5] and its malignant/benign status.[4] The bronchoscopist-associated factors include the apparatuses used and the bronchoscopist's skills and experience.[6]

At present, bronchoscopy for peripheral pulmonary lesions is performed using a bronchoscope with an external diameter of approximately 5 to 6 mm under x-ray fluoroscopy. Bronchoscopists mentally reconstruct the three-dimensional (3D) bronchial arrangement based on two-dimensional (2D) planar axial slices of CT, performed before the procedure, and select a bronchial path. A major problem with this method is difficulty in the guidance for the bronchoscope and its accessories. Bronchial path selection during the examination and at the same time maintaining the position of the bronchoscope along with its accessories in desired location under fluoroscopic guidance require time and skills. In addition, because the range of bronchoscope advancement is limited to around the subsegmental branches, biopsy instruments must be guided by fluoroscopy for a long distance from these proximal branches to the peripheral lesion. Therefore, the diagnostic yield depends on the bronchoscopist's experience and skill.[6]

To overcome these challenges, the use of a bronchoscope with a reduced external diameter (ultrathin bronchoscope) could be beneficial. In particular, because the ultrathin bronchoscope [7] can be advanced close to the lesion, guidance of the biopsy instruments is easier. In addition, the ultrathin bronchoscope can be negotiated to the difficult-to-reach areas of the endobronchial tree,[8] thus, it could be useful for the diagnosis of small peripheral pulmonary lesions.[9,10] However, because the number of bronchial branching increases as the bronchoscope advances further into the periphery, the path to the lesion is difficult to identify within the limited examination time even if bronchial branching is directly visible. In addition, endobronchial examination by itself does not provide the direction to the peripheral lesion. Intuitive bronchial path selection based on CT data is inaccurate even at the third- to fourth-generation bronchus levels,[11] and therefore cannot be applied to the levels of bronchi reached and observed by the ultrathin bronchoscope. In recent years, CT fluoroscopy has allowed real-time confirmation of the positions of the bronchoscope, sampling instruments, and the lesion, and has been useful for the diagnosis of small

Department of Pulmonary Medicine and Bronchoscopy, Gifu Prefectural General Medical Center, 4-6-1 Noishiki, Gifu, 500-8717, Japan
E-mail address: asano-fm@ceres.ocn.ne.jp

Clin Chest Med 31 (2010) 75–85
doi:10.1016/j.ccm.2009.08.007

peripheral lesions.[10,12,13] However, because the radiation exposure dose and the procedure time are significantly increased, path selection before the bronchoscopy is important.

Virtual bronchoscopic navigation (VBN) is a method in which bronchial path to the peripheral lesion is produced from virtual bronchoscopy (VB) images and used as a guide to navigate the bronchoscope. Because the bronchial branching pattern on VB images is similar to real bronchoscopic images, the bronchoscope can be advanced close to the target lesion according to the bronchial path to the lesion displayed on VB images. In addition, a system has been developed and applied that allows the automatic production of VB images of the bronchial path and their simultaneous display with real bronchoscopic images for navigation. VBN has been used in combination with CT-guided ultrathin bronchoscope, x-ray fluoroscopic bronchoscopy, and endobronchial ultrasonography with a guide sheath (EBUS-GS), and has been reported to reduce the examination time and increase the diagnostic yield. Its clinical application has also been reported. In this report, the author discusses VBN and the automatic VBN system, reviews the published literature, and describes its usefulness and limitations.

VIRTUAL BRONCHOSCOPY

Helical CT provides 3D serial volume data. VB is a method for a 3D fly-through display of the border between the bronchial lumen and the bronchial wall viewed from the bronchial lumen, as if it were observed using a bronchoscope.[14]

There are various 3D display methods. MPR (Multi Planner Reconstruction) can display any cross-sectional image. In addition to 2D planar axial slices, 3D observation of sagittal and coronal MPR images is useful in gaining an understanding of the lung structure including the airway.[15,16] However, branching structures along the bronchial path to the target are difficult to show in a single cross-sectional image. In addition, although cross-sectional images of the path can be displayed by curved multiplanar reconstruction (CMPR), the direct use of this data for the guidance of the bronchoscope is difficult. CT bronchoscopy is a method for the 3D display of the external appearance of the bronchial tree, but cannot be directly used for bronchoscopy. On the other hand, VB images reflect the actual anatomic findings[17] and provide useful data for the guidance of the bronchoscope, such as the bronchial branching pattern viewed from the bronchial lumen (ie, the size and shape of the entrance

to the bronchi at the branching site, the branching angle, and bronchial arrangement after branching).

Compared with real bronchoscopy, VB is noninvasive and has no adverse effects except radiation exposure. VB allows the display of areas peripheral to stenotic areas, and also the display of extramural structures simultaneously with endobronchial images using the volume rendering method.[18] Therefore, VB has been used for the evaluation of airway stenosis,[19,20] tracheal/bronchial injury, endobronchial malignancy,[21] airway lesions in children with attention to exposure dose,[22] foreign bodies in the airway,[23] and postoperative bronchial complications.[24] VB is also used for the education of bronchoscopists,[25,26] transbronchial needle aspiration (TBNA),[27] stent placement,[28] and the planning of interventions,[14,29] such as brachytherapy and laser photoresection.

However, conventional CT and software have demonstrated limitations in the visualization of the bronchi peripheral to the segmental bronchi, showing reduced consistency with actual anatomic findings.[19,30] Therefore, the clinical use of VB is limited to the central bronchi.

In recent years, multidetector CT has allowed physicians to obtain finer isotropic voxel data, reduce respiratory and cardiac motion artifacts, and facilitate more detailed and accurate three-dimensional CT reconstruction. In addition, because of recent advances in computers, real-time display of arbitrary endobronchial images has become possible.[31,32]

VIRTUAL BRONCHOSCOPY NAVIGATION

Virtual bronchoscopy navigation is a VB method clinically applicable to arrive at the peripheral lesions. Virtual images of the bronchial path to the lesion are produced and used for navigation at the time of advancing the bronchoscope.[33] In the case that the author first reported, virtual images up to the tenth-generation bronchus comprising the bronchial pathway to the target were displayed simultaneously with real images, and an ultrathin bronchoscope (external diameter, 2.8 mm) could be advanced along the path to the target. Since this report, various studies on the usefulness of VBN have been published. Note that in articles published using Japanese nomenclature, including this article, all subsegmental bronchi, even those after repeated branchings as in the lower lobe, are regarded as third-generation bronchi and the number of further peripheral branchings is added to calculate the bronchial generation.[34,35] Therefore, when articles in Japan are compared with those in Western countries, attention should be paid to the fact that the generation of the bronchi is seemingly lower in the former group of studies.

VBN can be performed using software attached to the CT system in each institution, but there are certain issues that need to be addressed. First, the level of anatomic detail visualized by VB depends on the obtained volume data. Therefore, performing CT imaging under conditions appropriate for each purpose is important. CT conditions (ie, parameters associated with good volume data) differ among CT systems. However, in general, good volume data are obtained by minimizing collimation and overlapping the image reconstruction by at least 50%.[16,32]

The second issue is that VB findings depend on the threshold value selected to differentiate between the airway wall and lumen. In particular, in the peripheral airway, inappropriate selection of the threshold leads to a lack of bronchial branchings or holes in the bronchial wall imaging, resulting in apparent branchings where there are none.[20,36] Therefore, inappropriate thresholds may cause the bronchoscope to be guided to the wrong bronchi. It is important to select appropriate threshold values while confirming the presence or absence of branchings on axial, sagittal, and coronal images, and this requires experience. Because the production of VB images also depends on experience,[32] it is desirable that bronchoscopists themselves produce VB images or compare them with each cross-sectional image for confirmation.

The third issue is that caution should also be taken regarding the rotation procedure at the time of bronchoscope insertion. Unlike the virtual bronchoscope, the tip of the real bronchoscope can only be moved up or down, so that appropriate rotation is always necessary at the time of insertion. When the bronchoscope is rotated, the real image shifts slightly from the virtual image. The bronchial branching pattern includes many bifurcations into two bronchi of similar sizes. When the bronchoscope is rotated 90° or more, mistakes tend to be made identifying the bronchus into which the bronchoscope should be advanced. Such a bifurcation pattern continues to the peripheral area. Therefore, unless both images are made to be consistent at each branching as the bronchoscope is advanced, the risk of disorientation is high.[37]

VIRTUAL BRONCHOSCOPY NAVIGATION SYSTEM

To overcome the issues mentioned earlier and for the widespread use of the system, a VBN system (Bf-NAVI; KGT, Olympus Medical Systems, Tokyo, Japan) was developed and introduced for clinical use. This system is characterized by the automatic production of VB images along the bronchial path[38] and the display of VB synchronized with real images for bronchoscopic navigation.[39]

Bronchoscopists perform the following functions: (1) Input of digital imaging and communication in medicine (DICOM) data of CT into the system. A slice thickness of CT less than or equal to 1 mm (0.5 mm if possible) is desirable. (2) Setting of the starting point in the trachea. An appropriate threshold is automatically adjusted, and bronchi to peripheral areas are extracted. (3) Setting of the target and the terminal point. While observing short-axis, sagittal, and coronal images, bronchoscopist select the lesion and the bronchus closest to it as the target and terminal point, respectively. Because the extracted bronchi are indicated in blue, the bronchi involved with the lesion are clearly observed all the way up to the proximal area on the monitor confirming that each branching is extracted. When the extraction is inadequate, manual extraction of the bronchi can be added (**Fig. 1**). When the target and terminal point are determined, the path to the terminal point is automatically searched and displayed. (4) Path confirmation. When the point in the path is moved from the starting to the terminal point, each corresponding cross-sectional image is displayed and the branching and extraction status in the path are reconfirmed. The path is also displayed in the bronchial tree (**Fig. 2**). When the path is determined, VB images along the path are automatically produced. (5) Thumbnail registration. While VB images are moved from the starting to terminal point, the bronchus for the insertion of the bronchoscope at each bronchial branching is marked and registered as a thumbnail (**Fig. 3**). The time required from the insertion of DICOM data of CT into the system to the completion of thumbnail registration is approximately 15 minutes, of which 6.5 minutes are used for manual setting and confirmation. The median range of the production of VB images using this system is the sixth-generation bronchi.[40]

VBN is performed while displayed VB images of the target bronchus are synchronized with real images by image rotation, advancement, and retreat. Concretely, the VB image that diverges from the real image because of the rotation at the time of bronchoscope insertion is made consistent with the real image using the rotation function. Subsequently, the VB image is advanced to the next bronchial branching and the bronchoscope is similarly advanced. This procedure is repeated. Because the bronchus to which the bronchoscope is advanced is displayed on the VB image at each branching, the bronchoscope is advanced to the target based on this display

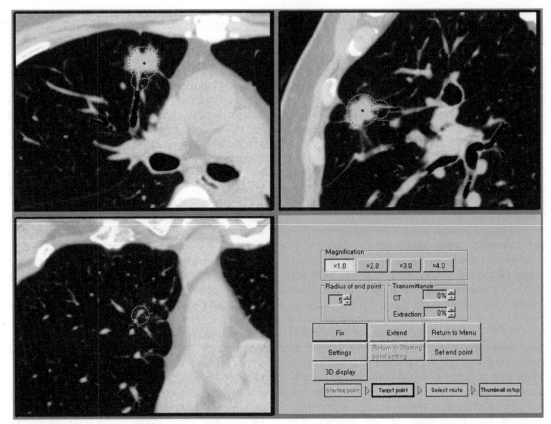

Fig. 1. VBN system setting of the target and terminal point. A small solitary lesion in the peripheral area of the right S3 is shown. The lesion is set as a target (*large circular dotted line*) while observing axial, sagittal, and coronal images. The terminal point (*small circle*) is set at the peripheral end of the extracted involved bronchus indicated in blue.

(**Fig. 4**). When branchings are lost during broncho-scopic advancement, VB images are redisplayed, or a thumbnail at each branching is provided as a reference. The direction of the lesion is displayed on the image and can also be referred to. Because the bronchoscope is advanced according to VB images indicating the target, even inexperienced bronchoscopists can guide the bronchoscope to the target in a short time. The time required for the guidance to the target bronchus is approximately 2 minutes.[39] This system can also be used for educational purposes, such as for illustrating the bronchial branching pattern.

VALIDATION STUDIES FOR THE DIAGNOSIS OF PERIPHERAL LESIONS

In VBN, biopsy instruments reaching the lesion itself cannot be confirmed; therefore, VBN is used in combination with CT, x-ray fluoroscopy, or EBUS. In the published studies on VBN and its system for the diagnosis of peripheral pulmonary lesions, the outline and characteristics of each combination were found to be as follows (**Table 1**).

CT-guided Ultrathin Bronchoscopy

CT-guided bronchoscopy allows the accurate confirmation of biopsy instruments even in the lesions that cannot be observed by fluoroscopy and is useful for the diagnosis of peripheral pulmonary lesions.[10,12,13]

Asano and colleagues[37] performed CT-guided ultrathin bronchoscopy under VBN in 36 peripheral pulmonary lesions. Using VB images produced to the 6.1-generation bronchi (on average), the 6.9-generation bronchi (on average) could be observed using the ultrathin bronchoscope. Because VB images accurately reflected the actual bronchial branching pattern, the ultrathin bronchoscope could be guided along the planned path toward the lesion in 30 (83.3%) of the cases without using x-ray fluoroscopy.

Shinagawa and colleagues[41] used a similar method for 26 peripheral pulmonary lesions less

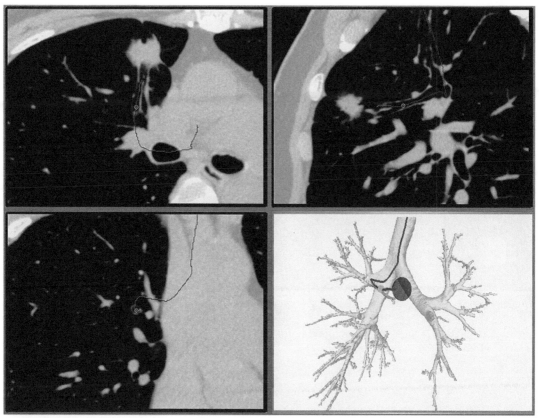

Fig. 2. Path display. After an automatic search for the path, the path (*red line*) to the terminal point is shown on each cross-sectional image. The left lower figure shows the bronchial tree, and the purple circle indicates the target.

than 2 cm in diameter, and could make a diagnosis in 17 (65.4%). The mean time to the first biopsy was 13.0 minutes, and the mean examination time was 29.3 minutes. In their study, more peripheral VB images were produced by a method[42] using the pulmonary arteries running along the bronchi.

Using the VBN system, Asano and colleagues[39] performed CT-guided ultrathin bronchoscopy in 38 peripheral pulmonary lesions less than or equal to 3 cm in diameter, and could guide the bronchoscope to the expected path without using x-ray fluoroscopy in 36 lesions (94.7%). The arrival of biopsy instruments at the lesion could be confirmed by CT in 33 lesions, and diagnosis was possible in 31 (81.6%). The median time required to use the system was 2.6 minutes, and the total examination time was 24.9 minutes. It is of note that the biopsy instrument arrival rate and diagnostic yield were high (96.4 and 89.3%, respectively) in 28 lesions showing bronchial involvement than otherwise.

Shinagawa and colleagues[43] performed CT-guided ultrathin bronchoscopy using the VBN system in 71 lesions less than 2 cm in diameter. The diagnostic yield was high (70.4%) but did not differ from the previous study at their institution. They stated that this was because of a higher percentage of benign cases considered to be associated with a low diagnostic yield. Although the comparison was retrospective, the mean time to the first biopsy was 8.5 minutes and the total examination time was 24.5 minutes, showing significant decreases in time from the previous study.

Shinagawa and colleagues[44] analyzed 85 lesions (<2 cm) by combining the two studies,[41,43] and reported that the location of the lesion (left superior segment of the lower lobe, S6) contributed to the diagnostic yield, and the diagnostic yield was high in lesions for which the ultrathin bronchoscope could be advanced to areas peripheral to the fifth-generation bronchi and those showing an involved bronchus or pulmonary artery.

When these reports are summarized, the diagnostic yield by CT-guided ultrathin bronchoscopy combined with VBN was 65.4% to 86.1% in all lesions and 65.4% to 80.8% in lesions less than 2

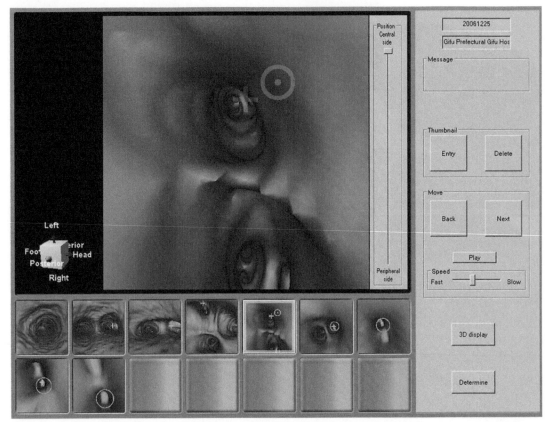

Fig. 3. VB image production, thumbnail registry. VB images of the path are automatically produced. While VB images are peripherally advanced, the bronchus for insertion is marked (*cross*) at each branching and registered as a thumbnail (lower area of the figure). The circle indicates the direction of the target.

cm in diameter. Although the comparison is retrospective, the usefulness of the VBN system has been confirmed. VBN is associated with a high-diagnostic yield and may be useful when diagnosis is impossible by other combinations of methods. On the other hand, the problems of the combination include radiation exposure caused by the CT, the cost of the use of the CT room, and the small size

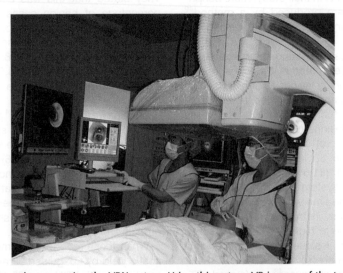

Fig. 4. Navigational bronchoscopy using the VBN system. Using this system, VB images of the target bronchus are displayed in comparison with real bronchoscopic images. Based on these images, the bronchoscope is advanced to the target.

Table 1
Diagnosis of pulmonary peripheral lesions using VBN

Authors	Years	References	VBN System	External Diameter of the Bronchoscope (mm)	Confirmation of Arrival	No. of Examined Lesions	No. of Diagnosed Lesions	Diagnostic Yield (%)	No. of Lesions <2 cm	No. of Diagnosed Lesions <2 cm	Diagnostic Yield for Lesions <2 cm (%)
1. Asano et al	2002	37	Not used	2.8	CT and x-ray fluoroscopy	36	31	86.1	26	21	80.8
2. Shinagawa et al	2004	41	Not used	2.8	CT fluoroscopy	26	17	65.4	26	17	65.4
3. Asahina et al	2005	49	Not used	4.0, 5.3	EBUS	30	19	63.3	18	8	44.4
4. Asano et al	2006	39	Used	2.8	CT and x-ray fluoroscopy	38	31	81.6	26	21	80.8
5. Shinagawa et al	2007	43	Used	2.8	CT fluoroscopy	71	50	70.4	71	50	70.4
6. Tachihara et al	2007	45	Used	2.8, 5.2	X-ray fluoroscopy	96	60	62.5	77	42	54.5
7. Asano et al	2008	38	Used	4.0	EBUS	32	27	84.4	15	11	73.3
8. Asano et al	2008	40	Used	4.0	EBUS	99	80	80.8	58	44	75.9
Summary						428	315	73.6	317	214	67.5

of the sample collected. Therefore, proper case selection is important and the combined use of all cytologic specimens may be important.

X-ray Fluoroscopy

Tachihara and colleagues[45] used the VBN system in 96 peripheral pulmonary lesions less than or equal to 3 cm in diameter and reported diagnostic yields of 62.5% in all lesions and 54.5% in lesions less than or equal to 2 cm in diameter, respectively, and an examination time of 24.1 minutes. The diagnostic yield did not significantly differ among lesions located in the central, intermediate, and peripheral regions.

VBN under x-ray fluoroscopy was reported only in the present study. However, because bronchoscopy under x-ray fluoroscopy is readily and widely performed, further studies on its usefulness are necessary.

Endobronchial Ultrasonography with a Guide Sheath

Regarding bronchoscopy for peripheral pulmonary lesions, EBUS has recently been reported to be useful for evaluating the location of the lesion.[46,47] EBUS-GS is a method in which arrival at the lesion is confirmed using an ultrasound probe with a guide sheath, and the lesion is biopsied through the guide sheath placed at the lesion.[48]

Asahina and colleagues[49] performed EBUS-GS under VBN in 30 peripheral pulmonary lesions less than or equal to 3 cm in diameter. As a result, 24 lesions (80%) were visualized by EBUS and 19 (63.3%) could be diagnosed. The diagnostic yield did not differ among bronchoscopists.

Asano and colleagues[38] performed EBUS-GS using a VBN system and a thin bronchoscope (external diameter, 4.0 mm; forceps channel, 2.0 mm) in 32 peripheral pulmonary lesions. VB images to a median of the fifth-generation bronchi could be produced and the branchings in VB images were in agreement with those in the real images in all cases. The median observation range using a thin bronchoscope was the fifth-generation bronchi. EBUS allowed the visualization of 30 lesions (93.8%), of which 27 could be diagnosed (84.4%). In this study, unlike Asahina's study, no curette-type instrument was used to lead the guide sheath. However, even in lesions less than or equal to 3 cm, 91.4% could be visualized and the diagnostic yield was 79.2%. These results suggest that most lesions can be visualized without the guidance of the EBUS probe if the bronchi leading to the lesion are correctly selected to the fifth-generation bronchi by a thin bronchoscope.

To objectively confirm the usefulness of the VBN system, Asano and colleagues[40] performed a multicentered, joint randomized study: Virtual Navigation in Japan (V-NINJA) bronchoscopic trial. Two hundred subjects who had peripheral pulmonary lesions less than or equal to 3 cm in diameter were randomized into two groups with and without using the VBN system (VBN and non-VBN groups, respectively) and performed biopsy using EBUS-GS. A thin bronchoscope was guided using the VBN in the VBN group and axial CT images in the non-VBN group. In the VBN group, VB images could be produced to the fourth- to twelfth-(median, sixth-) generation bronchi, and the rate of agreement with real images was 98%. The diagnostic yield in the VBN group (80.8%, 80/99) was significantly higher than that in the non-VBN group (67.4%, 64/95) at $P<.05$. The time until the initiation of the biopsy and the examination time (median, 8.1 and 24 minutes, respectively) were significantly shortened in the VBN compared with the non-VBN group $P<.05$.

When these reports are summarized, the diagnostic yield using VBN in combination with EBUS-GS is 63.3% to 84.4% in all lesions and 44.4% to 75.9% in lesions less than 2 cm in diameter. This method requires an EBUS system, but this system is inexpensive and simple. In addition, this combination is applicable to lesions that cannot be visualized by fluoroscopy, is accurate, and allows collection of multiple samples from the lesion. It is possible that the combination of a VBN system, a thin bronchoscope, and EBUS-GS will become the routine examination method for peripheral pulmonary lesions.

APPLICATION TO TREATMENT

VBN is applicable to not only for the diagnostic purposes but it can also be used for therapeutic purposes. Asano and colleagues[50,51] performed CT-guided transbronchial marking to clarify the location of the lesion and the resection range at the time of thoracoscopic surgery. The subjects consisted of 23 individuals who had 31 lesions showing a pure ground-glass opacity pattern less than or equal to 1 cm in diameter. The lesion could not be confirmed in any case under x-ray fluoroscopy. After an ultrathin bronchoscope was guided to a median of the sixth-generation bronchus under VBN, a site near the lesion was marked using a special catheter under CT guidance. The median distance from the barium marker and lesion was 4 mm, and marking within 1 cm was possible in 27 lesions. The required time was 23.5 minutes per subject. Seven subjects had multiple lesions and three of them had bilateral lesions. However, no complication was observed in any subject. Thoracoscopic partial resection was performed after 22 days or less, and the lesion, together with the barium marker, could be resected in all subjects. This method causes no complications, such as pneumothorax and hemorrhage, which are often observed with the percutaneous method. The procedure could be readily performed and can be used for multiple lesions. In addition, the resection range can be three-dimensionally indicated by multiple markings.

ADVANTAGES AND LIMITATION OF VIRTUAL BRONCHOSCOPIC NAVIGATION

When the results of the studies discussed earlier are summarized, the diagnostic yield is 73.6% for peripheral pulmonary lesions and 67.5% for those less than 2 cm in diameter (see **Table 1**). The diagnostic yield is affected not only by the size of the lesion but also by the type of disease, location, and presence/absence of bronchial involvement. Therefore, direct comparison is difficult, but the diagnostic yield was high compared with the current diagnostic yield (34%) according to ACCP Guidelines. One advantage of VBN is the improvement in the diagnostic yield. However, to confirm that this improvement is also observed by VBN used in combination with methods other than EBUS, randomized studies are necessary. VBN facilitates the guidance of the bronchoscope to the peripheral lesions. As a result, a high diagnostic yield may be achieved irrespective of the skill or experience of the bronchoscopist. VBN is a safe method in which the bronchoscope is guided by looking at the real image and the virtual image and no complications of VBN itself have been reported. In addition, because VBN requires no special apparatus except software, the cost is not generally prohibitive.

A limitation is that arrival at the lesion cannot be confirmed by VBN itself, unlike electromagnetic navigation.[52,53] Its combination with fluoroscopy, CT, or EBUS is necessary to confirm localization of the lesion. If a thin or ultrathin bronchoscope is used, its guidance to a site near the lesion is possible. Therefore, in most patients, the guidance of biopsy instruments is not necessary.

FUTURE PROSPECTS OF VIRTUAL BRONCHOSCOPIC NAVIGATION

The VBN system currently used is simple and practical but requires manual adjustment of VB to real images. A method for automatic adjustment has been developed.[54,55] As a clinical application, McLennan and colleagues[56] used a system allowing the real-time display of VB images showing the location of the lesion and path information on real images for TBNA biopsy of the mediastinal lymph nodes, and showed its usefulness. Merritt and colleagues[57] in a phantom study reported the usefulness of this system for peripheral lesions. For peripheral lesions, there are limitations, such as respiration-associated movements and difficulty in acquiring a good visual field. However, if a function for the automatic adjustment of VB to real images is added to the VBN system, the system will become easier to use. Because VBN is a useful method to support bronchoscopy for peripheral lesions, its widespread acceptance is unavoidable.

SUMMARY

Virtual bronchoscopic navigation is a method for the guidance of a bronchoscope to peripheral lesions using VB images of the bronchial path. Irrespective of the bronchoscopist's skill level, the bronchoscope can be readily guided to the target in a short time. In addition, a system to automatically search for the bronchial path to the target has been developed and clinically applied; this system produces VB images of the path to the fourth- to twelfth- (median, sixth-) generation bronchi, and displays the VB images simultaneously with real bronchoscopic images. VBN has been used in combination with CT-guided ultrathin bronchoscopy, x-ray fluoroscopic bronchoscopy, and endobronchial ultrasonography with a guide sheath; the diagnostic yields for lesions less than 2 cm in diameter in these examinations have been reported to be 65.4% to 80.8%, 54.5%, and 44.4% to 75.9%, respectively (total, 67.5%). A randomized study showed VBN improved the diagnostic yield and decreased the total examination time. VBN is used not only for diagnosis but also for treatment, such as marking in thoracoscopic surgery. VBN is a useful method supporting bronchoscopy for peripheral lesions, and its widespread use is likely.

ACKNOWLEDGMENTS

I express deep gratitude to the late Dr Koichi Yamazaki and to Dr Naofumi Shinagawa (First Department of Internal Medicine, Hokkaido University School of Medicine), Dr Takashi Ishida (Department of Pulmonary Medicine, Fukushima Medical University), Dr Hiroshi Moriya (Department of Radiology, Sendai Kousei Hospital), Dr Masaki Anzai (Department of Pulmonary Medicine, University of Fukui, Faculty of Medical Sciences), Dr Yoshihiko Matsuno and Dr Akifumi Tsuzuku (Department of

Pulmonary Medicine, Gifu Prefectural General Medical Center) for their collaboration.

REFERENCES

1. Kaneko M, Eguchi K, Ohmatsu H, et al. Peripheral lung cancer: screening and detection with low-dose spiral CT versus radiography. Radiology 1996; 201(3):798–802.

2. Rivera MP, Mehta AC. Initial diagnosis of lung cancer: ACCP evidence-based clinical practice guidelines (2nd edition). Chest 2007;132(Suppl 3):131S–48S.

3. Chechani V. Bronchoscopic diagnosis of solitary pulmonary nodules and lung masses in the absence of endobronchial abnormality. Chest 1996;109(3): 620–5.

4. Baaklini WA, Reinoso MA, Gorin AB, et al. Diagnostic yield of fiberoptic bronchoscopy in evaluating solitary pulmonary nodules. Chest 2000;117(4):1049–54.

5. Naidich DP, Sussman R, Kutcher WL, et al. Solitary pulmonary nodules. CT-bronchoscopic correlation. Chest 1988;93(3):595–8.

6. Minami H, Ando Y, Nomura F, et al. Interbronchoscopist variability in the diagnosis of lung cancer by flexible bronchoscopy. Chest 1994;105(6):1658–62.

7. Tanaka M, Takizawa H, Satoh M, et al. Assessment of an ultrathin bronchoscope that allows cytodiagnosis of small airways. Chest 1994;106(5):1443–7.

8. Asano F, Kimura T, Shindou J, et al. Usefulness of CT-guided ultrathin bronchoscopy in the diagnosis of peripheral pulmonary lesions that could not be diagnosed by standard transbronchial biopsy. J Jpn Soc Bronchol 2002;24(2):80–5 [in Japanese].

9. Saka H. Ultra-fine bronchoscopy: biopsy for peripheral lesions. Nippon Rinsho 2002;60(Suppl 5): 188–90 [in Japanese].

10. Asano F, Matsuno Y, Komaki C, et al. CT-guided transbronchial diagnosis using ultrathin bronchoscope for small peripheral pulmonary lesions. Nihon Kokyuki Gakkai Zasshi 2002;40(1):11–6 [in Japanese].

11. Dolina MY, Cornish DC, Merritt SA, et al. Interbronchoscopist variability in endobronchial path selection: a simulation study. Chest 2008;133(4):897–905.

12. Wagner U, Walthers EM, Gelmetti W, et al. Computer-tomographically guided fiberbronchoscopic transbronchial biopsy of small pulmonary lesions: a feasibility study. Respiration 1996;63(3):181–6.

13. Kobayashi T, Shimamura K, Hanai K. Computed tomography- guided bronchoscopy with an ultrathin fiberscope. Diagn Ther Endosc 1996;2:229–32.

14. Vining DJ, Liu K, Choplin RH, et al. Virtual bronchoscopy. Relationships of virtual reality endobronchial simulations to actual bronchoscopic findings. Chest 1996;109(2):549–53.

15. Ravenel JG, McAdams HP, Remy-Jardin M, et al. Multidimensional imaging of the thorax: practical applications. J Thorac Imaging 2001;16(4):269–81.

16. Boiselle PM, Reynolds KF, Ernst A. Multiplanar and three-dimensional imaging of the central airways with multidetector CT. AJR Am J Roentgenol 2002; 179(2):301–8.

17. Rodenwaldt J, Kopka L, Roedel R, et al. 3D virtual endoscopy of the upper airway: optimization of the scan parameters in a cadaver phantom and clinical assessment. J Comput Assist Tomogr 1997;21(3):405–11.

18. Amorico MG, Drago A, Vetruccio E, et al. Tracheobronchial stenosis: role of virtual endoscopy in diagnosis and follow-up after therapy. Radiol Med 2006; 111(8):1064–77.

19. Hoppe H, Dinkel HP, Walder B, et al. Grading airway stenosis down to the segmental level using virtual bronchoscopy. Chest 2004;125(2):704–11.

20. De Wever W, Vandecaveye V, Lanciotti S, et al. Multidetector CT-generated virtual bronchoscopy: an illustrated review of the potential clinical indications. Eur Respir J 2004;23(5):776–82.

21. Fleiter T, Merkle EM, Aschoff AJ, et al. Comparison of real-time virtual and fiberoptic bronchoscopy in patients with bronchial carcinoma: opportunities and limitations. AJR Am J Roentgenol 1997;169(6):1591–5.

22. Sorantin E, Geiger B, Lindbichler F, et al. CT-based virtual tracheobronchoscopy in children–comparison with axial CT and multiplanar reconstruction: preliminary results. Pediatr Radiol 2002;32(1):8–15.

23. Adaletli I, Kurugoglu S, Ulus S, et al. Utilization of low-dose multidetector CT and virtual bronchoscopy in children with suspected foreign body aspiration. Pediatr Radiol 2007;37(1):33–40.

24. McAdams HP, Palmer SM, Erasmus JJ, et al. Bronchial anastomotic complications in lung transplant recipients: virtual bronchoscopy for noninvasive assessment. Radiology 1998;209(3):689–95.

25. Colt HG, Crawford SW, Galbraith O 3rd. Virtual reality bronchoscopy simulation: a revolution in procedural training. Chest 2001;120(4):1333–9.

26. Ost D, DeRosiers A, Britt EJ, et al. Assessment of a bronchoscopy simulator. Am J Respir Crit Care Med 2001;164(12):2248–55.

27. McAdams HP, Goodman PC, Kussin P. Virtual bronchoscopy for directing transbronchial needle aspiration of hilar and mediastinal lymph nodes: a pilot study. AJR Am J Roentgenol 1998;170(5):1361–4.

28. Ferretti GR, Thony F, Bosson JL, et al. Benign abnormalities and carcinoid tumors of the central airways: diagnostic impact of CT bronchography. AJR Am J Roentgenol 2000;174(5):1307–13.

29. Liewald F, Lang G, Fleiter T, et al. Comparison of virtual and fiberoptic bronchoscopy. Thorac Cardiovasc Surg 1998;46(6):361–4.

30. Lacasse Y, Martel S, Hebert A, et al. Accuracy of virtual bronchoscopy to detect endobronchial lesions. Ann Thorac Surg 2004;77(5):1774–80.

31. Summers RM, Shaw DJ, Shelhamer JH. CT virtual bronchoscopy of simulated endobronchial lesions:

effect of scanning, reconstruction, and display settings and potential pitfalls. AJR Am J Roentgenol 1998;170(4):947–50.

32. Neumann K, Winterer J, Kimmig M, et al. Real-time interactive virtual endoscopy of the tracheobronchial system: influence of CT imaging protocols and observer ability. Eur J Radiol 2000;33(1):50–4.

33. Asano F, Matsuno Y, Matsushita T, et al. Transbronchial diagnosis of a pulmonary peripheral small lesion using an ultrathin bronchoscope with virtual bronchoscopic navigation. J Bronchol 2002;9:108–11.

34. Oho K, Amemiya R. Anatomy of the bronchus. In: Oho K, Amemiya R, editors. Practical fiberoptic bronchoscopy. 2nd edition. Tokyo: IGAKU-SHOIN; 1984. p. 27–33 [in Japanese].

35. Fujisawa T, Tanaka M, Saka H, et al. Report by the Bronchus Nomenclature Working Group. J Jpn Soc Bronchol 2000;22:330–1 [in Japanese].

36. Seemann MD, Seemann O, Luboldt, et al. Hybrid rendering of the chest and virtual bronchoscopy [corrected]. Eur J Med Res 2000;5(10):431–7.

37. Asano F, Matsuno Y, Takeichi N, et al. Virtual bronchoscopy in navigation of an ultrathin bronchoscope. J Jpn Soc Bronchol 2002;24(6):433–8 [in Japanese].

38. Asano F, Matsuno Y, Tsuzuku A, et al. Diagnosis of peripheral pulmonary lesions using a bronchoscope insertion guidance system combined with endobronchial ultrasonography with a guide sheath. Lung Cancer 2008;60(3):366–73.

39. Asano F, Matsuno Y, Shinagawa N, et al. A virtual bronchoscopic navigation system for pulmonary peripheral lesions. Chest 2006;130(2):559–66.

40. Asano F, Yamazaki K, Ishida T, et al. Usefulness of virtual bronchoscopic navigation in transbronchial biopsy for small pulmonary peripheral lesions: a multi-center, randomized trial. In: Programs and abstracts of the 15th World Congress for Bronchology. Tokyo. 2008:32.

41. Shinagawa N, Yamazaki K, Onodera Y, et al. CT-guided transbronchial biopsy using an ultrathin bronchoscope with virtual bronchoscopic navigation. Chest 2004;125(3):1138–43.

42. Onodera Y, Omatsu T, Takeuchi S, et al. Enhanced virtual bronchoscopy using the pulmonary artery: improvement in route mapping for ultraselective transbronchial lung biopsy. AJR Am J Roentgenol 2004;183(4):1103–10.

43. Shinagawa N, Yamazaki K, Onodera Y, et al. Virtual bronchoscopic navigation system shortens the examination time–feasibility study of virtual bronchoscopic navigation system. Lung Cancer 2007;56(2): 201–6.

44. Shinagawa N, Yamazaki K, Onodera Y, et al. Factors related to diagnostic sensitivity using an ultrathin

bronchoscope under CT guidance. Chest 2007; 131(2):549–53.

45. Tachihara M, Ishida T, Kanazawa K, et al. A virtual bronchoscopic navigation system under X-ray fluoroscopy for transbronchial diagnosis of small peripheral pulmonary lesions. Lung Cancer 2007; 57(3):322–7.

46. Herth FJ, Ernst A, Becker HD. Endobronchial ultrasound-guided transbronchial lung biopsy in solitary pulmonary nodules and peripheral lesions. Eur Respir J 2002;20(4):972–4.

47. Shirakawa T, Imamura F, Hamamoto J, et al. Usefulness of endobronchial ultrasonography for transbronchial lung biopsies of peripheral lung lesions. Respiration 2004;71(3):260–8.

48. Kurimoto N, Miyazawa T, Okimasa S, et al. Endobronchial ultrasonography using a guide sheath increases the ability to diagnose peripheral pulmonary lesions endoscopically. Chest 2004;126(3): 959–65.

49. Asahina H, Yamazaki K, Onodera Y, et al. Transbronchial biopsy using endobronchial ultrasonography with a guide sheath and virtual bronchoscopic navigation. Chest 2005;128(3):1761–5.

50. Asano F, Matsuno Y, Ibuka T, et al. A barium marking method using an ultrathin bronchoscope with virtual bronchoscopic navigation. Respirology 2004;9(3): 409–13.

51. Asano F, Shindoh J, Shigemitsu K, et al. Ultrathin bronchoscopic barium marking with virtual bronchoscopic navigation for fluoroscopy-assisted thoracoscopic surgery. Chest 2004;126(5):1687–93.

52. Schwarz Y, Greif J, Becker HD, et al. Real-time electromagnetic navigation bronchoscopy to peripheral lung lesions using overlaid CT images: the first human study. Chest 2006;129(4):988–94.

53. Gildea TR, Mazzone PJ, Karnak D, et al. Electromagnetic navigation diagnostic bronchoscopy: a prospective study. Am J Respir Crit Care Med 2006;174(9):982–9.

54. Mori K, Deguchi D, Sugiyama J, et al. Tracking of a bronchoscope using epipolar geometry analysis and intensity-based image registration of real and virtual endoscopic images. Med Image Anal 2002; 6(3):321–36.

55. Higgins WE, Helferty JP, Lu K, et al. 3D CT-video fusion for image-guided bronchoscopy. Comput Med Imaging Graph 2008;32(3):159–73.

56. McLennan G, Ferguson JS, Thomas K, et al. The use of MDCT-based computer-aided pathway finding for mediastinal and perihilar lymph node biopsy: a randomized controlled prospective trial. Respiration 2007;74(4):423–31.

57. Merritt SA, Gibbs JD, Yu KC, et al. Image-guided bronchoscopy for peripheral lung lesions: a phantom study. Chest 2008;134(5):1017–26.

Flexible Bronchoscopy and its Role in the Staging of Non–Small Cell Lung Cancer

Felix J.F. Herth, MD, DSc, FCCP*, Ralf Eberhardt, MD

KEYWORDS
- Flexible bronchoscopy • Transbronchial needle aspiration
- Endobronchial ultrasound • Electromagnetic navigation

The first ever bronchoscopy was performed in 1887 by Gustav Killian of Freiburg, Germany.[1] During the early years of the development of bronchoscopy, the indications for the procedure were primarily therapeutic: removal of foreign bodies and dilation of strictures from tuberculosis and diphtheria. In the early part of the twentieth century, Chevalier Jackson, the father of American bronchoesophagology, further advanced bronchoscopic techniques and designed modern rigid bronchoscopes.[2] Again, the primary indication was often therapeutic.

The flexible bronchoscope was developed in the late 1960s by Ikeda[3] and has become the mainstay investigation in the evaluation of patients suspected of lung cancer. It is used mainly as a diagnostic tool providing tissue to determine the histologic type of tumor. Bronchoscopy also has a role in disease staging and an extended role in delivering therapeutic modalities. Flexible bronchoscopy (FB) is easier to perform and is safe and well tolerated by patients. The requirement of only a moderate sedation makes it an acceptable outpatient procedure. It has almost completely replaced rigid bronchoscopy in the initial assessment. The development of video bronchoscopes has the added advantage of facilitating teaching and rendering the procedure more interesting for the observers in the bronchoscopy suite.

The flexibility of the bronchoscope allows the operator to inspect most of fourth order and often up to sixth order bronchi. In addition, the operator may directly assess mucosal details, such as color and vascularity. Relative contraindications to the procedure are few and include hypoxemia refractory to supplemental oxygen, intractable bleeding diathesis, severe pulmonary hypertension, cardiovascular instability, and acute hypercapnia.[4]

FB is safe with a complication rate of 0.12% and a mortality rate of 0.04%.[5] The dangers of hemorrhage and pneumothorax relate to the biopsy procedure used and are discussed later. In all patients, the bronchoscope causes a temporary increase in airflow obstruction, which may result in hypercapnia.[6] Inappropriate sedation with benzodiazepines or opiates increases the likelihood of respiratory complications and high-risk patients could be identified by prior measurement of arterial blood gases.[5–7] Supplemental oxygen should be provided and patients monitored throughout the procedure with pulse oximetry. Cardiac monitoring should be used for those patients with a history of ischemic heart disease and resuscitation equipment immediately available.

Although FB has largely replaced rigid bronchoscopy in the initial assessment of the patient, the rigid scope has advantages in certain situations.[8] It may provide more accurate information regarding the endobronchial location of a tumor before resection. Additionally, manipulation of the scope allows assessment of the mobility of the proximal airways providing an indirect

Department of Pneumology and Critical Care Medicine, Thoraxklinik, University of Heidelberg, Amalienstrasse 5, D-69126 Heidelberg, Germany
* Corresponding author.
E-mail address: felix.herth@thoraxklinik-heidelberg.de (F.J.F. Herth).

Clin Chest Med 31 (2010) 87–100
doi:10.1016/j.ccm.2009.08.006

evaluation of mediastinal nodal involvement. Airway obstruction is less and the rigid scope may be preferable in exploring patients with tracheal narrowing in whom the flexible scope may produce critical airway narrowing. It provides superior suction, facilitating the assessment and biopsy of potentially hemorrhagic lesions and the debulking of large tumors.[8–10] In addition, many physicians are now acquiring skills in this technique to facilitate endobronchial laser therapy and stent placement.[11]

THE DIAGNOSTIC YIELD OF FB

The expected diagnostic yield from FB depends on the location and the size of the lesion. Central endobronchial lesions yield the highest diagnostic return (>90%), whereas small peripheral lesions often prove more elusive unless more demanding and time-consuming techniques are used. The question of which combination of cytologic and histologic procedures provides the optimum diagnostic yield has not been conclusively answered but probably depends on the expertise available in any individual center. The routine techniques include bronchial washings, brushings, and biopsies but these may be augmented by the use of transbronchial needle aspiration (TBNA) and bronchoalveolar lavage (BAL).[12]

More than 70% of lung carcinomas can be approached with FB and although the yield is dependent on operator's experience, a high level of diagnostic accuracy can be achieved by taking between three and five biopsy specimens and a combination of brushing, biopsy, and bronchial washes can expect to establish a diagnosis in more than 60% of cases.[6,7,13,14] When the tumor is visible but is intramural rather than endobronchial in distribution the diagnostic yield falls to 55% and is reduced further when the tumor lies beyond the bronchoscopist's vision.[6,7,12]

The main role of BAL in patients with lung cancer is the diagnosis of opportunistic infections, especially in patients undergoing chemotherapy. BAL may have an extended role, however, in the diagnosis of malignancy itself. A high diagnostic yield has been shown in the detection of pulmonary hematologic malignancies, primary bronchoalveolar cell carcinoma, and metastatic adenocarcinoma of the breast.[15–17]

Information on the role of BAL in the diagnosis of primary lung cancer remains sparse. Examination of BAL from 55 patients with a peripheral lung lesion demonstrated a diagnostic yield of around 30% with no false-positive results and only one instance of incorrect cell typing. Additionally, in combination with bronchial washings and postbronchoscopy sputum analysis BAL increased the yield to 56%.[18] Examination of BAL in 162 patients with malignant lung infiltrates revealed improved sensitivity in cases of bronchoalveolar cell carcinoma (93%) and lymphangitic carcinomatosis (83%). Forty-five percent of non-Hodgkin lymphoma could be detected and immunocytochemistry is of value in identification and classification.[19]

BAL is safe; bleeding and pneumothorax are uncommon and the fever and transient loss of lung function reported are rarely serious and there is no need for fluoroscopy. Furthermore, the diagnostic yield is high in diseases other than cancer, such as pulmonary tuberculosis. Advances in cell and molecular biology may complement the technique of BAL to improve the rate of tumor diagnosis in peripheral lesions (particularly adenocarcinoma) and may also provide a useful tool to explore the molecular mechanisms governing the genesis of lung cancer.[20–22]

VISIBLE ENDOBRONCHIAL LESIONS

Central tumors can present as exophytic mass lesions, with partial or total occlusion of the bronchial lumen, as peribronchial tumors with extrinsic compression of the airway, or with submucosal infiltration of tumor. The changes with peribronchial tumors or with submucosal infiltration are often subtle. The airways should be examined closely for characteristic changes, such as erythema, loss of bronchial markings, and nodularity of the mucosal surface. Central lesions are usually sampled with a combination of bronchial washes, bronchial brushings, and endobronchial biopsies. The yield of endobronchial biopsies is highest for exophytic lesions, with a diagnostic yield of approximately 90%.[23–25] Three to four biopsies are likely adequate in this situation. Attempts should be made to obtain the biopsies from areas of the lesion that seem viable (**Fig. 1**).

For submucosal lesions, TBNA can be performed by inserting the needle into the submucosal plane at an oblique angle, and in patients with peribronchial disease and extrinsic compression, the needle should be passed through the bronchial wall into the lesion.[26,27] It is particularly frustrating when apparently adequate biopsy specimens from visible endobronchial disease fail to achieve a diagnosis (**Fig. 2**). Reasons for this include the presence of surface necrosis or the presence of crush artifact (particularly common with samples from small cell carcinoma). In these circumstances, TBNA may improve diagnostic yield.[28,29]

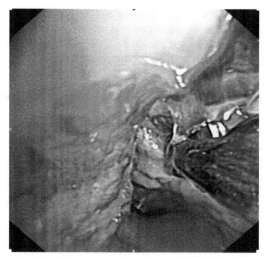

Fig. 1. Endobronchial biopsy from a lesion in the right main bronchus.

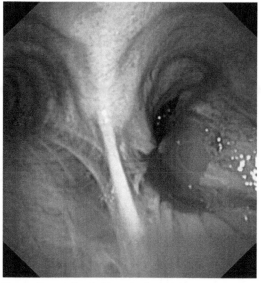

Fig. 3. Tumor in right main bronchus, reaching the level of the main carina.

Regarding the T (T, N, M classification) staging, FB may allow the operator to determine that the tumor is beyond resection. Pointers to inoperability include paralysis of a vocal cord, tumor to the level of the right tracheobronchial junction or to within 2 cm of the left tracheobronchial junction, and definite carinal or tracheal involvement (**Fig. 3**).

PERIPHERAL LUNG LESIONS

Peripheral lesions are usually sampled with a combination of bronchial wash, brushes,

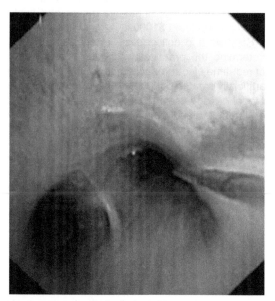

Fig. 2. TBNA needle before passing the bronchial wall in case of an endobronchial compression of the distal trachea.

transbronchial biopsy (TBBx), and TBNA. The diagnostic yield of bronchoscopy for peripheral lesions depends on a number of factors, including lesion size, the distance of the lesion from the hilum, and the relationship between the lesion and bronchus. The yield of bronchoscopy for lesions smaller than 3 cm varies from 14% to 50% compared with a diagnostic yield of 46% to 80% when the lesion is larger than 3 cm.[13,30,31] The presence of a bronchus sign on chest CT predicts a much higher yield of bronchoscopy for peripheral lung lesions. In these cases, fluoroscopic guidance should be used to ensure proper positioning of the diagnostic accessory (**Fig. 4**). Fluoroscopy increases the diagnostic yield from TBBx in focal lung lesions but it is time-consuming, requires experience, and is not universally available. If the disease process is diffuse, however, such as in lymphangitic carcinomatosis, yields are similar whether or not fluoroscopy is used.[32] Indeed, TBBx may be regarded as the procedure of choice for lymphangitic carcinomatosis. Complications from TBBx include pneumothorax and hemorrhage but these are generally low and rarely serious.

In situations where bronchial biopsies cannot be obtained examination of bronchial washings may still yield useful information and often provide complementary information.[25,33] It is often prudent to perform all types of sampling procedure to maximize the yield.[12]

Several studies have demonstrated that TBNA may be used to obtain diagnostic tissue from peripheral lesions. Typical results report an

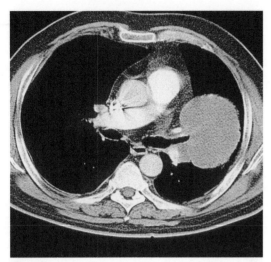

Fig. 4. Positive bronchus sign in a peripheral lung lesion in the left upper lobe.

increase in the diagnostic yield from percentage figures in the mid thirties up to the high sixties.[12,34–36] As with TBBx, the size of the peripheral lesion seems to be important, although this is not a feature of all studies. Optimum yields are provided by using a combination of diagnostic techniques. TBNA may represent an alternative to TBBx when the airway externally compressed to such a degree that it is not possible to negotiate the biopsy forceps.

The need to work-up and manage pulmonary nodules and masses is encountered with increasing frequency in chest medicine. In patients with such nodules, the diagnostic procedure is usually performed as a TBBx under fluoroscopic guidance. This commonly performed procedure is associated with a low yield in coin lesions smaller than 3 cm or fluoroscopically invisible lesions.[25,37] Nodules that are too small to be visualized by conventional fluoroscopy during the procedure pose a particular problem and usually require further, often surgical, biopsy procedures. Promising new technologies, such as electromagnetic navigation and endobronchial ultrasound (EBUS), may help overcome the limitations.

ELECTROMAGNETIC NAVIGATION

The electromagnetic navigation system is a device that assists in localizing and placing endobronchial accessories (eg, forceps, brush, and needle) in the desired areas of the lung. The system uses low-frequency electromagnetic waves, which are emitted from an electromagnetic board placed under the bronchoscopy table mattress. A 1-mm diameter, 8-mm long

sensor probe mounted on the tip of a flexible metal cable constitutes the main assembly of the device (locatable guide). Once the probe is placed within the electromagnetic field, its position in the X, Y, and Z planes, and its orientation (roll, pitch, and yaw movements), are captured by the electromagnetic navigation system. This information is then displayed on a monitor in real time (**Fig. 5**). The locatable guide also has an added feature that allows its distal section to be steered 360 degrees. The fully retractable probe is incorporated into a flexible catheter (serving as an extended working channel), which once placed in the desired location creates an easy access for bronchoscopic accessories. The computer software and monitor allow the bronchoscopist to view the reconstructed three-dimensional CT scans of the object's anatomy in coronal, sagittal, and axial views together with superimposed graphic information depicting the position of the sensor probe.

There are still some major limitations to the technique. For planning, a CT scan is necessary with a special protocol (1-mm cuts and tight overlay). For the planning of the procedure, use of the electromagnetic navigation bronchoscopy (ENB) software is required. The planning can be done even on the system or on a special dedicated laptop before the procedure; the planning needs some time, up to 10 minutes even in trained hands. The whole procedure time is prolonged compared with a traditional diagnostic bronchoscopy with fluoroscopy; but equal to that required by the CT-guided percutaneous needle aspiration. The locatable guide is a single-use device and costs between $500 and $1000.

Schwarz and colleagues[38] performed a trial to determine the practicality, accuracy, and safety of real-time electromagnetic navigation in locating artificially created peripheral lung lesions in a swine model. No adverse effects, such as pneumothorax or internal bleeding, were encountered in any animal in this study. Schwarz and colleagues[38] concluded that real-time electromagnetic positioning technology, coupled with previously acquired CT scans, is an accurate technology that can augment standard bronchoscopy to assist in reaching peripheral lung lesions and performing biopsies. Based on the results of Schwarz and colleagues,[38] Becker and colleagues[39] performed a pilot study in humans. They examined the use of the system in 30 consecutive patients presenting for endoscopic evaluation of lung nodules and masses. The lesion size in this population varied from 12 to 106 mm but was specifically not controlled for in this early trial. Evaluation was possible in 29 patients, and in 20

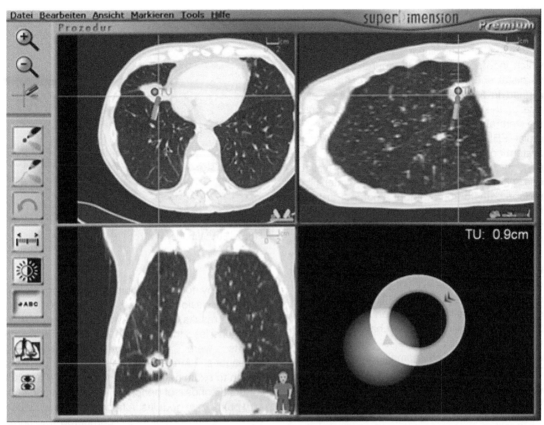

Fig. 5. Navigation screen during an electromagnetic navigation procedure. In the right lower lobe the relation from the sensor is seen.

patients a definitive diagnosis was established, with no complications related to the navigation device. In an uncontrolled study, again Schwarz and colleagues[40] confirmed that the procedure was safe and added only an average of 15 minutes to the time of a conventional bronchoscopy. Successful diagnostic biopsies were obtained in 69% of patients. A follow-up study of 60 patients,[41,42] published in 2006, successfully reached the target lesion in 100% of cases. Bronchoscopy with electromagnetic navigation diagnosed 80.3% of the lesions, 74% of the peripheral lesions, and 100% of the lymph nodes. Of the lesions, 57% were less than 2 cm in size. Diagnostic yield did not differ significantly based on the size of the lesion. The accuracy of ENB navigation has been proved in animal studies and against fluoroscopically[40,41] verified reference points in humans. Nevertheless, all preceding diagnostic studies using ENB also used fluoroscopy to guide biopsies. The role of ENB as a stand-alone technology is still unproved and concerns remain that biopsy instruments may dislodge an accurately positioned extended working channel when replacing the sensor probe.

Eberhardt and colleagues[42] examined the yield of ENB without fluoroscopy in the diagnosis of peripheral lung lesions and solitary pulmonary nodules. Ninety-two peripheral lung lesions were biopsied in the 89 subjects. The diagnostic yield of ENB was 67%, which was independent of lesion size. The mean navigation error was 9 ± 6 mm; range was 1 to 31. When analyzed by lobar distribution, there was a trend toward a higher ENB yield in diagnosing lesions in the right middle lobe (88%). Eberhardt and colleagues[42] concluded that ENB could be used as a stand-alone bronchoscopic technique without compromising diagnostic yield or increasing pneumothorax risk. This may result in sizable time saving and avoids radiation exposure. Makris and colleagues[43] confirmed these results. In 40 patients all target lesions but one was reached and the overall diagnostic yield was 62.5% (25 of 40). Also, the French group summarized that electromagnetic navigation–guided bronchoscopy has the potential to improve the diagnostic yield of transbronchial biopsies without further fluoroscopic guidance and may be useful in early diagnosis of lung cancer, particularly in non-operable patients.

EBUS

Two different types of EBUS systems are available in the market. The linear EBUS bronchoscope, which incorporates the ultrasound transducer at its distal end, uses a fixed array of transducers aligned in a curvilinear pattern. Because of the size of the scope, the system is usable only in the central airways. For the peripheral lung the radial EBUS must be used. The radial EBUS system consists of a mechanical radial miniprobe (**Fig. 6**). Two types of miniprobe are available, one with a notch at the tip for a water-fillable balloon catheter, one without a notch. Particularly with the notch type, ultrasonography can be performed using the balloon method; the balloon is inflated at the distal end of the probe after the probe has been inserted into the working channel. The balloon method makes possible easy delineation of ultrasound images even at sites where it is difficult to retain defecated water. The limitation is the size; with the balloon sheath an endoscope with 2.8 mm or larger diameter channel has to be used. The notchless probe is smaller (1.7 mm) and can also be used in smaller bronchoscopes. The 20-MHz frequency is commonly used, although 12- and 30-MHz probes are also available.

For use in the peripheral lung, most commonly the probe is placed through a guide sheath in the working channel of the bronchoscope. After localization of the lesion (**Fig. 7**), the bronchoscope is kept in place at the nearest visible subsegmental carina, and the miniprobe removed. Through the guide sheath, the forceps are guided to the lesion (**Fig. 8**). By using the guide sheath, EBUS-guided TBBx can be performed without losing the position of the nodule. The initial studies were performed without the guide sheath but most recently the use of the guide sheath is considered as the technique of choice. The feasibility trial of EBUS-guided TBBx[44] without the use of fluoroscopy showed that EBUS can provide an alternative to

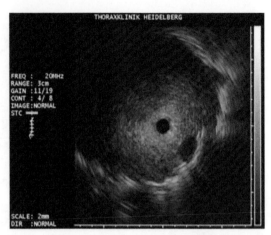

Fig. 7. EBUS image of a coin lesion.

fluoroscopy for image guidance in biopsies for peripheral lesions. In the study, a trend toward superior results with EBUS was particularly strong in lesions less than 3 cm in diameter. The same results were shown by Shirakawa and colleagues.[45] After the feasibility trial, investigators began to examine the use of EBUS as an adjunct for the diagnosis of peripheral lung lesion and solitary pulmonary nodules. A large prospective study by Paone and colleagues[46] compared traditional TBBx with EBUS for peripheral lesions. They found that EBUS-guided bronchoscopy had a sensitivity of 0.83 for lesions greater than 3 cm in size and 0.75 for lesions less than 3 cm in size; compared with the traditional TBBx EBUS also showed promise when used for nodules less than 3 cm in size. These types of lesion are often difficult to

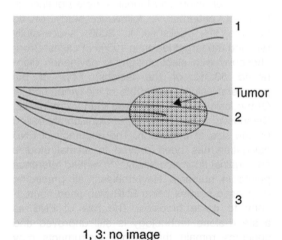

1, 3: no image

Fig. 8. The theoretical background of an EBUS-guided TBBx.

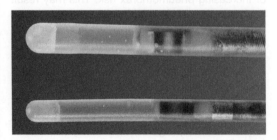

Fig. 6. The endobronchial miniprobe for peripheral lung biopsy.

visualize fluoroscopically for TBBx, and conventional bronchoscopy has a low diagnostic yield in such settings.

Most of the published studies used radiographic fluoroscopy, with radiation exposure for both the patient and medical staff. This result is in line with the study by Herth and colleagues[47] including only peripheral pulmonary lesions less than 30 mm and reporting a diagnostic yield of 87% for EBUS-guided TBBx without the need for radiographic equipment or radiation exposure.

For lesions less than 20 mm, the yield of EBUS-guided detection and pathologic diagnosis decreased fewer than 30% yield.[48] By contrast, Japanese groups have reported diagnostic yields of 53% and 72%, respectively, for lesions less than 20 mm using EBUS-guided TBBX with a catheter sheath and under radiographic fluoroscopy.[49,50] More recently, a Japanese group performed EBUS-guided TBBX using virtual bronchoscopic navigation and detected 67% of lesions less than 20 mm on EBUS, resulting in a diagnostic yield of 44%.[51] The limitation to the systems is a significant learning curve, and methods of physician training and education still need to be established. EBUS lacks a navigational system, however, and requires the operator to maneuver the bronchoscope blindly to the lesion with the knowledge of prior radiologic investigations, such as CT scans.

Biopsies using ENB have not always resulted in a diagnosis despite accurate navigation in most cases to within 10 mm of the target center. Respiratory variations causing larger than anticipated navigation errors and dislodgement of the extended working channel when biopsy instruments were introduced may account for this lower than expected diagnostic yield. ENB lacks a means to directly visualize lesions before biopsy. The role of combining EBUS with ENB to gain the benefits and minimize the limitations of either technique has never been reported. Eberhardt and colleagues[52] performed a prospective randomized controlled trial comprising three arms with EBUS only, ENB only, and combined EBUS-ENB to test this hypothesis. Of the 120 patients recruited, 118 had a definitive histologic diagnosis and were included in the final analysis. The diagnostic yield of the combined procedure (88%) was greater than either EBUS (69%) or electromagnetic navigation alone (59%; $P = .02$). The group concluded that combined EBUS and electromagnetic navigation improves the diagnostic yield of flexible bronchoscopy in peripheral lung lesions without compromising safety.

MEDIASTINAL STAGING
TBNA

The first description of sampling mediastinal lymph nodes through the tracheal carina using a rigid bronchoscope was by Schieppati,[53,54] an Argentinean physician who presented the technique at the Argentine Meeting of Bronchoesophagology in 1949. In 1978, Wang and colleagues[55] demonstrated that with this technique it was also possible to sample paratracheal nodes. In 1979, Oho and colleagues[56] introduced a flexible needle that could be used through a bronchofiberscope and in 1983, Wang and coworkers[57,58] pointed out the diagnostic possibility of the method in staging of lung cancer and developed new types of needles. Subsequent publications highlighted its use in the diagnosis of endobronchial and peripheral lesions and the ability of TBNA to provide a diagnosis even in the absence of endobronchial disease, in a nonsurgical fashion, confirmed its usefulness to bronchoscopists (**Fig. 9**).[59–61]

Operators have reported the use of 21- and 22-gauge cytology needles and 19-gauge histology needles.[62] Samples are provided by rinsing the needle with a small volume of normal saline and collecting the "flush solution" for analysis. Although TBNA is not widely used, it seems to improve the diagnostic yield when sampling from visible endobronchial, submucosal, and peripheral lesions. Additionally, the technique may detect mediastinal disease potentially allowing the operator to diagnose and stage a lung tumor in one procedure performed under local anesthetic.

TBNA may be used to sample lymph nodes that lie immediately adjacent to the trachea and major bronchi. Care must be taken to perform TBNA before inspection of the distal airways and other sampling procedures because contamination with exfoliated malignant cells is a recognized

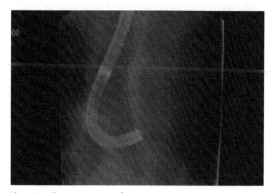

Fig. 9. Fluoroscopy of a TBNA in the left distal trachea.

cause of false-positive results. Studies have reported sensitivity rates of between 43% and
83% and positive predictive values of 89% to
100%.[63–68] Use of a 19-gauge needle provides
greater sensitivity than a 22-gauge needle but
a combination of samples provides the best
yields.[62,69] Although the positive predictive value
is high (often 100%) the negative predictive value
is low and does not obviate the requirement for
further surgical staging.[59–69] A potential limitation
of mediastinal lymph node staging with TBNA is
that it is a blind procedure. The technique may
be combined with that of EBUS by the minip-
robes.[70,71] The numerous papers on TBNA performed in the last few years confirm the safety of
the procedure. No cases of mortality related to
TBNA have been described. The rare complications reported are pneumothorax,[72] pneumomediastinum,[73] hemomediastinum,[74] bacteremia,[75]
and pericarditis.[76] None of these complications
determined clinical major consequences. One of
the major complications of TBNA is the possible
severe damage to the working channel of the
scope.[61]

Endoesophageal Ultrasound with Fine-needle Aspiration

EUS fine-needle aspiration (FNA) is a relatively
new method first described in 1991.[77] Since then
several studies have been published and it has
been demonstrated that generally all lesions out-
lined by EUS may be punctured, and even small
lesions down to the size of 5 mm may be
diagnosed.[78]

EUS-FNA is performed with the aid of esophagoscopy and a biopsy needle is passed through
the working channel of the endoscope, through
the esophageal wall and guided ultrasonographi-
cally toward the lesion of interest in the mediastinum (**Fig. 10**). The procedure is performed
under local anesthesia and moderate sedation.
This method gives an excellent overview of mediastinal structures, including a good access to the
paraesophageal space, the aorticopulmonary
window, the subcarinal region, and the region
around the left atrium (level 4, 5, and 7).[79–81] EUS
has the advantage of being noninvasive, safe,
and cost effective.[82] An area anterior to the air-
filled trachea, however, cannot be visualized. The
echoendoscope is initially introduced up to the
level of celiac axis and gradually withdrawn
upward for a detailed mediastinal imaging.
Because the ultrasound waves are emitted parallel
to the long axis of the endoscope, the entire needle could be visualized approaching a target in
the sector-shaped sound field. Pulse-wave

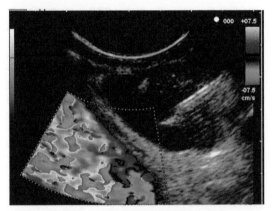

Fig. 10. EUS procedure of an enlarged lymph node
(4 left). The vessel is seen by the color Doppler flow.

Doppler ultrasonography imaging is performed,
whenever vascular structures are suspected in
the pathway of the needle or adjacent to it, to
correct the target line if necessary.[81] The needle
is advanced through the wall of the esophagus
and guided into the target lesion. The central stylet
is removed, and a special 10-mL syringe attached
to the hub of the needle to apply suction as the
needle is moved back and forth within the mass.
The suction is released slowly, and the needle
assembly removed out of the biopsy channel.
One to two needle passes are made to obtain
adequate tissue.[83,84]

Visual assessment of mediastinal lymph nodes
by EUS gave various observers sensitivity of 0.54
to 0.75, specificity of 0.71 to 0.98, positive predictive values of 0.46 to 0.77, and negative predictive
values of 0.85 to 0.93, in a total number of patients
studied being more than 1000.[85]

These studies varied widely with regard to the
number of examined mediastinal lymph node
levels, visual criteria for malignancy, and patient
population characteristics. Compared with CT,
the detection rate of malignant lymph nodes was
higher with EUS, with less false-positive results.[86]
EUS can assess mediastinal lymph nodes at most
levels, particularly at levels 4 left, 5, 7, 8, and 9, and
metastasis in the left adrenal gland. Levels 1, 2, 3,
and 4 right are not always assessable, because of
interference by air in the larger airways.[79,81] When
enlarged, however, detection is easier.[78,85] Properties of lymph nodes indicating possible malignancy are a hypoechoic core, sharp edges,
round shape, and a long axis diameter exceeding
10 mm.[85] Signs of benignancy are a hyperechoic
core (fat); central calcification (old granulomatous
disease); ill-defined edges; and a long and narrow
shape.[86,87] False-negative results may have been
introduced by an occasional poor lymph node

sampling during EUS-FNA (sampling only the most suspicious nodes). Many outcomes have been supported by not only clinical but also surgical follow-up. Despite these drawbacks, the clinical impact of EUS-FNA is illustrated by a change in the management of non–small cell lung cancer patients after EUS-FNA in 66% of the patients, or cancellation of 68% and 49% of the scheduled mediastinoscopies and thoracotomies, respectively. According to Hunerbein and colleagues,[83] EUS-FNA made an unexpected diagnosis of malignancy in 30% of the procedures. In two studies with decision-analysis models, EUS-FNA was shown to be less expensive compared with mediastinoscopy for the assessment of the entire mediastinum or only for subcarinal lymph nodes.[79,88,89] Barawi and colleagues[90] prospectively studied the incidence of complications associated with EUS-FNA. In 842 mediastinal EUS-FNA procedures, one infection, two hemorrhages, and one inexplicable transient hypotension were reported.

EUS-FNA is contraindicated in patients with a Zenker diverticulum or bleeding tendency.[91] FNA of a cystic mediastinal lesion should be avoided, or when necessary be preceded by prophylactic antibiotics.[92]

Real-time EBUS with TBNA

Lymph node staging is also the main indication for use of the new EBUS-TBNA scope. An ultrasound transducer integrated into a bronchoscope with a separate working channel potentially increases the yield of TBNA by allowing direct visualization of needle placement within the area of interest. A special ultrasonic puncture bronchoscope by integrating a convex probe at the tip of the FB has been developed. With this bronchoscope direct TBNA under real-time convex probe EBUS (EBUS-TBNA-bronchoscopy) guidance is now possible (**Fig. 11**).

EBUS-TBNA is performed by direct transducer contact with the wall of the trachea or bronchus. When a lesion is identified, a 22-gauge full-length steel needle is introduced through the biopsy channel of the endoscope. Power Doppler examination may be performed before the biopsy to avoid inadvertent puncture of mediastinal vessels. Under real-time ultrasonic guidance the needle is placed in the lesion (**Fig. 12**). Suction is applied with a syringe, and the needle is moved back and forth inside the lesion.[93]

Endobronchial, ultrasound-guided, TBNA (EBUS-TBNA) has been available for more than 5 years. A growing body of research supports its usefulness in airway assessment and procedure

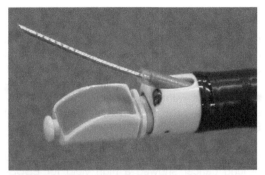

Fig. 11. The tip of the EBUS-TBNA scope with the ultrasound system. The TBNA needle is inserted.

guidance, especially since the availability of positron emission tomography scanning.[94–97] EBUS-TBNA has access to all of the mediastinal lymph node stations accessible by mediastinoscopy and N1 nodes. The largest trial reported the results of using the method in 502 patients[98]; 572 lymph nodes were punctured, and 535 (94%) resulted in a diagnosis. Biopsies were taken from all reachable lymph node stations (2l, 2r, 3, 4r, 4l, 7, 10r, 10l, 11r, and 11l). Mean (SD) diameter of the nodes was 1.6 cm (0.36 cm) and the range was 0.8 to 3.2 cm. Sensitivity was 92%, specificity was 100%, and the positive predictive value was 93%. Like in all other trials no complications occurred. The Danish-German group[99] examined in addition the accuracy of EBUS-TBNA in sampling nodes less than 1 cm in diameter. Among 100 patients, 119 lymph nodes with a size between 4 and 10 mm were detected and sampled. Malignancy was detected in 19 patients but missed in 2 others; all diagnoses were confirmed by surgical findings. The mean (SD) diameter of the punctured lymph nodes was 8.1 mm. The sensitivity of EBUS-TBNA for detecting malignancy was 92.3%, the specificity was

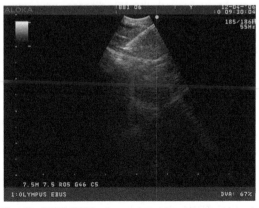

Fig. 12. EBUS-TBNA of an enlarged mediastinal lymph node. The needle is clearly visible within the node.

100%, and the negative predictive value was 96.3%. No complications occurred. They summarized that EBUS-TBNA can sample even small mediastinal nodes, avoiding unnecessary surgical exploration in one of five patients who have no CT evidence of mediastinal disease. Potentially operable patients with clinically nonmetastatic non–small cell lung cancer may benefit from presurgical EBUS-TBNA biopsies and staging.

A study comparing EBUS-TBNA, CT, and positron emission tomography for lymph node staging of lung cancer showed a high yield for EBUS-TBNA.[100] Altogether, 102 potentially operable patients with proved (N = 96) or radiologically suspected (N = 6) lung cancer were included in the study. CT, positron emission tomography, and EBUS-TBNA were performed before surgery for the evaluation of mediastinal and hilar lymph node metastasis. The sensitivities of CT, positron emission tomography, and EBUS-TBNA for the correct diagnosis of mediastinal and hilar lymph node staging were 76.9%, 80%, and 92.3%; the specificities were 55.3%, 70.1%, and 100%; and the diagnostic accuracies were 60.8%, 72.5%, and 98%, respectively. EBUS-TBNA was proved to have high sensitivity and specificity, compared with CT or positron emission tomography, for mediastinal staging in patients with potentially resectable lung cancer.

Restaging of the mediastinum is another area of growing interest for the treatment strategy of lung cancer. In cases of advanced lymph node stage lung cancer, induction chemotherapy before surgical resection is an option. Mediastinoscopy is considered the gold standard for staging the mediastinum. Remediastinoscopy can be technically difficult, however, and is not commonly performed. The ability to perform multiple, repeat biopsies using EBUS-TBNA allows restaging of the mediastinum after the introduction of chemotherapy. A group of 124 consecutive patients with tissue-proved IIIA-N2 disease who were treated with induction chemotherapy underwent mediastinal restaging by EBUS-TBNA. The sensitivity, specificity, positive predictive value, negative predictive value, and diagnostic accuracy of EBUS-TBNA for mediastinal restaging following induction chemotherapy were 76%, 100%, 100%, 20%, and 77%, respectively.

EBUS–TBNA is an accurate, minimally invasive test for mediastinal restaging of patients with non–small cell lung cancer. Because of the low negative predictive value, however, tumor-negative findings should be confirmed by surgical staging.[101]

EBUS-TBNA also can be used for the diagnosis of intrapulmonary nodules and mediastinal and hilar lymph nodes. The limitation is the reach of EBUS-TBNA, which depends on the size of the bronchus. Usually the EBUS-TBNA can be inserted as far as the lobar bronchus. Lung tumors located adjacent to the airway within reach of EBUS-TBNA can be diagnosed with EBUS-TBNA. Tournoy and colleagues[102] have reported their experience for this indication. In 60 patients who had an initial nondiagnostic bronchoscopy, they were able to establish the definitive diagnosis in 77% without any complication.

Complications related to the procedure are rare and similar to those of conventional TBNA including bleeding from major vessels, pneumomediastinum, mediastinitis, pneumothorax, bronchospasm, and laryngospasm. Authors have not encountered any major complications related to EBUS-TBNA. Although EBUS has enabled the bronchoscopist to see beyond the airway, one must be aware of the possible complications related to the procedure.[103,104]

Rapid On-site Evaluation

Rapid on-site evaluation (ROSE) is comparable with the intraoperative frozen-section examination. The technique requires the cytopathologist and the pathology technician to process and interpret the stained wet film of the aspirate immediately and report the result to the bronchoscopist. Several studies have shown that ROSE reduces the incidence of inadequate specimens, an important cause of nondiagnostic TBNA aspirates.[105–108]

Davenport[109] studied the value of ROSE in 73 aspirates and compared the results with 134 specimens processed routinely. The aspirates were obtained from the mediastinal lymph nodes and the peripheral lung nodules. With ROSE, the proportion of aspirates showing malignant cells increased from 31% to 56%. The proportion of the inadequate negative specimens dropped from 56% to 18%. The negative aspirate with ROSE had a higher negative predictive value than that of routinely prepared specimens. In a recent prospective study, Diette and colleagues[110] evaluated TBNA aspirates with ROSE in 81 of 204 cases. The overall diagnostic yield was 81% when ROSE was used compared with a 50% yield when specimens were processed in the usual manner. Multivariate analysis showed that ROSE was an independent predictor of a positive aspirate for malignant cells with an odds ratio of 4.5. The mean number of needle attempts was slightly greater with ROSE. The concordance between the preliminary diagnosis made in the bronchoscopy suite and the final diagnosis was reached after subsequent review of material in the cytopathology laboratory was 87%, indicating that the on-site evaluation of needle aspirate is fairly accurate but not perfect.

Although ROSE seems to improve the diagnostic yield of TBNA, its cost-effectiveness remains unclear. Successful use of ROSE requires services of an expert cytopathologist. Many pathologists do not favor ROSE because of the extra time and effort involved. The reimbursement from a third party payor for these services is highly variable. Presently, the decision to use ROSE remains institution-specific.

SUMMARY

Technologic advances in bronchoscopy continue to improve the ability to perform minimally invasive, accurate evaluations of the tracheobronchial tree and to perform an ever-increasing array of diagnostic, staging, therapeutic, and palliative interventions. The role of both old and new diagnostic bronchoscopy will continue to evolve as further improvements are made in bronchoscopes, accessory equipment, and imaging technologies. The major challenge is the adoption of the many new bronchoscopic techniques into routine clinical practice. There is a need for well-designed studies to delineate the appropriate use of these interventions and to better define their limitations and cost effectiveness.

REFERENCES

1. Killian G. Ueber directe bronchoscopie. MMW 1898;27:844–7.
2. Jackson CH. The life of Chevalier Jackson: an autobiography. New York: Macmillan; 1938.
3. Ohata M. History and progress of bronchology in Japan. JJSB 1998;20:539–46.
4. Barlési F, Doddoli C, Greillier L, et al. Bronchoscopy in the diagnosis of lung cancer: an evaluation of current practice. Rev Mal Respir 2006;23:17–26.
5. Becker HD, Shirakawa T, Tanaka F, et al. Transbronchial lung biopsy in the immunocompromised patient. Eur Respir Mon 1998;9:193–208.
6. Mazzone P, Jain P, Arroliga AC, et al. Bronchoscopy and needle biopsy techniques for diagnosing and staging of lung cancer. Clin Chest Med 2002;23(1):137–58.
7. El-Bayoumi E, Silvestri GA. Bronchoscopy for the diagnosis and staging of lung cancer. Semin Respir Crit Care Med 2008;29(3):261–70.
8. Wahidi MM, Herth FJ, Ernst A. State of the art: interventional pulmonology. Chest 2007;131(1):261–74.
9. Herth FJF, Ernst A. Innovative bronchoscopic diagnostic techniques: endobronchial ultrasound and electromagnetic navigation. Curr Opin Pulm Med 2005;11(4):278–81.
10. Folch E, Mehta AC. Airway interventions in the tracheobronchial tree. Semin Respir Crit Care Med 2008;29(4):441–52.
11. Herth FJF, Eberhardt R. Interventional bronchoscopy. Minvera Pneumol 2004;43:189–201.
12. Gasparini S, Ferrety M, Such E, et al. Integration of transbronchial and percutaneous approach in the diagnosis of peripheral pulmonary nodules or masses: experience with 1027 consecutive cases. Chest 1995;108:131–7.
13. Govert JA, Dodd LG, Kussin PS, et al. A prospective comparison of fiberoptic transbronchial needle aspiration and bronchial biopsy for bronchoscopically visible lung carcinoma. Cancer 1999;87:129–34.
14. Govert JA, Kopita JM, Matehar D, et al. Cost-effectiveness of collecting cytologic specimens during fiberoptic bronchoscopy for endoscopically visible lung tumors. Chest 1996;109:451–6.
15. De Gracia J, Bravo C, Miravitalles M, et al. Diagnostic value of bronchoalveolar lavage in peripheral lung cancer. Am Rev Respir Dis 1993;147:649–52.
16. Fabin E, Nagy M, Meszaros G. Experiences with bronchial brushing method. Acta Cytol 1975;19:320–1.
17. Fedullo AJ, Ettensohn DB. Bronchoalveolar lavage in the lymphangitic spread of adenocarcinoma to the lung. Chest 1985;87:129–31.
18. Semenzato G, Spatafora M, Feruglio C, et al. Bronchoalveolar lavage and the immunology of lung cancer. Lung 1990;168:1041–9.
19. Rennard SI. Bronchoalveolar lavage in the diagnosis of cancer. Lung 1990;168:1035–40.
20. Garg S, Handa U, Mohan H, et al. Comparative analysis of various cytohistological techniques in diagnosis of lung diseases. Diagn Cytopathol 2007;35(1):26–31.
21. Emad A, Emad V. The value of BAL fluid LDH level in differentiating benign from malignant solitary pulmonary nodules. J Cancer Res Clin Oncol 2008;134(4):489–93.
22. Azoulay E, Schlemmer B. Diagnostic strategy in cancer patients with acute respiratory failure. Intensive Care Med 2006;32(6):808–22.
23. Wilson RW, Frazier AA. Pathological-radiological correlations: pathological and radiological correlation of endobronchial neoplasms: part II, malignant tumors. Ann Diagn Pathol 1998;2(1):31–4.
24. Simoff MJ. Endobronchial management of advanced lung cancer. Cancer Control 2001;8(4):337–43.
25. Schreiber G, McCrory DC. Performance characteristics of different modalities for diagnosis of suspected lung cancer: summary of published evidence. Chest 2003;123(Suppl 1):115S–28S.

26. Dasgupta A, Jain P, Minai OA, et al. Utility of transbronchial needle aspiration in the diagnosis of endobronchial lesions. Chest 1999;115:1237–41.

27. Dasgupta A, Mehta AC. Transbronchial needle aspiration: an underused diagnostic technique. Clin Chest Med 1999;20:39–51.

28. Gasparini S. Evolving role of interventional pulmonology in the interdisciplinary approach to the staging and management of lung cancer: bronchoscopic mediastinal staging of lung cancer. Clin Lung Cancer 2006;8(2):110–5.

29. Horsley JR, Miller RE, Amy RWM, et al. Bronchial submucosal needle aspiration performed through the fiberoptic bronchoscope. Acta Cytol 1984;28:211–7.

30. Gasparini S. Bronchoscopic biopsy techniques in the diagnosis and staging of lung cancer. Monaldi Arch Chest Dis 1997;4:392–8.

31. Hanson RR, Zavala DC, Rhodes ML, et al. Transbronchial biopsy via flexible fiberoptic bronchoscope: result in 164 patients. Am Rev Respir Dis 1976;114:67–72.

32. Pisani RJ, Wright AJ. Clinical utility of bronchoalveolar lavage in immunocompromised hosts. Mayo Clin Proc 1992;67(3):221–7.

33. Cortese DA, McDougall JC. Biopsy and brushing of peripheral lung cancers with fluoroscopic guidance. Chest 1979;75:141–5.

34. Yung RC. Tissue diagnosis of suspected lung cancer: selecting between bronchoscopy, transthoracic needle aspiration, and resectional biopsy. Respir Care Clin N Am 2003;9(1):51–76.

35. Liam CK, Pang YK, Poosparajah S. Diagnostic yield of flexible bronchoscopic procedures in lung cancer patients according to tumour location. Singapore Med J 2007;48(7):625–31.

36. Ellis JH Jr. Transbronchial biopsy via the fiberoptic bronchoscope: experience with 107 consecutive cases and comparison with bronchial brushing. Chest 1975;68:524–32.

37. Baaklini WA, Reinoso MA, Gorin AB, et al. Diagnostic yield of fiberoptic bronchoscopy in evaluating solitary pulmonary nodules. Chest 2000;117(4):1049–54.

38. Schwarz Y, Mehta AC, Ernst A, et al. Electromagnetic navigation during flexible bronchoscopy. Respiration 2003;70:516–22.

39. Becker HD, Herth F, Ernst A, et al. Bronchoscopic biopsy of peripheral lung lesions under electromagnetic guidance. J Bronchol 2005;12:9–13.

40. Schwarz Y, Greif J, Becker HD, et al. Real-time electromagnetic navigation bronchoscopy to peripheral lung lesions using overlaid CT images: the first human study. Chest 2006;129:988–94.

41. Gildea TR, Mazzone PJ, Karnak D, et al. Electromagnetic navigation diagnostic bronchoscopy: a prospective study. Am J Respir Crit Care Med 2006;174:982–9.

42. Eberhardt R, Anantham D, Herth FJF, et al. Electromagnetic navigation diagnostic bronchoscopy in peripheral lung lesions. Chest 2007;131:1800–5.

43. Makris D, Scherpereel A, Leroy S, et al. Electromagnetic navigation diagnostic bronchoscopy for small peripheral lung lesions. Eur Respir J 2007;29(6):1187–92.

44. Herth F, Ernst A, Becker H. Endobronchial ultrasound-guided transbronchial lung biopsy in solitary pulmonary nodules and peripheral lesions. Eur Respir J 2002;20:972–4.

45. Shirakawa T, Imamura F, Hamamoto J, et al. Usefulness of endobronchial ultrasonography for transbronchial lung biopsies of peripheral lung lesions. Respiration 2004;71:260–8.

46. Paone G, Nicastri E, Lucantoni G, et al. Endobronchial ultrasound-driven biopsy in the diagnosis of peripheral lung lesions. Chest 2005;128:3551–7.

47. Herth FJ, Becker HD, Ernst A, et al. Endobronchial ultrasound-guided transbronchial lung biopsy in fluoroscopically invisible solitary pulmonary nodules: a prospective trial. Chest 2006;129:147–50.

48. Dooms CA, Verbeken EK, Becker HD, et al. Endobronchial ultrasonography in bronchoscopic occult pulmonary lesions. J Thorac Oncol 2007;2:121–4.

49. Kurimoto N, Miyazawa T, Okimasa S, et al. Endobronchial ultrasonography using a guide sheath increases the ability to diagnose peripheral pulmonary lesions endoscopically. Chest 2004;126:959–65.

50. Kikuchi E, Yamazaki K, Sukoh N, et al. Endobronchial ultrasonography with guide-sheath for peripheral pulmonary lesions. Eur Respir J 2004;24:533–7.

51. Asahina H, Yamazaki K, Onodera Y, et al. Transbronchial biopsy using endobronchial ultrasonography with a guide sheath and virtual bronchoscopic navigation. Chest 2005;128:1761–5.

52. Eberhardt R, Anantham D, Ernst A, et al. Multimodality bronchoscopic diagnosis of peripheral lung lesions: a randomized controlled trial. Am J Respir Crit Care Med 2007;176:36–41.

53. Schieppati E. La puncion mediastinal a traves del espolon traqueal. Rev Asoc Med Argent 1949;663:497–9.

54. Schieppati E. Mediastinal lymph nodes puncture through the tracheal carina. Surg Gynecol Obstet 1958;107:243–6.

55. Wang KP, Terry PB, Marsh B. Bronchoscopic needle aspiration biopsy of paratracheal tumors. Am Rev Respir Dis 1978;118:17–21.

56. Oho K, Kato H, Ogawa I, et al. A new needle for transfiberoptic bronchoscope use. Chest 1979;76:492.

57. Wang KP, Marsh BR, Summer WR, et al. Transbronchial needle aspiration for diagnosis of lung cancer. Chest 1981;80:48–50.

58. Wang KP, Terry PB. Transbronchial needle aspiration in the diagnosis and staging of bronchogenic carcinoma. Am Rev Respir Dis 1983;127:344–7.

59. Wang KP, Britt EJ, Haponik EF, et al. Rigid transbronchial needle aspiration biopsy for histological specimens. Ann Otol Rhinol Laryngol 1985;94:382–5.

60. Schenk DA, Bower JH, Bryan CL, et al. Transbronchial needle aspiration staging of bronchogenic carcinoma. Am Rev Respir Dis 1986;134:146–8.

61. Dasgupta A, Mehta AC, Wang KP. Transbronchial needle aspiration. Semin Respir Crit Care Med 1997;18:571–81.

62. Schenk DA, Chambers SL, Derdak S, et al. Comparison of the Wang 19 gauge and 22 gauge needles in the mediastinal staging of lung cancer. Am Rev Respir Dis 1993;147:1251–8.

63. Salazar AM, Westcott JL. The role of transthoracic needle biopsy for the diagnosis and staging of lung cancer. Clin Chest Med 1993;14:99–110.

64. Jain P, Arroliga A, Mehta AC. Cost-effectiveness of transbronchial needle aspiration in the staging of lung cancer. Chest 1996;110:24s.

65. Wang KP, Haponik EF, Gupta PK, et al. Flexible transbronchial needle aspiration: technical considerations. Ann Otol Rhinol Laryngol 1984;93:233–6.

66. Shure D, Fedullo PF. The role of transcarinal needle aspiration in the staging of bronchogenic carcinoma. Chest 1984;86:693–6.

67. Utz JP, Ashok MP, Edell ES. The role of transcarinal needle aspiration in the staging of bronchogenic carcinoma. Chest 1993;104:1012–6.

68. Chin R Jr, McCain TW, Lucia MA, et al. Transbronchial needle aspiration in diagnosing and staging lung cancer. How many aspirates are needed? Am J Respir Crit Care Med 2002;166:377–81.

69. Gasparini S, Zuccatosta L, De Nictolis M. Transbronchial needle aspiration of mediastinal lesions. Monaldi Arch Chest Dis 2000;1:29–32.

70. Herth FJ, Becker HD, Ernst A. Ultrasound-guided transbronchial needle aspiration: an experience in 242 patients. Chest 2003;123:604–7.

71. Herth F, Becker HD, Ernst A. Conventional vs endobronchial ultrasound-guided transbronchial needle aspiration: a randomized trial. Chest 2004;125(1):322–5.

72. Wang KP, Brower R, Haponik EF, et al. Flexible transbronchial needle aspiration for staging of bronchogenic carcinoma. Chest 1983;84:571–6.

73. Harrow EM, Abi-Saleh W, Blum J, et al. The utility of transbronchial needle aspiration in the staging of bronchogenic carcinoma. Am J Respir Crit Care Med 2000;161:601–7.

74. Talebian M, Recanatini A, Zuccatosta L, et al. Hemomediastinum as a consequence of transbronchial needle aspiration. J Bronchol 2004;11:178–80.

75. Witte MC, Opal SM, Gilbert JG, et al. Incidence of fever and bacteraemia following transbronchial needle aspiration. Chest 1986;89:85–7.

76. Sterling BE. Complication with a transbronchial histology needle. Chest 1990;98:783–4.

77. Schuder G, Isringhaus H, Kubale B, et al. Endoscopic ultrasonography of the mediastinum in the diagnosis of bronchial carcinoma. Thorac Cardiovasc Surg 1991;39:299–303.

78. Vilmann P. Endoscopic ultrasonography-guided fine-needle aspiration biopsy of lymph nodes. Gastrointest Endosc 1996;43:S24–9.

79. Vilmann P. Endoscopic ultrasound-guided fine-needle biopsy in Europe. Endoscopy 1998;30:161–2.

80. Wiersema MJ, Vilmann P, Giovannini M, et al. Endosonography-guided fine-needle aspiration biopsy: diagnostic accuracy and complication assessment. Gastroenterology 1997;112:1087–95.

81. Vilmann P, Hancke S, Henriksen FW, et al. Endosonographically-guided fine needle aspiration biopsy of malignant lesions in the upper gastrointestinal tract. Endoscopy 1993;25(8):523–7.

82. Aabakken L, Silvestri GA, Hawes RH, et al. Cost-efficacy of endoscopic ultrasonography with fine-needle aspiration vs. mediastinotomy in patients with lung cancer and suspected mediastinal adenopathy. Endoscopy 1999;31:707–11.

83. Hunerbein M, Ghadimi BM, Haensch W, et al. Transesophageal biopsy of mediastinal and pulmonary tumors by means of endoscopic ultrasound guidance. J Thorac Cardiovasc Surg 1998;116:554–9.

84. Claussen M, Annema JT, Welker L, et al. Endoscopic ultrasound-guided fine-needle aspiration in pulmonary medicine. Pneumologie 2004;58(6):435–42.

85. Micames CG, McCrory DC, Pavey DA, et al. Endoscopic ultrasound-guided fine-needle aspiration for non-small cell lung cancer staging: a systematic review and metaanalysis. Chest 2007;131(2):539–48.

86. Fritscher-Ravens A, Sriram PV, Bobrowski C, et al. Mediastinal lymphadenopathy in patients with or without previous malignancy: EUS-FNA-based differential cytodiagnosis in 153 patients. Am J Gastroenterol 2000;95:2278–84.

87. Chang KJ, Erickson RA, Nguyen P. Endoscopic ultrasound (EUS) and EUS-guided fine-needle aspiration of the left adrenal gland. Gastrointest Endosc 1996;44:568–72.

88. Annema JT, Hoekstra OS, Smit EF, et al. Towards a minimally invasive staging strategy in NSCLC: analysis of PET positive mediastinal lesions by EUS-FNA. Lung Cancer 2004;44(1):53–60.

89. Hawes RH, Gress FG, Kesler KA, et al. Endoscopic ultrasound versus computed tomography in the evaluation of the mediastinum in patients with non-small-cell lung cancer. Endoscopy 1994;26:784–7.

90. Barawi M, Gottlieb K, Cunha B, et al. A prospective evaluation of the incidence of bacteremia associated with EUS-guided fine-needle aspiration. Gastrointest Endosc 2001;53:189–92.

91. Rabe KF, Welker L, Magnussen H. Endoscopic ultrasonography (EUS) of the mediastinum: safety, specificity, and results of cytology. Eur Respir J 1998;12:974.

92. Annema JT, Veselic M, Versteegh MI, et al. Mediastinitis caused by EUS-FNA of a bronchogenic cyst. Endoscopy 2003;35(9):791–3.

93. Herth FJF, Krasnik M, Yasufuku K, et al. Endobronchial ultrasound-guided transbronchial needle aspiration: how I do it. J Bronchol 2006;13(2):84–91.

94. Krasnik M, Vilmann P, Larsen SS, et al. Preliminary experience with a new method of endoscopic transbronchial real time ultrasound guided biopsy for diagnosis of mediastinal and hilar lesions. Thorax 2003;58(12):1083–6.

95. Yasufuku K, Chhajed PN, Sekine Y, et al. Endobronchial ultrasound using a new convex probe: a preliminary study on surgically resected specimens. Oncol Rep 2004;11(2):293–6.

96. Yasufuku K, Chiyo M, Sekine Y, et al. Real-time endobronchial ultrasound-guided transbronchial needle aspiration of mediastinal and hilar lymph nodes. Chest 2004;126:122–8.

97. Rintoul RC, Skwarski KM, Murchison JT, et al. Endobronchial and endoscopic ultrasound-guided real-time fine-needle aspiration for mediastinal staging. Eur Respir J 2005;25:416–21.

98. Herth FJ, Eberhardt R, Vilmann P, et al. Real-time endobronchial ultrasound guided transbronchial needle aspiration for sampling mediastinal lymph nodes. Thorax 2006;61(9):795–8.

99. Herth FJ, Ernst A, Eberhardt R, et al. Endobronchial ultrasound-guided transbronchial needle aspiration of lymph nodes in the radiologically normal mediastinum. Eur Respir J 2006;28:910–4.

100. Yasufuku K, Nakajima T, Motoori K, et al. Comparison of endobronchial ultrasound, positron emission tomography, and computed tomography for lymph node staging of lung cancer. Chest 2006;130:710–8.

101. Herth FJ, Annema JT, Eberhardt R, et al. Endobronchial ultrasound with transbronchial needle aspiration for restaging the mediastinum in lung cancer. J Clin Oncol 2008;26:3346–50.

102. Tournoy KG, Rintoul RC, van Meerbeeck JP, et al. EBUS-TBNA for the diagnosis of central parenchymal lung lesions not visible at routine bronchoscopy. Lung Cancer 2009;63:45–9.

103. Herth FJ, Rabe KF, Gasparini S, et al. Transbronchial and transoesophageal (ultrasound-guided) needle aspirations for the analysis of mediastinal lesions. Eur Respir J 2006;28:1264–75.

104. Herth FJ, Eberhardt R. Actual role of endobronchial ultrasound (EBUS). Eur Radiol 2007;17(7):1806–12.

105. Uchida J, Imamura F, Takenaka A, et al. Improved diagnostic efficacy by rapid cytology test in fluoroscopy-guided bronchoscopy. J Thorac Oncol 2006;1(4):314–8.

106. Baram D, Garcia RB, Richman PS. Impact of rapid on-site cytologic evaluation during transbronchial needle aspiration. Chest 2005;128(2):869–75.

107. Gasparini S. It is time for this 'ROSE' to flower. Respiration 2005;72(2):129–31.

108. Omiya H, Nagatomo I, Yamamoto S, et al. Rapid staining with the modified Gill-Shorr method for reliable, rapid bronchoscopic diagnosis. Acta Cytol 2006;50(4):444–6.

109. Davenport RD. Rapid on-site evaluation of transbronchial aspirates. Chest 1990;98:59–61.

110. Diette GB, White P Jr, Terry P, et al. Utility of onsite cytopathology assessment for bronchoscopic evaluation of lung masses and adenopathy. Chest 2000;117:1186–90.

Interventional Bronchoscopy from Bench to Bedside: New Techniques for Central and Peripheral Airway Obstruction

Septimiu D. Murgu, MD, Henri G. Colt, MD*

KEYWORDS

- Central airway obstruction • Tracheal stenosis
- Expiratory central airway collapse • Bronchial thermoplasty
- Bronchoscopic lung volume reduction

Scientific and technological innovations are the principal change agents responsible for revolutionary health care and prevention practices. Elements leading to technological innovation, defined as the transformation of knowledge into new products, processes, systems, and services, warrant exploration. To translate new technologies into productivity and improved health care–related outcomes, they must be deployed and integrated into common medical practice. Their deployment requires knowledge transfer from researchers to practitioners in the field.

Interest in interventional bronchoscopy is growing, and could increase dramatically in the near future given the increased recognition of benign and malignant causes of central airway obstruction (CAO)[1] and potentially useful minimally invasive procedures for common pulmonary disorders such as asthma and chronic obstructive pulmonary disease (COPD).[2,3] Bronchoscopists no longer simply need to prove the efficacy of a few robust interventional techniques. An era is

beginning when interventional bronchoscopists will be able to apply the principles of scientific and technological discoveries to address not only the symptoms but also the basic foundations of medical illness itself.

This article discusses how basic scientific concepts, based on a greater understanding of airway physiology, support the development and dissemination of multidimensional classification systems for tracheal stenosis, expiratory central airway collapse (ECAC), and innovative interventional bronchoscopic procedures for patients with asthma and COPD.

CAO

CAO is caused by various disorders, the description of which has been for the most part subjective, using empirical severity criteria that have not been validated physiologically.[4] Patients with different degrees of airway narrowing have different functional limitations,[5] and the extent and location of

Financial disclosures: The authors have no financial disclosures and no conflicts of interest related to the content of this article.

Parts of this article were presented by Dr Colt during the Pasquale Ciaglia Memorial Lecture, American College of Chest Physicians Meeting in Philadelphia, 2008.

University of California, Irvine Medical Center, Pulmonary Division, 101 The City Drive South, The City Tower, Suite 400, ZOT 4095, Orange, CA 92868-3217, USA

* Corresponding author.

E-mail address: hcolt@uci.edu (H.G. Colt).

Clin Chest Med 31 (2010) 101–115
doi:10.1016/j.ccm.2009.09.002

airway abnormalities affect the therapeutic decision-making process.[1] A classification system based on a common language and sound scientific physiologic principles is needed so that investigators can stratify patients, analyze and interpret data, and compare populations over time.[6] CAO could thus be classified based on descriptive qualitative factors such as histology, mechanism, dynamics, and quantitative factors such as functional impairment, severity of airway narrowing, and extent of airway abnormalities (**Fig. 1**).

Tracheal Stenosis

Functional status

The ability to accurately and reproducibly assess symptoms such as dyspnea in this patient population is important for providing patient care based on the efficacy of different treatment strategies. A recently validated tool is the Medical Research Council (MRC) dyspnea scale.[7] One study found the MRC dyspnea scale highly sensitive to the presence of varying degrees of tracheal stenosis. Strong correlations were noted between the severity of the stenosis and the MRC grade. There were also significant, but weaker correlations between the MRC scale and preoperative ventilatory physiology variables, supporting the notion that dyspnea perception is related to, but not completely determined by changes in pulmonary

physiology.[8] These findings are similar to observations made in patients with COPD, which also demonstrate a strong correlation between the MRC scale and disability, despite weaker correlations between the MRC scale and measures of ventilatory function such as forced expiratory volume in the first second of expiration (FEV_1) and peak expiratory flow (PEF).[9]

Severity of airway narrowing

Severity criteria, other than empirical estimates, have been evaluated in physiologic studies using computer-based modeling of tracheal strictures. These have shown that the work of breathing depends on the degree of pressure drop along a stenosis.[10] This pressure drop depends on the degree of stenosis but also on the flow velocity through the stenotic lesion: $[\Delta P = k\, V^2((R/r)^2 - 1)^2]$, where ΔP is the pressure drop, K is a constant, R is the radius of the normal lumen, r is the radius of the stenosis, and V is the flow velocity (**Fig. 2**A). The effect of normal triangular glottic narrowing is known to be of the same order as that of a 50% circumferential constriction in a computer-based model.[11] The pressure drop across the stricture doubles when a 70% stenosis is observed.[10] In addition, it seems that, at 50% obstruction, patients are usually symptomatic with exertion, whereas at 70% obstruction they become symptomatic at rest, based on simulation using different

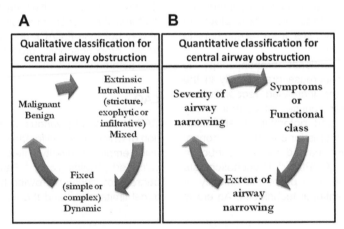

A   **B**

Fig. 1. (*A*) Qualitative criteria for classifying CAO. Based on histology, CAO is malignant or benign; based on mechanism of obstruction, CAO can be classified as extrinsic compression, intraluminal (stricture, exophytic, or infiltrative), or mixed (a combination of extrinsic compression and intraluminal obstruction). Based on dynamic features, CAO is fixed, in which there is airflow limitation during inspiration and expiration (ie, idiopathic subglottic stenosis), or dynamic, in which there is limitation to flow during a certain respiratory phase (ie, tracheomalacia). The stenosis is considered simple if there is only 1 cartilaginous ring involved (<1 cm in length) and no associated chondritis/cartilaginous collapse. The stenosis is complex if it is multilevel (at least 2 rings) or if there is associated chondritis/cartilaginous collapse. (*B*) Quantitative criteria for classifying CAO. Based on severity, the CAO is labeled as mild, moderate, or severe (cutoff values depend on the form of CAO: fixed or dynamic). Functional class can be objectively evaluated by applying 1 of the validated scales (ie, WHO functional class). The extent of airway narrowing refers to the location and distribution of the abnormal airway segment.

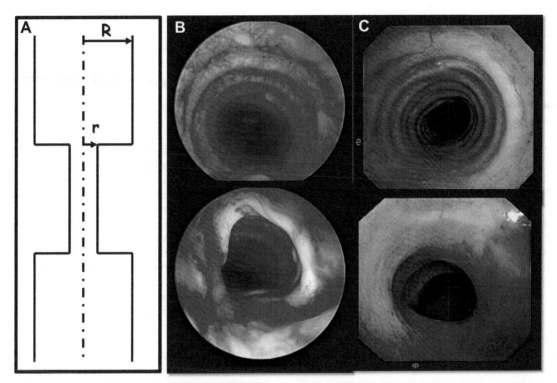

Fig. 2. (*A*) Tracheal stricture. Symptoms depend on the degree of pressure drop along a stenotic lesion. The pressure drop depends on the severity of airway narrowing (radius) but also on the flow velocity through the stenotic lesion, based on the formula: $\Delta P = kV^2((R/r)^2-1)^2]$, where ΔP is the pressure drop, K is a constant, R is the radius of the normal lumen, r is the radius of the stenosis, and V is the flow velocity. (*B*) Symptomatic patient with active lifestyle and with idiopathic subglottic stenosis resulting in 50% obstruction. (*C*) Asymptomatic patient with sedentary lifestyle and with idiopathic subglottic stenosis resulting in 50% obstruction. The variability in flow velocity through the stenosis explains why patients with similar degrees of airway narrowing have different degrees of functional impairment. Patients with active lifestyles have increased flow velocity, greater pressure drop across the stenotic area, and increased work of breathing.

flow rates.[10] The variability in flow velocity through the stenotic area explains why patients with similar degrees of airway narrowing have different degrees of functional impairment, and why patients with active lifestyles have increased flow velocity, a greater pressure drop across the stenotic area, and increased work of breathing (**Fig. 2**B, C).

There are 2 widely used staging systems of tracheal stenosis: the Myer-Cotton and McCaffrey systems.[12,13] The Myer-Cotton system, based on the degree of airway narrowing, uses cutoff values of 50% and 70% narrowing to define grade I (<50%), grade II (51%–70%), and grade III (71%–99%) stenosis. Investigators found that the location and extent (which might be defined as the distributive length of the abnormal airway segment) of the lesions do not affect the grade of stenosis, thus justifying severity criterion as an independent parameter in a classification system. Based on available physiologic data, cutoff values used in the Myer-Cotton classification seem appropriate. The system also includes a grade IV stenosis in which no lumen is detected (100% narrowing). Myer-Cotton grade IV is obviously not compatible with life in nontracheostomized patients, and is rare.[7] The McCaffrey system classifies stenoses based on their location and on the extent of airway involvement.[13]

Extent of the abnormality

From a flow limitation perspective, the severity of airway narrowing seems to depend greatly on the extent of airway narrowing.[10] Long stenoses show a modest difference in pressure profiles, with a slightly smaller magnitude of total pressure drop, than short weblike stenoses of comparable narrowing. Furthermore, the extent of stenosis does not seem to correlate with clinical data such as age, duration of intubation, or previous surgery.[14] Extent is important to types of treatment, prognosis, and risk for recurrence.

In patients with strictures less than 1 cm in length, for example, good results are often achieved after bronchoscopic therapy, although open surgical laryngotracheal resection with primary end-to-end anastomotic reconstruction is viewed as preferable in patients who are operable.[15–17] However, surgical treatment of strictures 4 cm and longer are often associated with anastomotic complications consisting of granulation, stenosis, or dehiscence. Open surgery becomes less desirable or impossible in these cases.[18] Some classification systems from the surgical literature account for the extent and location of the stenosis,[13,19,20] whereas systems proposed in the medical literature seem to be limited to location only.[4] The most commonly used system for describing the extent of the lesion and shown to predict outcome, is that described by McCaffrey.[13] Based on this system, stenosis is stage I if it is confined to the subglottis or trachea and less than 1 cm long, stage II if stenosis is isolated to the subglottis or trachea and more than 1 cm long, stage III if the tracheal/subglottic lesions do not involve the glottis, and stage IV if the lesions involve the glottis with vocal cord fixation and paralysis. Contrary to the Myer-Cotton system,[12] the McCaffrey system addresses the extent and location as the predominant predictors of outcome. Another step toward creating a multidimensional system was attempted by Anand and colleagues,[21] who reviewed the treatment of

tracheal stenosis, mostly postintubation cases, and characterized stenoses based on severity, location, length, and number of stenoses. The investigators divided severity into 3 grades: mild (<70%), moderate (71%–90%), and severe (>90%). Locations were defined as glottic, cervical, or thoracic. Lengths were divided into less than 1 cm, 1 to 3 cm, and more than 3 cm.[21]

Although tracheal resection with primary repair often provides curative treatment in patients with tracheal stenosis, the surgically resectable length is restricted to 30% of the total airway length in children, and a maximum of about 4 to 6 cm in adults.[22] Replacement of longer sections would be feasible if a safe, functional tracheal replacement could be developed. Pioneering work in this field is promising, as demonstrated recently by Macchiarini and colleagues,[23] who were able to produce a cellular, tissue-engineered airway with mechanical properties that allow normal functioning, free from the risks of rejection.

Morphology

The literature on tracheal stenosis includes various morphologic descriptions such as "A-shaped," triangular, concentric, circumferential, weblike, complex, and eccentric (**Fig. 3**).[4,24,25] Morphology might affect flow dynamics, symptoms, and

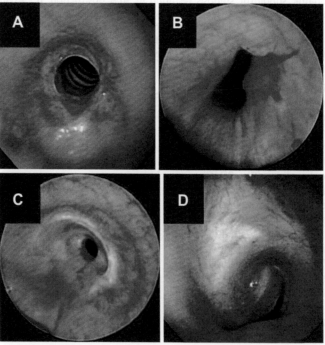

Fig. 3. Morphologic types of tracheal stenosis. (*A*) Circumferential (concentric) simple, idiopathic subglottic stenosis. (*B*) Triangular (A-shaped) simple, post-tracheostomy tracheal stenosis. (*C*) Hourglass, complex, postintubation tracheal stenosis. (*D*) Triangular (A-shaped), complex post-tracheostomy tracheal stenosis with cartilaginous collapse (malacia).

response to certain therapeutic interventions. Strictures with associated chondritis and malacia, for example, have been shown to predict poor results and failure of endoscopic treatment.[17] The annotation "+ m" should therefore probably be included to describe the morphology of tracheal stenosis when there is associated malacia.[26]

Completely circumferential strictures were shown to have poorer outcomes, requiring more interventions, than eccentric lesions.[17,24] The shape of airway narrowing affects flow velocity and pressure drops in a computer modeling study of tracheal flow.[11] The triangular glottal aperture shifts the laryngeal airflow toward the posterior wall, generating 2 pairs of counter-rotating secondary vortices downstream from the glottis. Circular or elliptical apertures, on the other hand, generate only 1 pair of vortices. However, differences in pressure drop are dominated by the cross-sectional area more than by the shape of the glottis.[11]

Certain abnormal morphologies are characteristic. For instance, post-tracheostomy tracheal strictures are typically triangular or A-shaped.[25] A stenosis with chondromalacia is due to ischemic damage and mechanical effects induced by prolonged intubation or tracheostomy. Chondromalacia results from extensive degeneration of cartilage with irregular borders of inner perichondrium. However, in idiopathic tracheal stenosis, there is normal cartilage with smooth inner and outer perichondrium, associated with extensive keloidal fibrosis and dilation of mucus glands, which is uncommon in most cases of chondromalacia. Studies have shown that immunohistochemical staining for estrogen and progesterone receptors is positive in fibroblast cells in most cases of idiopathic tracheal stenosis, leading some investigators to suggest that this entity is a form of fibromatosis.[25]

This correlation between morphology and pathogenesis has potential therapeutic implications. In a study of excised specimens from intubation and stent-related tracheal and subglottic stenoses, for example, high-level expression of TGF-β1, deposition of the extracellular matrix (ECM) and a dose-dependent in vitro proliferation of human fibroblasts were noted even in the presence of mitomycin C.[27] Proliferation of the fibrotic subepithelium is not the main mechanism responsible for airway narrowing in intubation or stent-related tracheal stenosis, which could be a reason why response to mitomycin C has been variable among studies.[28,29] Pharmacologic therapy for this specific entity should therefore probably address the inhibition of profibrotic cytokines such as TGF-β1 and the deposition of ECM in subglottic and tracheal stenoses, rather than the subepithelial proliferation of fibroblasts.[27]

ECAC

Functional status
Patients with ECAC have pure tracheobronchomalacia (TBM), characterized by softening of the airway cartilage, or excessive dynamic airway collapse (EDAC) in which an exaggerated protrusion of the posterior membrane into the airway lumen results in a decrease in the cross-sectional area of more than 50%, or both.[5] Both conditions can cause significant dyspnea, cough, inability to clear secretions, and even respiratory failure.[30,31] Occasionally, malacia and EDAC are incidental findings on bronchoscopy performed for various reasons. The authors consider that the effect of these findings on a patient's functional status needs to be considered when committing these patients to therapeutic alternatives such as continuous positive airway pressure (CPAP), stent insertion, or surgery.[32] Although the best tool to assess the functional status in patients with ECAC remains to be determined, several scales have been used in retrospective and prospective studies. Patients with ECAC were shown to improve their dyspnea, quality of life, and functional status after airway stent insertion or membranous tracheoplasty as assessed by the World Health Organization (WHO) functional status scoring system, modified St George respiratory questionnaires, a baseline dyspnea index (BDI)/ transitional dyspnea index (TDI), the American Thoracic Society (ATS) dyspnea score, or Karnofsky performance scales (KPS).[33–36]

A thorough functional assessment before and after therapeutic intervention is also warranted to objectively assess response to treatment and to determine whether any lack of improvement after therapy is due to progression of coexistent disease or is a result of treatment failure. In part, this is because patients with ECAC may have several comorbidities, such as asthma and COPD.[33–35] Functional status should be objectively documented, along with the other descriptive and stratification parameters of ECAC.[5] A recent prospective study in children with TBM showed that the malacic site and the severity of the abnormality might not exert a dose effect on rates, risks, and severity of illness assessed by the validated Canadian Acute Respiratory Illness and Flu Scale,[37] suggesting that functional status may be a parameter independent of extent and severity of airway collapse. Although 7 classification systems have been proposed for patients with ECAC over the last 45 years,[31] only recently has functional status been included as a separate independent criterion.[5] Because the improvements in functional status seen in several studies were not associated with improvements in pulmonary function as measured by FEV_1,[34,35] other physiologic parameters, such as markers of hyperinflation, should perhaps also be included in a multidimensional classification system.[38]

Severity of airway narrowing

The quantification of the severity of airway collapse remains empirical,[31] and a correlation between the degrees of severity, functional status, and pulmonary physiology remains to be determined. During normal exhalation there is a certain degree of physiologic dynamic airway collapse (DAC) that reduces the airway lumen by a maximum of 40%.[39] A reduction of 50% or more has traditionally been considered abnormal.[40] However, different classification systems use different cutoff values, such as 50% or 80% narrowing, to define abnormal collapse during exhalation.[31] Furthermore, some investigators estimate narrowing during tidal exhalation, whereas others estimate it during forced exhalation or coughing maneuvers.[31] Although cutoff values for defining mild, moderate, and severe obstruction remain to be determined, and might depend on the impact of airway narrowing on flow limitation, several investigators propose that airway collapse should be defined as mild if greater than 50%/less than 75%, moderate if greater than 75%/less than 100%, and severe if 100%.[5,31]

However, the bronchoscopic assessment of airway caliber is usually a subjective estimate that depends on the technique and experience of the bronchoscopist, the position in which the procedure is performed (supine or sitting), the use of sedation or respiratory maneuvers, and whether the bronchoscope and its accessories, such as open biopsy forceps or measurement calipers, are used.[41] These facts might explain why clinicians may use nonbronchoscopic assessments of airway collapse, such as physiologic measures or radiographic imaging.[42] Spirometry and flow-volume loops are nonspecific.[43] Multidetector computed tomography (CT) with three-dimensional reconstructions is used to quantify the degree of airway collapse and to identify the relationship of the airways with the adjacent mediastinal structures, thus potentially identifying the cause of the abnormal airway collapse.[44] Disadvantages include the difficulty in image acquisition in dyspneic, comatose, or uncooperative patients, airway narrowing mimicked by secretions and

blood clots, radiation delivery, and the need for costly computer hardware and an experienced radiologist.[41] Dynamic magnetic resonance imaging (MRI) avoids the radiation exposure and administration of potentially nephrotoxic contrast agents. This technique has been used to quantify the degree of airway collapse, but experience is limited.[45]

There are also several morphometric bronchoscopy techniques with which to objectively quantify the degree of airway narrowing in adult patients with CAO.[41] These consist of software processing methods whereby bronchoscopic digital images are analyzed to measure airway lumen diameter. Modalities using freely available software and calculated indices measure airway caliber more simply than previously proposed labor-intensive image calibration and distortion correction techniques.[41]

Extent of the abnormality

The extent of ECAC applies to the location and distribution of the abnormal airway segment as seen at bronchoscopy. The extent of the collapse affects management. Focal tracheomalcia, as seen after tracheostomy, can be cured by tracheal sleeve resection.[46] However, diffuse severe malacia, as seen in relapsing polychondritis, is not amenable to surgery, and stent insertion might be the only alternative for severely symptomatic patients. Diffuse and severe EDAC has been successfully treated by membranous tracheoplasty.[34]

Four of the 7 available classification systems addressed extent of the disease,[5,31] but descriptions remain subjective. In an attempt to provide an accurate extent criterion, a recently proposed system used in clinical studies described the extent as: normal, no airway abnormality; focal, the abnormality is present in 1 main or lobar bronchus or 1 tracheal region (upper, mid- or lower); multifocal, the abnormality is present in 2 contiguous, or at least 2 noncontiguous, regions; and diffuse, an abnormality present in more than 2 contiguous regions.[5,33,47]

Morphology

Several forms of ECAC are described in the literature, depending on the morphology of the airway lumen during expiration.[31] At least 7 terms have been used to describe ECAC, but it remains unclear which terms refer to the collapse of the posterior membrane or to the cartilaginous collapse.[31] EDAC refers to bulging of the posterior membrane within the airway lumen during exhalation, as is seen in some patients with COPD or asthma.[31,32,48] The cartilage is intact in this process. TBM refers to softening of the cartilaginous airway structures and has 3 different morphologies. When the lateral walls are weakened, the configuration during exhalation is that of a saber sheath. If the anterior wall is weakened, the airway lumen takes the shape of a crescent. If anterior and lateral cartilaginous wall are involved, as in patients with relapsing polychondritis, narrowing is circumferential and often accompanied by edema (**Fig. 4**). The distinction between these 2 entities, which may occur separately or together, is important because the 2 processes might be different not only from a morphology perspective, but each may also have a distinct physiopathology and airway wall structure, and each might be amenable to various, yet different, treatment modalities.[31,49]

ASTHMA
Pathophysiology and Rationale for Bronchoscopic Treatment

Remodeling is a term that refers to changes in the size, mass, or number of tissue components that occur during growth or in response to injury and inflammation.[50,51] Remodeling may be appropriate during normal lung development and in response to acute injury, or inappropriate, when it is chronic and associated with abnormally altered tissue structure or function.[50] It is not necessarily a secondary phenomenon that occurs late in the disease process. This process might begin early in the development of asthma and may occur in parallel with, or even be required for, the establishment of persistent inflammation. As part of this remodeling, smooth muscle mass increases significantly.[50] Remodeling tends to occur in airways larger than 2 mm in diameter, and seems to be increased in older patients and in patients with a longer duration of hyperreactive airways disease.[52] Because airway smooth muscle (ASM) contractility determines airway narrowing, blocking the ASM contractility has been a primary focus of antiasthma treatment. However, this approach is not satisfactory in approximately 10% of patients with asthma who have poor control and who account for 50% of asthma-related health care costs.[53]

In normal airways, smooth muscle provides structural support, helps regulate gas exchange, and contributes to mucus clearance, defense mechanisms, and cough.[53] Although smooth muscle also might be vestigial, resulting from lung development, and not play an important role,[54] there is evidence that implicates smooth muscle in the pathogenesis of airway inflammation

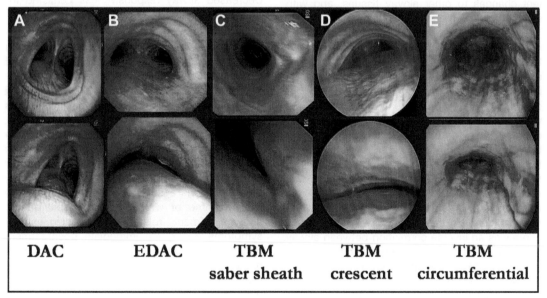

| DAC | EDAC | TBM saber sheath | TBM crescent | TBM circumferential |

Fig. 4. Morphologic types of ECAC. (*A*) Normally, during exhalation there is a certain degree of DAC that reduces the airway lumen by a maximum of 40%. (*B*) EDAC is due to bulging of the posterior membrane within the airway lumen during exhalation that narrows the lumen by 50% or more. The cartilage is intact in this process. (*C*) TBM refers to softening of the airway cartilaginous structures. When the lateral walls are weakened, the configuration during exhalation is that of a saber sheath. (*D*) If the anterior wall is weakened, the airway lumen takes the shape of a crescent. (*E*) If anterior and lateral cartilaginous walls are involved, this has been called the circumferential type.

and remodeling, and points to interactions with bronchial epithelium and nerves.[53] The benefit of current asthma treatments, including bronchodilators, inhaled corticosteroids, and anti-immunoglobin E (anti-IgE) antibody, may be due in part to their actions on ASM.[55,56] These 3 features (remodeling, inflammation, and hyperresponsiveness) lead to symptoms of asthma. Because ASM cells are the most important cells involved in airway hyperresponsiveness (AHR), and have been shown to be involved in remodeling and inflammation, several investigators propose that these cells should be targeted, rather than targeting inflammation or treating symptoms.[57]

Heat generated by radiofrequency (RF) energy can destroy smooth muscle, a concept applied clinically, especially in cardiology, to treat conduction defects, and in gynecology to treat endometrial hemorrhage.[58–60] The concept of treating airways with heat generated by RF energy is based on the supposition that blockade of the bronchial smooth muscle tone in asthmatic patients not responding optimally to conventional therapy could cause amelioration of chronic symptoms and reduce exacerbations.[61]

In the first animal study evaluating heat-related destruction of ASM, the investigators determined a dose of temperature-controlled RF energy capable of reducing the amount of functional ASM in the canine airway wall, with limited persistent changes to other airway tissues, and with subsequent decreased airway responsiveness. The treatment temperatures chosen were in the range used in RF electrosurgical tissue coagulation (55, 65, and 75°C).[61] Airway responsiveness data, reported as percent change in diameter after local methacoline challenge, showed significant differences in the groups treated at 65 and 75°C with respect to the control group. This study validated the temperature of 65°C as efficient for bronchial thermoplasty. Histopathologic examination showed that ASM in the untreated airway was normal, and ASM in the airway treated at 65°C was reduced throughout the circumference of the treated airway. The parenchyma, epithelium, and mucous glands in the treated airway are normal. There was an inverse correlation between airway responsiveness and percentage of airway circumference containing altered ASM, which means that this technique of reducing the muscle mass might have clinical significance. As an addition to the previous study, more recent animal data show that reducing the amount of functional smooth muscle with bronchial thermoplasty leads to increased airway size in relaxed and contracted states over a normal range of inflation pressures and at different lung volumes.[62]

Bronchial Thermoplasty: Technique and Results

During bronchial thermoplasty, an expandable basket with 4 electrode arms is opened to make circumferential contact with the airway wall. The catheter fits through the 2-mm working channel of a standard 5-mm fiber-optic bronchoscope and has an expandable 4-electrode basket with heating and temperature-sensing elements for feedback control at the distal end. Airways greater than 3 mm in diameter are treated in sessions that last approximately 10 minutes per segment, maintaining target temperatures in each location for about 10 seconds. According to protocol, treatments are performed at 3-week intervals for a maximum of 3 treatments.[63]

The first human study included 9 patients treated before they underwent lung resection. The study confirmed the feasibility and general safety of the application of bronchial thermoplasty in the human airway, and showed that the histologically confirmed reduction in ASM seen in animal studies could be reproduced in humans.[64] Subsequently, a prospective, non-randomized study showed that bronchial thermoplasty was well tolerated and resulted in stable spirometry and significant improvement in number of symptom-free days compared with controls during a 12-week posttreatment period. Decreased airway responsiveness persisted for 2 years.[65]

The largest study published to date was performed in patients with persistent asthma requiring daily therapy with inhaled corticosteroids and long-acting β 2 agonists and who had a prebronchodilator FEV_1 of 60% to 85% of predicted, and a methacholine provocation test positive at less than 8 mg/mL.[66] Asthma control improved, particularly for patients with moderate and severe disease, and bronchial thermoplasty resulted in approximately 10 fewer mild exacerbations per subject per year in the treatment group. However, thermoplasty is associated with several adverse events, some of which require hospitalization, and are primarily related to worsening asthma symptoms during the immediate posttreatment period. Dyspnea, cough, and wheezing were noted in about 50% of treated patients. Although promising, there are several unanswered questions about bronchial thermoplasty. One pertains to identifying whether reducing ASM mass is truly the reason why the procedure works, or whether perhaps other effects on ASM, such as airway wall stiffening, loss of the continuity of bands of muscularis, or increased tethering by peribronchial lung parenchyma might also play a role. Another regards potential development of bronchiectasis or other lung damage over the long term. Ongoing studies might answer these questions.[67]

COPD
Pathophysiology and Rationale for Bronchoscopic Treatment

The enthusiasm for bronchoscopic treatment of emphysema derives almost entirely from experiences with open lung volume reduction surgery (LVRS). The National Emphysema Treatment Trial (NETT) study showed that patients with COPD and upper lobe disease who did not improve after pulmonary rehabilitation had the most favorable outcome with LVRS, compared with medical therapy alone.[68] However, LVRS is associated with an operative mortality rate of 4% to 7%, a morbidity rate of 30% to 50%, and an average hospital stay of 10 to 14 days. The mortality rate is even higher outside the NETT in cohort studies.[69,70]

The goal of LVRS is to remove the most emphysematous portions of the lungs, which usually results in removal of approximately 20% to 30% of lung tissue. With successful open LVRS, subjective and objective functional measures, composite measures, and physiologic measures of lung volumes (residual volume [RV], inspiratory capacity, and ventilatory capacity [VC]) and expiratory flows (FEV$_1$) improve in a meaningful way.[71]

Bronchoscopic lung volume reduction (BLVR) was developed to achieve the functional and survival benefit seen with LVRS in the NETT study, but without its associated morbidity, mortality, and cost. Presently, however, BLVR is still considered an experimental therapy, and the physiologic and clinical responses seem to be less durable than those of LVRS.[71] It is therefore reasonable to consider BLVR for the patients who refuse LVRS, or who are not candidates for LVRS but still qualify for trial participation.[71] Most bronchoscopic therapies for emphysema are associated with a pattern of response in which patients report feeling better. Subjective functional and composite outcomes have improved without any meaningful change in objective physiologic outcome measures. Indeed, physiologic changes are less than minimal clinically important difference standards,[71] and distinction from a placebo effect is difficult. Thus, attributing improvement to the intervention based on this pattern of response in the absence of a randomized, blinded, placebo-controlled comparison is not possible.

Three physiologic principles can be applied in the treatment of emphysema. These have given rise to 3 different bronchoscopic treatment techniques, none of which has yet proven to be consistently effective in providing durable clinical benefit. Although they share a common objective, these different principles are based on distinct technologies of which none is yet available for general clinical application. These are: (1) placement of endobronchial one-way valves designed to promote atelectasis by blocking inspiratory flow; (2) formation of airway bypass tracts using an RF catheter designed to facilitate emptying of damaged lung regions with long expiratory times; and (3) instillation of biologic adhesives designed to collapse and remodel the hyperinflated lung.

The resizing principle
Resection of lung tissue in emphysema was shown to improve overall function of the respiratory system, based on the "resizing principle."[72] This principle states that reducing the size of emphysematous lung produces space within the chest cavity for the remaining lung to expand and function during inspiration. A pattern of response is obtained in which there is reduction in static and dynamic RV, and associated improvement in elastic recoil.[71]

Based on this principle, one-way endobronchial valves and spigots were designed to cause lung collapse by promoting progressive deflation and adsorption atelectasis. Using these devices, built from biocompatible materials, air is allowed to leave, but not to enter, the damaged lung areas. The efficacy of these devices was demonstrated in cases similar to surgical lung volume reduction (LVR), mainly in patients with CT-proven heterogeneous emphysema, but findings were slightly different from those of the LVRS studies in which patients treated bilaterally did better than those treated unilaterally.[73,74] It seems that lobar collapse is facilitated if there is plenty of room for the contralateral lung to expand. In addition, patients with complete fissures are most likely to benefit because lobar collapse may be more successful. Because the fissures are more often complete on the left side than on the right, treating the left lung might result in better outcomes (VENT study: preliminary data presented at the American College of Chest Physicians [ACCP] meeting, Chicago, 2007).

Endobronchial valves: technique and results These bronchoscopic procedures are usually performed under general anesthesia, although cases can be done using moderate sedation. The general technique usually involves placement of a guidewire or loaded catheter into the target segmental bronchus, after which the one-way valve or spigot is ejected into position through the working channel of the bronchoscope.

In one recent article, health-related quality of life improved 6 months after treatment, but there was no improvement noted in physiologic measurements.[73] Even in the largest study performed to date, including 321 patients with severe bilateral heterogenous upper lobe predominant emphysema, FEV_1 improved by only 6% at 6 months (VENT study: preliminary data presented at ACCP meeting, Chicago 2007). A recent publication summarizing the broad experience using endobronchial valve therapy in 98 patients confirms wide variability in therapeutic response. Overall, the 98-patient cohort showed small improvements in physiologic parameters that failed to meet minimal clinical important difference criteria for FEV_1 (10%), VC (9%) or 6-minute walk distance (6MWD; 36 m) at 90-day follow-up. Subjective outcomes were not reported in this study.[74]

To date, clinical trials show that endobronchial valve therapy is capable of producing initial responses similar to those of LVRS in selected cases, but responses are variable, criteria for identifying responders are poorly defined, and benefits are often short lived.[71] The US Food and Drug Administration (FDA) recently found insufficient evidence of benefit to outweigh the risks of implanting these devices for the treatment of emphysema (http://www.medpagetoday.com/ProductAlert/DevicesandVaccines/12047; Accessed May 24, 2009).

However, even in the absence of changes in FEV_1, forced vital capacity (FVC), and RV, these devices can produce physiologic benefit by altering regional airflow impedance and reducing dynamic hyperinflation. Overall, valves seem safe, with a procedure-related mortality of approximately 1%. Morbidities include pneumonthorax, pneumonia, or exacerbations of COPD as a result of placement. In the VENT study, the valve group had higher rates of serious adverse events related to COPD than the control group (23% vs 10%, $P = .01$). They were also more likely to be hospitalized (39.7% vs 25.3%, $P = .024$). One major concern, in addition to the need for understanding more about the physiologic effects of these devices, is how placement might affect health care costs, because it seems, from some studies, that valve revisions are necessary in more than 50% of cases.[73] Furthermore, the future of this technology is questionable after the FDA rejected the Zephyr Endobronchial Valve (Emphasys Medical, Redwood City, CA) for emphysema based on results from the 80 million dollar VENT study.

Collateral ventilation

Another physiologic principle for treating emphysema is based on the mechanism of collateral ventilation. In young normal persons the resistance to collateral ventilation is high at functional residual capacity (FRC) and there is a negligible role for collateral channels in the distribution of ventilation. Thus, airflow leaves the lung unit through the same path as it came in (**Fig. 5**A). In emphysema, however, on inspiration, the regular airways can open, allowing inspiration through normal channels. On expiration, the collateral passageways provide escape pathways to bypass the collapsed small airways (**Fig. 5**B). This ability of gas to move from one part of the lung to another through nonanatomic pathways is greatly increased in emphysema, because of the extensive breakdown of alveolar walls and lobular septae. There is evidence from autopsy studies that

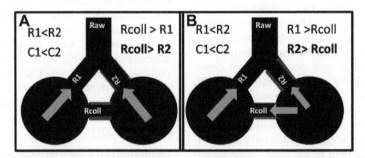

Fig. 5. Collateral ventilation principle. (A) In young normal persons, the resistance to collateral ventilation is high at FRC (Rcoll>R1 and R2) and there is a negligible role for collateral channels in the distribution of ventilation. Thus the airflow leaves the lung unit through the same path as it came in (*blue arrows*). (B) In emphysema, on inspiration, the regular airways can open, allowing inspiration through normal channels. On expiration, the collateral passageways provide escape pathways to bypass the collapsed small airways (R2>Rcoll). C, compliance; R, resistance; Rcoll, resistance through the collateral channel; thick red lines, increased resistance to flow; thin red lines, decreased resistance to flow.

the fissures are rarely complete in human lungs, and major defects in fissures were found in 30% of the lungs dissected.[75] Interlobar collateral ventilation occurs to a much greater extent in patients with radiologically homogeneous emphysema than in those with heterogeneous emphysema. Thus, heterogeneity of emphysema may be predictive of patients with a significantly reduced chance of interlobar collateral ventilation.[76] This becomes important in selecting patients for airway bypass systems, because the procedure may be more useful in patients with homogenous emphysema, contrary to endobronchial valve insertion, which seems more appropriate for patients with heterogenous emphysema.[71]

Airway bypass stents: technique and results Airway bypass stents were designed to reduce lung volume by altering flow dynamics (regional time constants) and airway closure, rather than by promoting lung collapse. They are noncollapsing, extra-anatomic stents connecting lung parenchyma to large airways that facilitate expiration and help alleviate some of the adverse consequences of dynamic hyperinflation. They do not promote atelectasis as valves do, but they do reduce lung volume by altering flow dynamics and allowing the lung units to empty.

Initial work applying this technique was performed in excised human emphysematous lungs removed at the time of lung transplantation.[77] The lungs were placed in an airtight ventilation chamber with the bronchus attached to a tube traversing the chamber wall, and attached to a pneumotachometer. A flexible bronchoscope was then inserted into the airway and an RF catheter was used to create a passage through the wall of 3 separate segmental bronchi into the adjacent lung parenchyma. An expandable stent, 1.5 cm in length and 3 mm in diameter, was then inserted through each passage. There was significant improvement in expiratory flow, which also correlated with the number of stents inserted.

Human studies have demonstrated improvement with placement of numerous stents, primarily in patients with evidence of homogenous emphysema and significant hyperinflation. In a study including 19 patients with a 6-month follow-up, there was immediate improvement in dyspnea score and lung physiology (FEV_1, FVC, and RV); however, this was not sustained at 30 days.[78] In a subset of patients (8 of 19) with homogeneous disease and marked baseline hyperinflation (total lung capacity [TLC]>133% predicted) there were marked reductions in RV (-1.1 L), improvements in VC ($+189$ mL), and improvements in dyspnea and health related quality of life (HRQOL).[78] These

results were reproduced in the largest study published to date, which included 35 patients. A median of 8 stents were required per patient to achieve physiologic and subjective improvements.[79] This fact raises questions about the cost of such interventions and their associated risks. Significant complications are seen in 5% of patients, and are mostly related to hemorrhage and pneumothorax. To avoid these, the insertion site can be examined using a Doppler probe to look for adjacent vascular structures. Many patients also develop acute exacerbations of COPD in the immediate postprocedure period.

There are still several questions that remain to be answered regarding airway bypass systems. How many stents are necessary? What is their ideal location and how should one determine that location? Furthermore, what is their long term effect? The long term stent patency seems to be a major limiting factor. In one study, control stents were all occluded at the first week of bronchoscopic follow-up.[80] In contrast, mitomycin C–treated stents had a prolonged patency, and the duration of patency was associated with the number of once-weekly topical mitomycin applications. Weekly application of topical mitomycin is not practical. Another study by the same investigators[81] evaluated paclitaxel-eluted stents, which were compared with 50 control stents in dogs. Sixty-five percent of drug-eluting stents were patent, compared with 0% of the control stents at 12 weeks. The investigators concluded that paclitaxel-eluting stents were safe and remain patent for at least 3 months. Human studies evaluating these drug-eluted stents have not yet been published.

Biologic remodeling
The third principle for treating emphysema is based on biologic remodeling. The goal is the same as for LVRS and endobronchial valves, namely to cause atelectasis. The treatment is intended to produce a permanent change in tissue configuration similar to LVRS, rather than reversible adsorption atelectasis. However, the site and mechanism of action are fundamentally different from endobronchial valve systems. The components polymerize distally at the target site to produce collapse and remodeling over several weeks. The agents act at the alveolar rather than the airway level. There is disruption of the epithelium with deactivation of surfactant to produce local atelectasis and modulation of the resultant inflammatory response. This process induces scarring and shrinkage of the hyperinflated lung in patients with heterogeneous upper lobe emphysema. At sites of treatment, there was extensive

collagen deposition, with collections of fibroblasts and mononuclear cells, consistent with organized scar tissue.[82]

Biologic remodeling sealants/systems: technique and results The initial work done by Ingenito and colleagues[82] was in an animal model of emphysema. An enzymatic primer solution was instilled in the hyperinflated lung to remove epithelial cells from the target region, and then a modified hydrogel scaffold was injected to promote fibroblast attachment and collagen synthesis. The TLC and RV were found to be significantly reduced in the treated animals, compared with controls.[82] Studies in sheep, and consideration of human lung anatomy, have indicated that each pulmonary subsegment represented 2% to 3% of TLC. Consequently, in terms of technique, biologic LVR performed at 2 subsegments is expected to reduce lung volume by only 4% to 6% of TLC, and was not anticipated to produce physiologic benefits. However, treatment at 4 subsegments has greater potential for a therapeutic impact resulting in LVR of 8% to 12%.

Clinical data are available in several abstracts and a couple of peer-reviewed manuscripts.[83,84] The inclusion and exclusion criteria are similar to those used for open LVRS. One difference from LVRS, but a similarity to endobronchial valves, is that treatment is usually unilateral. At low doses in patients with heterogeneous emphysema, the biologic system produces mild volume reduction and small changes in physiology and exercise capacity.[83] However, the overall response for all 6 patients was a pattern of response with failure to meet minimum clinically important difference (MCID) criteria for exercise capacity or physiologic parameters. In animal studies, there was no suggestion of pneumonitis, granuloma formation, residual foreign body material, or evidence of tissue necrosis or abscess formation at the treatment site. Although this human study seemed to be safe, the long-term durability and safety of this technique remained to be established. In the largest human study performed to date, which included 50 patients with upper lobe–predominant emphysema, spirometric improvements were documented at 6 months, but serious treatment-related complications were seen in 8% of patients and consisted of aspiration, pneumonia, and pulmonary embolism.[84]

SUMMARY

Several classification systems have been proposed for tracheal stenosis and ECAC. Some of the shortcomings of these systems include limited criteria, use of inconsistent definitions for abnormal stenosis and collapse, severity grades that vary among systems, exclusion of patients' functional status assessments, and the lack of clear delineation of the various morphologic types. Comparing the results of different bronchoscopic treatment modalities for CAO in different centers has, therefore, been difficult, and is mostly due to this lack of uniformity of classifications[4] and to the absence of a common language among bronchoscopists, otolaryngologists, and surgeons.

An ideal classification system should be developed to simply and reproducibly identify and characterize CAO among different centers. Such a system might lend itself to placing stenoses into a finite number of specific categories. Studies are ongoing not only to identify potential consensus regarding nomenclatures and descriptors but also to design and study a system that includes an assessment of the patient's functional status, extent of airway abnormality, morphologic types and severity of fixed airway stenosis or collapse that would allow quantitative analyses for outcome studies.

A multidimensional scoring system is likely to better predict outcomes than isolated variables. This superiority has been demonstrated in other disease states, such as COPD, for which the BODE index, a simple multidimensional grading system encompassing body mass index, degree of airflow obstruction, dyspnea, and exercise capacity, was shown to be better than FEV_1 alone at predicting risk of death from any cause.[85] For patients with CAO, a multidimensional classification system might offer not only a means with which to objectively assess disease states and outcomes but also might provide the benefit of a common language for physicians from different centers and disciplines. The importance of detailed and precise communication is evident in this field, as conservative medical treatments, minimally invasive procedures, and open surgery are now available to these patients.[21,22,33–36]

For peripheral airway obstruction, understanding the physiologic and pathologic basis for airflow limitation in patients with refractory asthma and COPD has led to the development of bronchoscopic procedures which alter airway wall structure or affect flow dynamics. These minimally invasive interventional procedures are enhancing the therapeutic armamentarium for patients with severe refractory obstructive ventilatory impairment, which until recently has been limited to pharmaceutical and open surgical techniques.

REFERENCES

1. Ernst A, Feller-Kopman D, Becker HD, et al. Central airway obstruction. Am J Respir Crit Care Med 2004; 169:1278–97.

2. Sahi H, Karnak D, Meli YM, et al. Bronchoscopic approach to COPD. COPD 2008;5:125–31.

3. Bel EH. "Hot stuff": bronchial thermoplasty for asthma. Am J Respir Crit Care Med 2006;173:941–2.

4. Freitag L, Ernst A, Unger M, et al. A proposed classification system of central airway stenosis. Eur Respir J 2007;30:7–12.

5. Murgu SD, Colt HG. Description of a multidimensional classification system for patients with expiratory central airway collapse. Respirology 2007;12: 543–50.

6. The WHO Family of International Classifications. Available at: http://www.who.int/classifications/en/. Accessed August 30, 2009.

7. Nouraei SA, Nouraei SM, Randhawa PS, et al. Sensitivity and responsiveness of the Medical Research Council dyspnoea scale to the presence and treatment of adult laryngotracheal stenosis. Clin Otolaryngol 2008;33:575–80.

8. Dyspnea. Mechanisms, assessment, and management: a consensus statement. American Thoracic Society. Am J Respir Crit Care Med 1999;159:321–40.

9. Bestall JC, Paul EA, Garrod R, et al. Usefulness of the Medical Research Council (MRC) dyspnoea scale as a measure of disability in patients with chronic obstructive pulmonary disease. Thorax 1999;54:581–6.

10. Brouns M, Jayaraju ST, Lacor C, et al. Tracheal stenosis: a flow dynamics study. J Appl Physiol 2007;102:1178–84.

11. Brouns M, Verbanck S, Lacor C. Influence of glottic aperture on the tracheal flow. J Biomech 2007;40: 165–72.

12. Myer CM, O'Connor DM, Cotton RT. Proposed grading system for subglottic stenosis based on endotracheal tube sizes. Ann Otol Rhinol Laryngol 1994;103:319–23.

13. McCaffrey TV. Classification of laryngotracheal stenosis. Laryngoscope 1992;102:1335–40.

14. Zagalo C, Santiago N, Grande NR, et al. Morphology of trachea in benign human tracheal stenosis: a clinicopathological study of 20 patients undergoing surgery. Surg Radiol Anat 2002;24:160–8.

15. Ashiku SK, Kuzucu A, Grillo HC, et al. Idiopathic laryngotracheal stenosis: effective definitive treatment with laryngotracheal resection. J Thorac Cardiovasc Surg 2004;127:99–107.

16. Valdez TA, Shapshay SM. Idiopathic subglottic stenosis revisited. Ann Otol Rhinol Laryngol 2002; 111:690–5.

17. Simpson GT, Strong MS, Healy GB, et al. Predictive factors of success or failure in the endoscopic management of laryngeal and tracheal stenosis. Ann Otol Rhinol Laryngol 1982;91:384–8.

18. Wright CD, Grillo HC, Wain JC, et al. Anastomotic complications after tracheal resection: prognostic factors and management. J Thorac Cardiovasc Surg 2004;128:731–9.

19. Lano CF Jr, Duncavage JA, Reinisch L, et al. Laryngotracheal reconstruction in the adult: a ten year experience. Ann Otol Rhinol Laryngol 1998;107: 92–7.

20. Grundfast KM, Morris MS, Bernsley C. Subglottic stenosis: retrospective analysis and proposal for standard reporting system. Ann Otol Rhinol Laryngol 1987;96:101–5.

21. Anand VK, Alemar G, Warren ET. Surgical considerations in tracheal stenosis. Laryngoscope 1992;102: 237–43.

22. Grillo HC. Tracheal replacement: a critical review. Ann Thorac Surg 2002;73:1995–2004.

23. Macchiarini P, Jungebluth P, Go T, et al. Clinical transplantation of a tissue-engineered airway. Lancet 2008;372:2023–30.

24. Roediger FC, Orloff LA, Courey MS. Adult subglottic stenosis: management with laser incisions and mitomycin-C. Laryngoscope 2008;118:1542–6.

25. Mark EJ, Meng F, Kradin RL, et al. Idiopathic tracheal stenosis: a clinicopathologic study of 63 cases and comparison of the pathology with chondromalacia. Am J Surg Pathol 2008;32:1138–43.

26. Murgu SD, Colt HG. A multidimensional classification for patients with benign central airway strictures. Chest 2008;134:10003.

27. Karagiannidis C, Velehorschi V, Obertrifter B, et al. High-level expression of matrix-associated transforming growth factor-beta1 in benign airway stenosis. Chest 2006;129:1298–304.

28. Rahbar R, Shapshay SM, Healy GB. Mitomycin: effects on laryngeal and tracheal stenosis, benefits, and complications. Ann Otol Rhinol Laryngol 2001; 110:1–6.

29. Eliashar R, Gross M, Maly B, et al. Mitomycin does not prevent laryngotracheal repeat stenosis after endoscopic dilation surgery: an animal study. Laryngoscope 2004;114:743–6.

30. Carden KA, Boiselle PM, Waltz DA, et al. Tracheomalacia and tracheobronchomalacia in children and adults: an in-depth review. Chest 2005;127: 984–1005.

31. Murgu SD, Colt HG. Tracheobronchomalacia and excessive dynamic airway collapse. Respirology 2006;11:388–406.

32. Murgu SD, Colt HG. Treatment of adult tracheobronchomalacia and excessive dynamic airway collapse: an update. Treat Respir Med 2006;5:103–15.

33. Murgu SD, Colt HG. Complications of silicone stent insertion in patients with expiratory central airway collapse. Ann Thorac Surg 2007;84:1870–7.

34. Majid A, Guerrero J, Gangadharan S, et al. Tracheobronchoplasty for severe tracheobronchomalacia: a prospective outcome analysis. Chest 2008;134: 801–7.

35. Ernst A, Majid A, Feller-Kopman D, et al. Airway stabilization with silicone stents for treating adult tracheobronchomalacia: a prospective observational study. Chest 2007;132:609–16.

36. Wright CD, Grillo HC, Hammoud ZT, et al. Tracheoplasty for expiratory collapse of central airways. Ann Thorac Surg 2005;80:259–66.

37. Masters IB, Zimmerman PV, Pandeya N, et al. Quantified tracheobronchomalacia disorders and their clinical profiles in children. Chest 2008;133:461–7.

38. Murgu SD, Colt HG. Tracheobronchoplasty for severe tracheobronchomalacia. Chest 2009;135: 1403–4.

39. Fraser RG. Measurements of the caliber of human bronchi in three phases of respiration by cinebronchography. J Can Assoc Radiol 1961;12:102–12.

40. Johnson TH, Mikita JJ, Wilson RJ, et al. Acquired tracheomalacia. Radiology 1973;109:576–80.

41. Murgu S, Colt HG. Morphometric bronchoscopy in adults with central airway obstruction: case illustrations and review of the literature. Laryngoscope 2009;119:1318–24.

42. Dörffel WV, Fietze I, Hentschel D, et al. A new bronchoscopic method to measure airway size. Eur Respir J 1999;14:783–8.

43. Miller RD, Hyatt RE. Evaluation of obstructing lesions of the trachea and larynx by flow-volume loops. Am Rev Respir Dis 1973;108:475–81.

44. Boiselle PM. Multislice helical CT of the central airways. Radiol Clin North Am 2003;41:561–74.

45. Faust RA, Remley KB, Rimell FL. Real-time, cine magnetic resonance imaging for evaluation of the pediatric airway. Laryngoscope 2001;111:2187–90.

46. Grillo HC. Surgical treatment of postintubation tracheal injuries. J Thorac Cardiovasc Surg 1979; 78:860–75.

47. Molina JL, Izikson R, Sivashankar S, et al. Spirometric features of patients with excessive dynamic expiratory central airway collapse. Chest 2008;134: s28002.

48. Park JG, Edell ES. Dynamic airway collapse: distinct from tracheomalacia. J Bronchol 2005;12:143–6.

49. Murgu S, Kurimoto N, Colt H. Endobronchial ultrasound morphology of expiratory central airway collapse. Respirology 2008;13:315–9.

50. Jeffery PK. Remodeling and inflammation of bronchi in asthma and chronic obstructive pulmonary disease. Proc Am Thorac Soc 2004;1:176–83.

51. Davies DE, Wicks J, Powell RM, et al. Airway remodeling in asthma: new insights. J Allergy Clin Immunol 2003;111:215–25.

52. Paré PD, Wiggs BR, James A, et al. The comparative mechanics and morphology of airways in asthma and chronic obstructive pulmonary disease. Am J Respir Crit Care Med 1991;143:1189–93.

53. Solway J, Irvin CG. Airway smooth muscle as a target for asthma therapy. N Engl J Med 2007;356:1367–9.

54. Mead J. Point: airway smooth muscle is useful. J Appl Physiol 2007;102:1708–11.

55. Bonacci JV, Schuliga M, Harris T, et al. Collagen impairs glucocorticoid actions in airway smooth muscle through integrin signalling. Br J Pharmacol 2006;149:365–73.

56. Grunstein MM, Hakonarson H, Leiter J, et al. IL-13-dependent autocrine signaling mediates altered responsiveness of IgE sensitized airway smooth muscle. Am J Physiol Lung Cell Mol Physiol 2002; 282:L520–8.

57. Zuyderduyn S, Sukkar MB, Fust A, et al. Treating asthma means treating airway smooth muscle cells. Eur Respir J 2008;32:265–74.

58. Manolis AS, Vassilikos V, Maounis TN, et al. Radiofrequency ablation in pediatric and adult patients: comparative results. J Interv Card Electrophysiol 2001;5:443–53.

59. Badhwar N, Kalman JM, Sparks PB, et al. Atrial tachycardia arising from the coronary sinus musculature: electrophysiological characteristics and long-term outcomes of radiofrequency ablation. J Am Coll Cardiol 2005;46:1921–30.

60. Friberg B, Persson BR, Willén R, et al. Endometrial destruction by hyperthermia–a possible treatment of menorrhagia. An experimental study. Acta Obstet Gynecol Scand 1996;75:330–5.

61. Danek CJ, Lombard CM, Dungworth DL, et al. Reduction in airway hyperresponsiveness to methacholine by the application of RF energy in dogs. J Appl Physiol 2004;97:1946–53.

62. Brown RH, Wizeman W, Danek C, et al. Effect of bronchial thermoplasty on airway distensibility. Eur Respir J 2005;26:277–82.

63. Cox PG, Miller J, Mitzner W, et al. Radiofrequency ablation of airway smooth muscle for sustained treatment of asthma: preliminary investigations. Eur Respir J 2004;24:659–63.

64. Miller JD, Cox G, Vincic L, et al. A prospective feasibility study of bronchial thermoplasty in the human airway. Chest 2005;127:1999–2006.

65. Cox G, Miller JD, McWilliams A, et al. Bronchial thermoplasty for asthma. Am J Respir Crit Care Med 2006;173:965–9.

66. Cox G, Thomson NC, Rubin AS, et al. Asthma control during the year after bronchial thermoplasty. N Engl J Med 2007;356:1327–37.

67. Asthma Intervention Research 2 (AIR2) Trial. Available at: http://www.clinicaltrial.gov/ct/show/ NCT00231114. Accessed August 30, 2009.

68. Fishman A, Martinez F, Naunheim K, et al. National Emphysema Treatment Trial Research Group. A randomized trial comparing lung-volume-reduction

surgery with medical therapy for severe emphysema. N Engl J Med 2003;348:2059–73.

69. Criner GJ, Cordova FC, Furukawa S, et al. Prospective randomized trial comparing bilateral lung volume reduction surgery to pulmonary rehabilitation in severe chronic obstructive pulmonary disease. Am J Respir Crit Care Med 1999;160:2018–27.

70. Geddes D, Davies M, Koyama H, et al. Effect of lung-volume-reduction surgery in patients with severe emphysema. N Engl J Med 2000;343:239–45.

71. Ingenito EP, Wood DE, Utz JP. Bronchoscopic lung volume reduction in severe emphysema. Proc Am Thorac Soc 2008;5:454–60.

72. Fessler HE, Permutt S. Lung volume reduction surgery and airflow limitation. Am J Respir Crit Care Med 1998;157:715–22.

73. Wood DE, McKenna RJ Jr, Yusen RD, et al. A multicenter trial of an intrabronchial valve for treatment of severe emphysema. J Thorac Cardiovasc Surg 2007;133:65–73.

74. Wan IY, Toma TP, Geddes DM, et al. Bronchoscopic lung volume reduction for end-stage emphysema: report on the first 98 patients. Chest 2006;129:518–26.

75. Kent EM, Blades B. Surgical anatomy of the pulmonary lobes. J Thorac Surg 1942;12:18.

76. Higuchi T, Reed A, Oto T, et al. Relation of interlobar collaterals to radiological heterogeneity in severe emphysema. Thorax 2006;61:409–13.

77. Lausberg HF, Chino K, Patterson GA, et al. Bronchial fenestration improves expiratory flow in emphysematous human lungs. Ann Thorac Surg 2003;75:393–7.

78. Macklem PT, Cardosa P, Snell G, et al. Airway bypass: a new treatment for emphysema [abstract]. Proc Am Thorac Soc 2006;167:A726.

79. Cardoso PF, Snell GI, Hopkins P, et al. Clinical application of airway bypass with paclitaxel-eluting stents: early results. J Thorac Cardiovasc Surg 2007;134:974–81.

80. Choong CK, Phan L, Massetti P, et al. Prolongation of patency of airway bypass stents with use of drug-eluting stents. J Thorac Cardiovasc Surg 2006;131:60–4.

81. Choong CK, Haddad FJ, Gee EY, et al. Feasibility and safety of airway bypass stent placement and influence of topical mitomycin C on stent patency. J Thorac Cardiovasc Surg 2005;129:632–8.

82. Ingenito EP, Berger RL, Henderson AC, et al. Bronchoscopic lung volume reduction using tissue engineering principles. Am J Respir Crit Care Med 2003;167:771–8.

83. Reilly J, Washko G, Pinto-Plata V, et al. Biological lung volume reduction: a new bronchoscopic therapy for advanced emphysema. Chest 2007;131:1108–13.

84. Criner GJ, Pinto-Plata V, Strange C, et al. Biologic Lung Volume Reduction in advanced upper lobe emphysema: phase 2 results. Am J Respir Crit Care Med 2009;179:791–8.

85. Celli BR, Cote CG, Marin JM, et al. The body-mass index, airflow obstruction, dyspnea, and exercise capacity index in chronic obstructive pulmonary disease. N Engl J Med 2004;350:1005–12.

Endoscopic Management of Emphysema

Armin Ernst, MD[a],*,
Devanand Anantham, MBBS, MRCP, FCCP[b]

KEYWORDS

- Emphysema • Chronic obstructive pulmonary disease
- Lung volume reduction surgery • Bronchoscopy
- Endoscopy • Airway bypass

Endoscopic techniques for the management of emphysema have evolved from the success of surgical treatment. Lung volume reduction surgery (LVRS) can potentially alter the natural history of chronic obstructive pulmonary disease (COPD). This procedure involves the surgical removal of 20% to 30% of each lung and targets the most emphysematous segments. Patients with heterogeneous upper lobe emphysema and a low baseline exercise capacity and those who are not at high surgical risk, that is, FEV_1 (forced expiratory volume in 1 second) greater than 20% and DLCO (diffusing capacity of the lung for carbon monoxide) greater than 20%, are identified as a subgroup within COPD, in whom improvements in exercise capacity and quality and quantity of life can be achieved.[1]

Airway narrowing and loss of elastic recoil cause expiratory airflow limitation in COPD. During exercise, increasing the respiratory rate shortens expiratory time, which results in air trapping. Air trapping reduces inspiratory capacity and limits ventilation (**Fig. 1**). Because of this restriction on inspiratory volumes, any increase in ventilation can be achieved only by further increasing respiratory rate, which in turn results in a vicious cycle of more air trapping. Air trapping and neuromechanical dissociation, that is, the disparity between respiratory efforts and ventilatory output, serve as the mechanistic links between exertion and dyspnea in COPD that are being targeted by LVRS.[2]

LVRS attempts to correct loss of elastic recoil by reducing the volume of the most damaged lung segments and allowing the remaining relatively less-damaged tissues to resize. Removing such dead space and eliminating parts of the emphysematous lung that have the longest expiratory time constants increases the exercise inspiratory capacity by reducing dynamic air trapping. The operating length of respiratory muscles is also normalized by restoring the normal dimensions of the diaphragm and chest wall.

Increased short-term mortality of about 5% and postoperative morbidity are the main limitations of LVRS.[1] The reported rate of intraoperative complications is 9% and that of postoperative complications is 58.7%, with elevated risks for reintubation (21.8%), arrthymias (18.6%), pneumonia (18.2%), readmission to the intensive care unit (11.7%), and tracheotomy (8.2%).[3] Air leaks with a median duration of 7 days were reported in 90% of patients.[4] The proportion of patients hospitalized, living in a nursing home or rehabilitation facility, or unavailable for interview in the National Emphysema Treatment Trial (NETT) study was 28.1% at 1 month and 14.3% at 2 months.[1] The price of this postoperative morbidity and mortality did not guarantee benefits. Only 30% of patients in the most favorable subgroup of COPD derived a clinically significant improvement in exercise capacity of more than 10 W, and 48% registered a greater

[a] Interventional Pulmonology, Beth Israel Deaconess Medical Center, Harvard Medical School, 330 Brookline Avenue, Boston, MA 02215, USA
[b] Department of Respiratory and Critical Care Medicine, Singapore General Hospital, Outram Road, Singapore 169608
* Corresponding author.
E-mail address: aernst@bidmc.harvard.edu (A. Ernst).

Clin Chest Med 31 (2010) 117–126
doi:10.1016/j.ccm.2009.08.001
0272-5231/10/$ – see front matter © 2010 Published by Elsevier Inc.

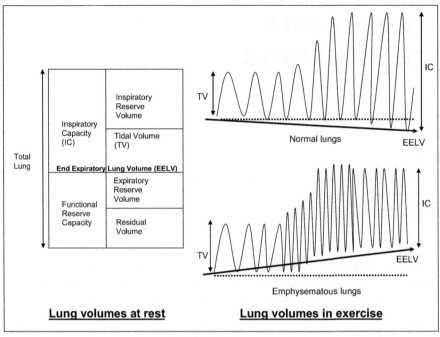

Fig. 1. Ventilatory limitation in patients with COPD during exercise because of air trapping that causes a reduction in inspiratory capacity.

than 8-point decrease in the St George Respiratory Questionnaire at 24 months.[1]

The extremely restrictive selection criteria for LVRS coupled with the relatively high mortality/morbidity and the associated costs in patients with even the lowest risk profile have been the impetus for developing less-invasive endoscopic modalities. Bronchoscopic lung volume reduction (BLVR) has pursued various approaches using a range of modalities, such as blockers, stents, valves, sealants, and implants. The physiologic basis of each modality is not identical and in some cases is distinct from conventional LVRS. The ideal indications also differ with some BLVR techniques targeting homogenous emphysema, whereas others target heterogeneous emphysema (**Box 1**).

ENDOBRONCHIAL BLOCKERS

The first published human data on BLVR reported the use of endobronchial blockers to occlude airways leading to emphysematous lung segments to cause resorption atelectasis. Silicone vascular balloons filled with radiopaque contrast were initially inserted bilaterally before custom-built stainless steel stents with a central occlusive biocompatible sponge were used.[5] However, the high rate of endobronchial blocker migration, postobstructive pneumonia, and need for repeat

endoscopic procedures have limited the further development of this technique.[5]

AIRWAY BYPASS

The creation of extra-anatomic bronchial fenestrations to deflate emphysematous lung parenchyma is called airway bypass. This technique relies on the presence of preexisting collateral ventilation. Collateral ventilation is defined as the ventilation of alveoli through anatomic channels that bypass the airways. These pathways include interalveolar

---

Box 1
Range of endoscopic modalities for the management of emphysema and target patient populations

Heterogeneous emphysema

    Endobronchial blockers

    Endobronchial valves

    Biologic sealants

Homogenous emphysema

    Airway bypass stents

Both homogenous and heterogeneous emphysema

    Airway implants or coils

pores, accessory bronchiole-alveolar connections, accessory respiratory bronchioles, and interlobar pathways across fissures.[6] Although collateral ventilation plays an insignificant role in normal lungs, these channels enable continued ventilation of severely obstructed areas in emphysema, where there is increased airflow limitation. The degree of collateral ventilation is also believed to correlate with the degree of homogeneity of emphysema.[7] In endoscopic airway bypass, low-resistance bronchial fenestrations allow trapped air to escape by bypassing obstructed airways, and consequently, emphysematous lung segments are drained via collateral ventilation.[8] Lung compliance is improved by reductions in resting dead space and dynamic hyperinflation. This improvement in lung compliance occurs without any actual change in pulmonary elastic properties and by simply increasing the inspiratory capacity available for gas exchange.[9]

Current airway bypass procedures are performed with the Exhale Emphysema Treatment System (Broncus Technologies, Inc, Mountain View, CA, USA) on patients with homogenous emphysema (Fig. 2). There are 3 steps that are performed via a flexible bronchoscope: (1) identification of an area of the segmental bronchi that is free from blood vessels using a Doppler probe, (2) fenestration of the airways, and (3) placement of a paclitaxel-eluting stent. Initial airway bypass

that used radiofrequency ablation to fenestrate the airways has been replaced by 25-G transbronchial needle puncture and balloon dilation. Paclitaxel is a mitotic inhibitor that prevents granulation tissue from obstructing the stent.

Published data on airway bypass is a multicenter, open-labeled study on 35 patients with homogenous emphysema who had bypass stents placed in both lungs.[10] A median of 8 stents, with a range of 2 to 12, were inserted. Efficacy data at 6 months were limited. Significant reductions were found in mean residual volume of 400 mL and dyspnea as measured on a modified Medical Research Council scale of 0.5 points.[10] No significant changes were recorded on spirometry, 6-minute walk, and St George Respiratory Questionnaire. The Exhale Airway Stents for Emphysema (EASE) study is a randomized, double-blind trial that recruited patients to clarify the efficacy of this technology.

One death from bleeding in the airways was reported with airway bypass procedures.[10] Data and safety monitoring board review of the fatal hemoptysis had the following recommendations, which were incorporated into subsequent procedures: placement of an endobronchial balloon blocker in the main bronchus and Doppler rescanning between fenestration by the transbronchial needle and stent deployment. Other patients had failure of stent implantation because of either the presence

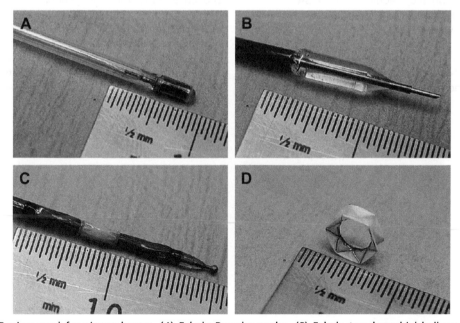

Fig. 2. Devices used for airway bypass. (A) Exhale Doppler probe. (B) Exhale transbronchial balloon dilation needle. (C) Exhale drug-eluting stent mounted on delivery catheter. (D) Exhale drug-eluting stent deployed. (*Reprinted from* Cardoso PF, Snell GI, Hopkins P, et al. Clinical application of airway bypass with paclitaxel-eluting stents: early results. J Thorac Cardiovasc Surg 2007;134(4):976; with permission from Elsevier.)[10]

of excessive peribronchial blood vessels or markedly increased airway wall thickness.[10] Postprocedure complications occurred in 22 of 37 (59%) cases, with COPD exacerbation in 32%, pneumomediastinum in 5%, and respiratory infection in 27%.[10] At follow-up bronchoscopy 6 months later, 69% of stents remained patent. Granulation tissue, radial traction by the surrounding airways, and secretions are the possible causes of stent occlusion.[11]

ENDOBRONCHIAL VALVES

Endobronchial valves are designed to exclude the worst affected emphysematous regions from ventilation and reduce dynamic air trapping. If segmental or lobar resorption atelectasis can be induced as an additional result, a physiologic effect similar to LVRS is expected. Therefore, patients with heterogeneous emphysema are suitable candidates for endobronchial valve therapy. Valves allow one-way flow of secretions and air out of an occluded pulmonary segment but prevent any distal flow. The ideal valve should be efficacious, easy to deploy, and readily removable to permit adjustments in position. These valves should also maintain patency, not migrate, and not compromise any future surgical interventions, such as LVRS or transplant.[12] Currently, 2 different endobronchial valve designs are being studied by Emphasys Medical, Inc, Redwood City, CA, USA, and Spiration, Inc, Redmond, WA, USA.

Emphasys technology uses a polymer, one-way duckbill valve (**Fig. 3**). The Zephyr valve has replaced the first-generation valves that were mounted on to a stainless steel cylinder attached to a self-expanding retainer. Zephyr valves are supported by a nitinol self-expanding tubular mesh retainer that is covered with a silicone membrane to form a seal between the valve and the bronchial wall. The valves are mounted on to a loading catheter and deployed via the working channel of a flexible bronchoscope. Deployment involves 2 stages: (1) an endoscopic measurement gauge is used to size the bronchial diameter before a valve of the equivalent size is chosen and (2) the loading catheter with the chosen valve is advanced to the target airway, and the valve is deployed by using an actuation handle. A perfectly positioned endobronchial valve can be visualized by bronchoscopy such that the proximal edge is sitting flush with the carina of the segmental bifurcation.

Spiration IBV valves have an umbrella-shaped nitinol framework comprising 6 support struts (**Fig. 4**). These struts are covered by a polyurethane membrane that seals the airways. Air and mucus can escape proximally around the edges of the membrane, but distal flow is limited. A central rod enables removal or repositioning of the valve. IBV valves are also deployed via a catheter loader through the working channel of a flexible bronchoscope after the airway orifice is endoscopically sized with a calibrated water-filled balloon.

The efficacy data for endobronchial valve therapy are inconclusive because all published studies were open-labeled trials with no control arms and had relatively short follow-up. The recently completed, but yet unpublished Endobronchial Valve for Emphysema Palliation Trial (VENT) study on Emphasys valves[13] and the currently recruiting Spiration IBV valve study aim to address these limitations. Data available on endobronchial valves describe procedures that were performed in 1 or both lungs with the intent of either lobar or nonlobar, that is, segmental,

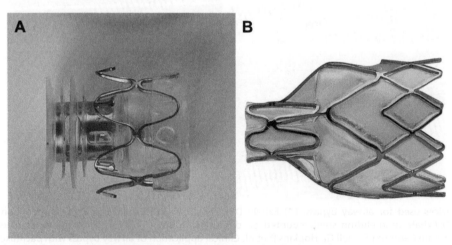

Fig. 3. (*A*) First-generation Emphasys valve. (*B*) Second-generation Zephyr valve.

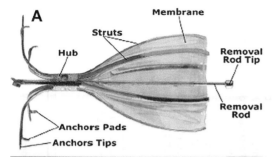

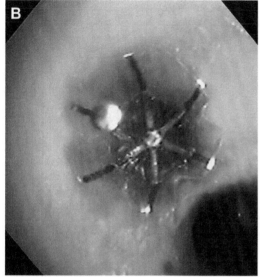

Fig. 4. (*A*) Intrabronchial valve and nomenclature. (*B*) Intrabronchial valve in an airway, as viewed with a flexible bronchoscope. (*Reprinted from* Wood DE, McKenna RJ Jr, Yusen RD, et al. A multicenter trial of an intrabronchial valve for treatment of severe emphysema. J Thorac Cardiovasc Surg 2007;133(1):73, e2; with permission from Elsevier.)[15]

exclusion using a wide variation in number of valves deployed (**Table 1**). The physiologic measures of improvements at 3 months were small. Minimal clinically important differences in FEV_1 were observed in 18% to 46% [12,14,15] and in 6-minute walk in 11% to 55% of patients.[12,14] The reported improvements in subjective parameters such as dyspnea and quality of life were more impressive. Up to 85% of patients reported a marked improvement in dyspnea at 30 days, and significant improvements on the St George Respiratory Questionnaire was a frequent finding.[14,16,17] Endobronchial valve therapy contrasts with LVRS in that patients who had unilateral lung intervention appeared to have better outcomes than those who had bilateral therapy.[12,18] The reasons for this interesting observation remain unknown.

Lobar atelectasis was not achieved in most patients, even with a lobar exclusion approach whereby all the bronchi to a target lobe are occluded with valves.[16,17] Incompleteness of fissures between lobes of the lung and collateral ventilation may have accounted for this finding. However, patients still recorded symptomatic benefits, which suggest that physiologic mechanisms besides improvements in lung compliance and chest wall dimensions may be in operation.[18,19] By occluding airways, valves increase resistance to airflow such that air is diverted to other relatively less emphysematous parts of the lung resulting in reduced dynamic air trapping. By excluding the most diseased parts of the lung from ventilation, physiologic dead space is reduced even in the absence of any atelectasis.[19] Therefore, FEV_1 or static lung volumes are unlikely to be the ideal measures of physiologic benefits of endobronchial valve therapy. This may explain the discrepancy between the limited gains in pulmonary function tests and the improvements in dyspnea. Other measures such as dynamic hyperinflation and composite scores such as the BODE index[19,20] may be more appropriate in future studies. Alternatively, subjective symptomatic improvements may be attributable to a placebo effect that can only be excluded in future studies that have appropriate control data.

Current data suggest that endobronchial valve therapy for emphysema is safer than LVRS (see **Table 1**). The reported mortality rate is approximately 1%, and hospital length of stay has been short with most patients discharged within 2 to 4 days.[12,14,15,21,22] The recorded death from endobronchial valve placement was attributed to postobstructive pneumonia. Postprocedure complications such as COPD exacerbations (6%–26%) and pneumothorax (7%–11%) were also reported.[12,14,15,21,22] The pneumothoraces occurred in patients who had an entire lobe successfully targeted for therapy.[12] During a lobar collapse, pleural adhesions may have caused visceral pleural tears and rapidly expanding bulla in adjacent lobes may have ruptured.[19] An ex vacuo phenomenon rather than an air leak may have also accounted for some of the pneumothoraces. Despite the single reported mortality, postobstructive pneumonia was not a commonly reported complication.

Technical challenges include difficulty in placement of endobronchial valves in some of the segmental bronchi in the upper lobes. When only moderate sedation is used instead of general anesthesia, respiratory movements and cough can impede accurate placement and adjustment of valves.[12,14] Hyperplastic granulation tissue proximal to the valves was also observed. This

Table 1
Summary of clinical data on endobronchial valve therapy in heterogeneous emphysema

Study	Target Population	Procedure	Outcomes at 3 Months Unless Otherwise Stated	Complications/LOS
Snell GI et al[21] Emphasys valves First generation Single center	n = 10 Age, 60 ± 6 y FEV$_1$, 0.7 ± 0.2 L (30 ± 11%)	Bilateral therapy Valves, 4–11 per patient Procedure duration, 115 ± 24.5 min (52–137 min)	Symptomatic improvement in 4 patients at 1 mo No change in radiology, FEV$_1$, or 6 MW at 1 mo	AECOPD, 2/10 (20%) Pneumothorax, 1/10 (10%) Pneumonia, 1/10 (10%) Mean LOS, 3.4 ± 2.1 d
Wan IY et al[12] Emphasys valves First generation Retrospective registry 9 centers in 7 countries	n = 98 Age, 63 ± 10 y FEV$_1$, 0.9 ± 0.3 L (30 ± 11%)	Unilateral, 64 (48 lobar and 16 nonlobar exclusion technique) Bilateral, 34 (21 lobar and 13 nonlobar exclusion technique) Valves, 4.0 ± 1.6 per patient	FEV$_1$ increase, 10.7 ± 26.2 % 6 MW increase, 23 ± 55.3% FEV$_1$ increase>15%, 45/98 (46%) 6 MW increase>15%, 54/98 (55%)	Death, 1/98 (1%) Pneumothorax, 3/98 (3%) BPF, 4/98 (4%) AECOPD. 17/98 (17%)

de Oliveira HG et al[15]
Longitudinal case series
Emphasys valves
First generation, 7
Second generation, 12
Single center
	n = 19
	Age, 68 ± 9 y
		Bilateral therapy, 8
		Right upper lobe, 11
		Procedure duration range,
		30–90 min
		Valves, 3.35 per patient
			FEV$_1$ increase>12%, 4/18 (22%)
			At 1 mo, 6/18 (33%) patients
			   had a 54 m improvement in 6 MW.
			Atelectasis, 2/19 (11%) patients
				AECOPD, 2/19 (11%)
				Pneumothorax, 2/19 (11%)
				Bronchial hypersecretion resulting in
				   valve removal, 1/19 (5%)
				LOS, 15/19 discharged from hospital
				   within 48 h

Wood DE et al[14]
Intrabronchial valves
from Spiration
5 centers
	n = 30
	Age, 64 ± 10 y
	FEV$_1$, 0.9 ± 0.3 L
	(31 ± 9%)
		Bilateral therapy
		Procedure duration, 65 ± 33
		min (15–125 min)
		Valves, 6.1 per patient
			SGRQ decrease>8, 10/28 (36%)
			FEV$_1$ increase>15%, 5/28 (18%)
			6MW increase>15%, 3/27 (11%)
			SGHQ at 6 mo, −6.8 ± 14.3
				AECOPD, 4/66 (6%)
				1 patient had postprocedure
				   bronchospasm, respiratory
				   distress, and myocardial
				   infarction.
				LOS, 27/30 patients discharged
				   within 2 d

Hopkinson NS et al[22],** Emphasys valves ** Overlap data 12 Single center	n = 19 Age, 58.7 ± 9 y FEV$_1$, 28 ± 12%	Unilateral therapy Valves inserted in staged manner 1–2 wk apart	Exercise testing* benefit in 9/19 (47%) * Endurance cycle ergometry at 80% maximal workload Atelectasis, 5/19 (26%)	Pneumothorax, 2/19 (11%) AECOPD, 5/19 (26%)

Mean data or proportions presented unless otherwise stated.
Abbreviations: AECOPD, acute exacerbation of COPD; BPF, bronchopleural fistula; LOS, hospital length of stay; SGHQ, St George Health Questionnaire; 6 MW, 6-minute walk.

granulation tissue may occlude the valves and prevent future removal, should the need arise.[14,15]

BIOLOGIC LUNG VOLUME REDUCTION

Biologic sealants (Aeris Therapeutics, Inc, Woburn, MA, USA) aim to reduce lung volume in heterogeneous emphysema by sealing off the most damaged areas. Unlike endobronchial valves or bypass, these sealants are designed to work at the alveolar level rather than in the airways. The mechanism of action involves resorption atelectasis from airway occlusion, subsequent airspace inflammation, and finally remodeling, which will lead to scarring and contraction of lung parenchyma. A mature scar and functional lung volume reduction can be expected within 6 to 8 weeks.[23] Collateral ventilation is unlikely to interfere with the formation of atelectasis because the sealant causes blockage of interalveolar and bronchiolar-alveolar collateral channels. This technology aims to achieve benefits by actual reductions in dead space and residual volume that is physiologically similar to LVRS.[24]

Biologic lung volume reduction is performed via flexible bronchoscopy, and the procedure time is about 6 to 12 minutes per bronchopulmonary subsegment.[23] After identifying a target region of emphysematous lung, the distal airways in this segment are collapsed by wedging the bronchoscope in the appropriate bronchial orifice and applying suction. Initially, 10 mL of a primer (5000 U porcine trypsin) is instilled via the bronchoscope working channel to deactivate surfactant and promote detachment of epithelial cells.[24] After 2 minutes, the primer is suctioned out and 10 mL of a cell culture media is used for wash out. A dual-lumen catheter (medical grade Pebax [Arkema, Colombes Cedex, France] construction with an outer diameter of 1.85 mm) is inserted through the working channel and advanced to within 2 cm of the distal end of the bronchoscope. A fibrinogen suspension and thrombin solution (1000 IU thrombin and 4.4 mg of calcium chloride) are then instilled simultaneously such that they are mixed in the lumen of the airways distal to the catheter tip. The fibrinogen suspension contains 266 mg of human fibrinogen, 9.3 mg of poly-L-lysine hydrobromide, 9.1 mg of shark sodium chondroitin sulfate, and 14 mg of tetracycline. After the delivery of the hydrogel, 60 mL of air is injected through the bronchoscope working channel to push the reagents distally. As the fibrinogen and thrombin mix, they polymerize into a hydrogel within 30 seconds. This hydrogel, which is biocompatible and biodegradable, serves as the sealant to effect biologic lung volume reduction.[23]

A phase 2, multicenter trial has assessed the safety and therapeutic dose of biologic lung volume reduction.[25] Bilateral therapy was instituted in 50 patients with upper lobe predominant emphysema. Eight bronchopulmonary subsegments were occluded either in a single endoscopic session or in a staged manner with 2 procedures. Patients were treated with either a low-dose therapy at 10 mL per subsegment of hydrogel or a high-dose therapy at 20 mL per subsegment. Serious adverse events were documented in 4 patients because of aspiration, pneumonia, pulmonary embolism, and severe pleurisy, with a subsequent fall secondary to analgesia. However, there were no documented fatalities. Procedure-related COPD exacerbations occurred in 22%, and 89% of patients had postoperative leucocytosis, fever, or malaise. The mean duration of hospitalization was approximately 2 days.

The primary efficacy endpoint of a significant reduction in gas trapping as measured by a decrease in residual volume (RV) or total lung capacity (TLC) at 3 months was met in both the low-dose and high-dose arms of the study.[25] However, this reduction was only sustained in patients receiving high-dose therapy at 6 months. Minimal clinically important differences at 6 months were identified in endpoints such as FEV_1 in 38% to 44%, 6-minute walk in 27%, and St George Respiratory Questionnaire in 32% to 46%. Spirometric improvements were greater in patients who received high-dose treatment. Radiologic evidence of remodeling correlated better with high-dose therapy than with low-dose therapy.

Therefore, biologic lung volume reduction appears safe, and a dose-dependent response was identified. To achieve the 20% to 30% of lung volume that is removed in LVRS, up to 12 subsegments may need to be sealed in future studies that assess efficacy.[24,26] Concerns also remain that any atelectasis may diminish with time because of metabolic dissolution of the hydrogel. Long-term follow-up data are required after treatment, and more stable formulations of sealant may be needed if these fears should materialize.[24]

AIRWAY IMPLANTS

Airway implants such as nitinol coils (PneumRx Inc, Mountain View, CA, USA) of 10 to 20 cm in length were designed to induce lung volume reduction in patients with either homogeneous or heterogeneous emphysema. These implants, which are straight when housed in the delivery catheter, coil up on deployment and tether the lung (**Fig. 5**). This is hoped to change the elastic

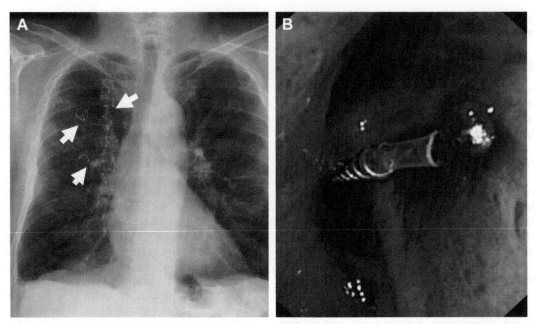

Fig. 5. Airway coil implants. (A) Chest radiograph view of deployed coil implants in the right upper lobe. (B) Endoscopic view of a deployed coil implant.

recoil and was shown to reduce lung volumes in explanted lungs.[27] The coils are inserted via flexible bronchoscopes under fluoroscopic guidance, with each insertion taking less than 2 minutes.[28] Preliminary safety data on 6 patients with either homogenous or heterogeneous emphysema have shown no evidence of pneumothorax, postobstructive pneumonia, or coil migration.[29] Bilateral lung volume reduction was attempted with coils inserted unilaterally at the initial setting and then placed in the contralateral lung 3 months later. Maximal reduction in lung volume occurred between 2 to 4 weeks after implantation and there is some suggestion of improvements in spirometry, exercise capacity, and quality of life.[28] Despite these promising results, concerns remain that the coils will cause bronchiectasis by distorting bronchi and pulmonary infarcts by kinking pulmonary vessels. If pleural adhesions are present, implanted coils can also be expected to cause visceral pleural tears and pneumothoraces. Therefore, more clinical data are needed to clarify the long-term safety and efficacy in defined patient populations.

ANESTHESIA FOR BLVR

Although most BLVR modalities can be performed under moderate or deep sedation, use of general anesthesia to maintain control over the airways and minimize coughing is still the current practice. The anesthetic challenges are similar in all techniques of BLVR because of the dual considerations of avoiding auto–positive end-expiratory pressure (PEEP) and the need to recover the patients rapidly after the procedure.[30] Auto-PEEP secondary to air trapping is a concern because of the degree of airflow obstruction secondary to emphysema. Obstruction of the endotracheal tube by the instruments being inserted to deploy the BLVR devices can also exacerbate auto-PEEP. Therefore, positive pressure ventilation with strict pressure limits (20 mm Hg), a low respiratory rate (10 breaths per minute), and a prolonged expiratory (inspiratory/expiratory ratio of 1:3) time is recommended.[30] Total intravenous anesthesia with propofol and remifentanil affords greater predictability and control. Unlike inhalational agents, this form of anesthesia does not depend on damaged, emphysematous lungs for either uptake or clearance. Remifentanil is rapidly metabolized and does not carry the risk of accumulation. These properties facilitate quick recovery of respiratory function postprocedure and avoid prolonged mechanical ventilation.

SUMMARY

BLVR, regardless of modality, appears to be safer than LVRS in terms of mortality and morbidity. This relatively better safety profile presents an attractive alternative to patients with COPD who are physiologically very fragile because of the severity of their lung disease and comorbid illnesses.

Efficacy data in the form of short-term, subjective improvement in dyspnea and quality of life are readily available from the currently published small, nonrandomized studies. This kind of data requires verification in larger studies that include a sham or placebo control group. Minimal clinically important differences in objective endpoints, such as spirometry and exercise capacity, were not a consistent finding in the current data. Differences in patient selection account for some of the heterogeneity of the results. Inclusion criteria for most BLVR studies have relied on the criteria used in the NETT trial, and refining patient selection to identify optimal candidates for individual BLVR modality will further improve outcomes in future. It is also hoped that the ongoing, larger randomized controlled trials will separate the therapeutic effect from the placebo effect of these endoscopic procedures.

There are other theoretical benefits of BLVR. LVRS causes peridiaphragmatic pleural scarring and can restrict diaphragm movement when lower lobe emphysema is treated. BLVR does not result in such scarring and may result in better postoperative functional outcomes. BLVR can also be performed via an endotracheal tube at the bedside of an intubated patient. Therefore, such an approach may enable stepwise and gradual therapy that may facilitate weaning of COPD patients from ventilators. BLVR modalities such as endobronchial valves are reversible and can be removed if nonbeneficial or if complications arise.

Although BLVR remains largely experimental and its benefits are unproven, the data that are emerging are promising. Perhaps in future, these endoscopic modalities can even be used in combination.[10] For example, endobronchial valves can target disease in heterogeneously diseased upper lobes, whereas airway bypass can aim to reduce hyperinflation in more homogenously affected lower lobes. BLVR may also serve as a bridge to LVRS or lung transplant. The evolution of these techniques coupled with the accumulating clinical experience aim to expand endoscopic technology such that most patients with severe COPD can in future be offered efficacious therapeutic options with far less risk of complications.

REFERENCES

1. Fishman A, Martinez F, Naunheim K, et al. A randomized trial comparing lung-volume-reduction surgery with medical therapy for severe emphysema. N Engl J Med 2003;348(21):2059–73.

2. O'Donnell DE. Hyperinflation, dyspnea, and exercise intolerance in chronic obstructive pulmonary disease. Proc Am Thorac Soc 2006;3:180–4.

3. DeCamp MM Jr, McKenna RJ Jr, Deschamps CC, et al. Lung volume reduction surgery: technique, operative mortality, and morbidity. Proc Am Thorac Soc 2008;5(4):442–6.

4. DeCamp MM, Blackstone EH, Naunheim KS, et al. NETT Research Group. Patient and surgical factors influencing air leak after lung volume reduction surgery: lessons learned from the National Emphysema Treatment Trial. Ann Thorac Surg 2006;82(1): 197–207.

5. Sabanathan S, Richardson J, Pieri-Davies S. Bronchoscopic lung volume reduction. J Cardiovasc Surg (Torino) 2003;44(1):101–8.

6. Cetti EJ, Moore AJ, Geddes DM. Collateral ventilation. Thorax 2006;61(5):371–3.

7. Higuchi T, Reed A, Oto T, et al. Relation of interlobar collaterals to radiological heterogeneity in severe emphysema. Thorax 2006;61(5):409–13.

8. Macklem PT. Collateral ventilation. N Engl J Med 1978;298(1):49–50.

9. Choong CK, Macklem PT, Pierce JA, et al. Airway bypass improves the mechanical properties of explanted emphysematous lungs. Am J Respir Crit Care Med 2008;178(9):902–5.

10. Cardoso PF, Snell GI, Hopkins P, et al. Clinical application of airway bypass with paclitaxel-eluting stents: early results. J Thorac Cardiovasc Surg 2007;134(4):974–81.

11. Rendina EA, De Giacomo T, Venuta F, et al. Feasibility and safety of the airway bypass procedure for patients with emphysema. J Thorac Cardiovasc Surg 2003;125(6):1294–9.

12. Wan IY, Toma TP, Geddes DM, et al. Bronchoscopic lung volume reduction for end-stage emphysema: report on the first 98 patients. Chest 2006;129(3):518–26.

13. Strange C, Herth FJ, Kovitz KL, et al. Design of the Endobronchial Valve for Emphysema Palliation Trial (VENT): a non-surgical method of lung volume reduction. BMC Pulm Med 2007;7:10.

14. Wood DE, McKenna RJ Jr, Yusen RD, et al. A multicenter trial of an intrabronchial valve for treatment of severe emphysema. J Thorac Cardiovasc Surg 2007;133(1):65–73.

15. de Oliveira HG, Macedo-Neto AV, John AB, et al. Transbronchoscopic pulmonary emphysema treatment: 1-month to 24-month endoscopic follow-up. Chest 2006;130(1):190–9.

16. Yim AP, Hwong TM, Lee TW, et al. Early results of endoscopic lung volume reduction for emphysema. J Thorac Cardiovasc Surg 2004;127(6):1564–73.

17. Venuta F, de Giacomo T, Rendina EA, et al. Bronchoscopic lung-volume reduction with one-way valves in patients with heterogenous emphysema. Ann Thorac Surg 2005;79(2):411–7.

18. Ingenito EP, Wood DE, Utz JP. Bronchoscopic lung volume reduction in severe emphysema. Proc Am Thorac Soc 2008;5(4):454–60.

19. Hopkinson NS. Bronchoscopic lung volume reduction: indications, effects and prospects. Curr Opin Pulm Med 2007;13(2):125–30.

20. Martinez FJ, Han MK, Andrei AC, et al. Longitudinal change in the BODE index predicts mortality in severe emphysema. Am J Respir Crit Care Med 2008;178(5):491–9.

21. Snell GI, Holsworth L, Borrill ZL, et al. The potential for bronchoscopic lung volume reduction using bronchial prostheses: a pilot study. Chest 2003; 124(3):1073–80.

22. Hopkinson NS, Toma TP, Hansell DM, et al. Effect of bronchoscopic lung volume reduction on dynamic hyperinflation and exercise in emphysema. Am J Respir Crit Care Med 2005;171(5):453–60.

23. Reilly J, Washko G, Pinto-Plata V, et al. Biological lung volume reduction: a new bronchoscopic therapy for advanced emphysema. Chest 2007;131(4):1108–13.

24. Ingenito EP, Tsai LW. Evolving endoscopic approaches for treatment of emphysema. Semin Thorac Cardiovasc Surg 2007;19(2):181–9.

25. Criner GJ, Pinto-Plata V, Strange C, et al. Biologic lung volume reduction in advanced upper lobe emphysema: phase 2 results. Am J Respir Crit Care Med 2009;179(9):791–8.

26. Pinto Plata V, Reilly J, Rafaely Y, et al. Biologic lung volume reduction for advanced emphysema. Chest 2006;130:121S.

27. Ost D, Ernst A, Maxfield R, et al. Evaluation of a bronchoscopically delivered non-valve implant that mechanically compresses diseased lung for the treatment of emphysema [abstract]. European Respiratory Society Congress 2008;192: 1588.

28. McKenna R, Ernst A, Maxfield R, et al. Novel implant device and procedure to compress lung parenchyma for the treatment of emphysema via bronchoscope [abstract]. European Respiratory Society Congress 2008;296:2825.

29. Herth F, Eberhardt R, Ernst A. Non-valve minimally invasive implantable device for the treatment of late stage homogeneous and heterogeneous emphysema—results of a feasibility trial [abstract]. European Respiratory Society Congress 2008;192: 1589.

30. Hillier JE, Toma TP, Gillbe CE. Bronchoscopic lung volume reduction in patients with severe emphysema: anesthetic management. Anesth Analg 2004;99(6):1610–4.

Bronchoscopic Management of Prolonged Air Leak

Douglas E. Wood, MD[a,b], Robert J. Cerfolio, MD[c,d], Xavier Gonzalez, MD[e], Steven C. Springmeyer, MD[e,f,*]

KEYWORDS

- Air leak • Bronchoscopy • Bronchial occlusion
- Bronchial valve • Endobronchial treatment
- Pneumothorax

A prolonged air leak is an important clinical problem and is generally a consequence of spontaneous pneumothorax caused by underlying lung disease; chest trauma, iatrogenic and otherwise; or pulmonary surgery, such as lung biopsy, segmentectomy, lung volume reduction, or anatomic resections when there are incomplete fissures separating the lobes of the lung. Prolonged air leaks after surgery have significant morbidity and increase costs.[1]

Primary spontaneous pneumothorax has an estimated incidence of 6 per 100,000 in men and 2 per 100,000 in women and rarely results in prolonged air leak.[2] Secondary spontaneous pneumothorax with chronic obstructive pulmonary disease (COPD) has a reported incidence of 26 per 100,000 per year.[3] These numbers have been extrapolated to estimate there are 4500 new cases of secondary pneumothorax per year in patients in the United States who have COPD.[4] With COPD and spontaneous pneumothorax, prolonged air leaks are more common with an incidence of approximately 20%.[5,6]

Prolonged air leaks are the most common complication after pulmonary resection[7] and have an average incidence of approximately 8% after segmental or wedge resection,[8] about 10% after lobectomy,[9] and 45% after lung volume reduction surgery (LVRS).[10]

CURRENT APPROACHES TO AIR LEAKS

Current management for prolonged air leaks include prolonged thoracostomy tube drainage (chest tube management); attempt at surgical repair; blood patch and pleurodesis.[11] If the air leak is manageable without chest tube suction and respiratory function is adequate, then outpatient management with a Heimlich valve attached to the chest tube is also feasible.[12,13] More recently, the use of self-contained portable chest tube drainage devices have been used over the Heimlich valve.[14] Although surgery may help to resolve an ongoing air leak, it is accompanied by significant morbidity, provides no assurance of correction, and in some cases creates the potential

Disclosures: Drs Wood and Cerfolio received support for research and consulting fees. Drs Gonzalez and Springmeyer are employees and stockholders of Spiration Inc.
^a Division of Cardiothoracic Surgery, Endowed Chair of Lung Cancer Research, University of Washington, Seattle, WA, USA
^b University of Washington Medical Center, 1959 NE Pacific, AA-115, Box 356310, Seattle, WA 98195 6310, USA
^c Section of Thoracic Surgery at University of Alabama at Birmingham, Birmingham, AL, USA
^d Department of Surgery, University of Alabama, 1900 University Boulevard, ZHR Building room 714, Birmingham, AL 35294, USA
^e Spiration Inc, 6675 185th Avenue NE, Redmond, WA 98052, USA
^f Division of Pulmonary and Critical Care Medicine, University of Washington, Seattle, WA, USA
* Corresponding author. Spiration Inc, 6675 185th Avenue NE, Redmond, WA 98052, USA.
E-mail address: sspringmeyer@spiration.com (S.C. Springmeyer).

Clin Chest Med 31 (2010) 127–133
doi:10.1016/j.ccm.2009.10.002
0272-5231/10/$ – see front matter

for an exacerbation of the problem in the creation of new areas of pulmonary injury. Timing and judgment to try surgical revision is very challenging, even for experienced thoracic surgeons, particularly in the presence of underlying lung disease. Infusion of autologous blood into the pleural space (blood patch) presumably helps to seal an air leak with the blood components that can initiate and support a fibrinous and inflammatory response and although many surgeons have adopted this as a therapy,[15] there is no substantive evidence that it results in earlier resolution of the air leak. Likewise, pleurodesis may indirectly impact an air leak by creating pleural symphysis and a localized inflammatory response, but data is lacking regarding its efficacy. In cases of a pleural space, pleurodesis is less likely to be effective and may be contraindicated. Unfortunately, no reliable and minimally invasive method is established for the management of prolonged air leaks.

CONSEQUENCES AND IMPACT OF AIR LEAKS

Prolonged air leaks may contribute directly to respiratory failure by increasing the work of breathing. Prolonged air leaks more often contribute to other complications that are associated with limited activity, continuing pain medications, and prolonged hospitalizations. These complications include pneumonia, deep venous thrombosis, pulmonary embolus, atelectasis, subcutaneous emphysema, empyema, deconditioning, and nosocomial infections.[7]

The presence of postoperative air leaks has a significant impact on the length of the hospital stay and complications. In 91 postoperative patients with pulmonary resection, the patients with air leak after 3 days had longer length of stay (mean of 9.4 days vs 5.4 days).[16] Similarly, in 552 postoperative patients after LVRS in the National Emphysema Treatment Trial, the patients with air leak had more complications (57% vs 30%, $P<.01$) and longer LOS (11.8 days vs 7.6 days, $P<.01$).[17]

DEFINITION, CLASSIFICATION, AND MEASUREMENT OF AIR LEAKS

The definition of prolonged air leak used in the literature is often 7 days or longer,[18] but others have been as short as 3 days.[16] There are three major factors to be considered for evaluating air leaks: the volume, duration, and trend of the leakage. For example, an air leak of larger volume, longer duration, and showing no improvement would exhibit a combination of factors that indicate a low likelihood of early resolution, and

therefore the need for an earlier intervention. Conversely, a small or moderate volume leak that is improving each day is likely to resolve spontaneously and does not warrant intervention. There are additional factors, such as patient comorbidities, that influence the decision to intervene with a prolonged air leak. However, a definition of prolonged air leak by duration alone is not adequate to capture the details needed for management decisions.

There are multiple ways to evaluate the volume of air leaks and most are simple and based on observing the water seal chamber. Most common in clinical use is a simple description, such as mild, moderate, or severe. This method lacks standardization and validation among observers. An alternative is the Cerfolio Classification System that is also based on observation, but is less subjective, is validated, and is reproducible among observers.[13] In this classification there are four categories based on the timing of the air leak in the respiratory cycle (**Box 1**), coupled with the grading or sizing of the air leak as measured by an air leak meter. More recently, several companies have developed commercially available digital devices that quantify the size of the air leak.[19]

BRONCHOSCOPIC APPROACHES TO AIR LEAKS

Different types of bronchoscopic approaches to treating air leaks have been tried over the years. This is not surprising because there are patients with prolonged air leaks that are poor surgical candidates or have already exhausted all the usual approaches. The challenge to the bronchoscopic approach is to localize the airways connected to the leak, followed by placement of an occluding device or substance. An ideal device or substance

---

Box 1
Four classifications of air leak in the Cerfolio System

1. Continuous (C): present throughout the respiratory cycle

   • Tends to be in patients receiving positive pressure ventilation

2. Inspiratory (I): present during the inspiration phase of the respiratory cycle

   • Like continuous air leaks, patients with this pattern are often on a ventilator

3. Expiratory (E): present only during expiratory phase of the respiratory cycle

4. Forced Expiration (FE): present only when patient coughs or forces exhalation

would (1) block distal air flow without stopping proximal decompression of air or secretions, (2) be easily and selectively placed, and (3) be removable or absorbable. Many different approaches were tried and there were sporadic reports of success, but an evidence-based guideline in 2001 by the American College of Chest Physicians (ACCP) provided good consensus that patients should not undergo bronchoscopic techniques to attempt to seal endobronchial sites of air leaks.[20] Guidelines and review articles after 2001 on treatment of spontaneous pneumothorax were silent on bronchoscopic approaches,[21,22] but there continued to be reports about the use of various agents with the bronchoscope. The history and agents used have recently been reviewed by Lois and Noppen.[23] **Box 2** is a partial list of the many devices, sealants, chemicals, or physical agents that have been reported to be tried by using a bronchoscope to treat air leaks.

The Watanabe Spigot (Novatech, Cedex, France) is the only bronchial blocker specifically made to reduce a persistent air leak by occluding the affected bronchus. The Watanabe spigot is a silicone plug that comes in multiple sizes (**Fig. 1**) and has been used for prolonged air leaks in Japan and the United States.[24,25] Watanabe and colleagues treated 60 patients and produced air leak reduction in 38% and stoppage in 40% using an average of 4.0 spigots per case.

BRONCHOSCOPIC LOCALIZATION OF THE AIRWAY LEADING TO THE LEAK

A bronchoscopic approach to stopping an air leak is dependent on identifying the airway leading to the leakage. The most common approach is to perform selective airway occlusion with a balloon catheter while observing the air coming through the chest tube for 20 to 30 seconds[24] or 1 to 3

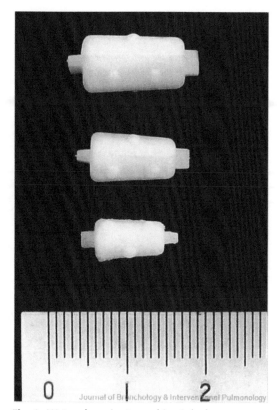

Fig. 1. Watanabe spigots used in air leak cases.

minutes.[26] There are multiple commercially available balloon catheters that are compatible with flexible bronchoscopes and can be used for this purpose. The balloon may allow the identification of a segment or subsegment that communicates with the leak. In some cases, cessation of the leak may be immediate and complete with test occlusion of a segmental or subsegmental airway, but it is common that sublobar occlusion will result in only a significant decrease in the air leak, rather than complete resolution. Test occlusion of adjacent segments may also have an effect showing that it is sometimes necessary to treat more than one segment or subsegment to maximize the outcome. However, it is generally preferable to test and treat at a sublobar level, avoiding occlusion of an entire lobe that is associated with lobar atelectasis.[27] In addition, blocking the ventilation to less tissue is going to have less impact on patients' work of breathing, especially when there is underlying lung disease.

BRONCHIAL VALVES FOR AIR LEAKS

Small, but encouraging trials with LVRS in the mid 1990s prompted the development of less invasive methods for lung volume reduction. Two companies, Emphasys Medical (**Fig. 2**) and Spiration

---

Box 2
Agents, chemicals, and objects used with a bronchoscope to stop air leaks

Glues or adhesives: fibrin, albumin, glutaraldehyde, or acrylic

Gel foam or cellulose

Ethanol

Antibiotics

Metal coils

Decalcified spongy calf bone

Watanabe spigots

Cautery

Laser

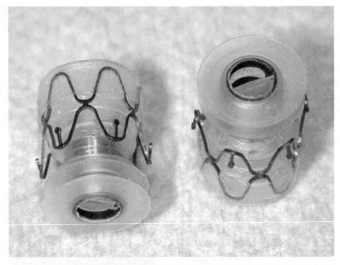

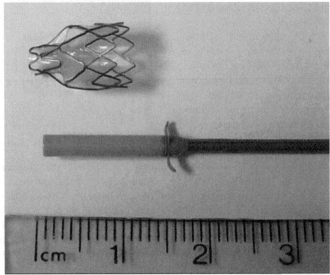

Fig. 2. The EBV valves used in air leak cases, classic and transcopic. The catheter for delivery is also shown with the transcopic valve.

(**Fig. 3**), began developing bronchial valves for blocking air flow to selected areas of lung to create lung volume reduction and redirect airflow to the less diseased lung parenchyma.[28,29] Spiration recognized in 2001 that a bronchial valve could be an effective and minimally invasive intervention for air leaks because the valve could reduce air flow through the leaking tissue, facilitating local tissue healing and spontaneous resolution (S. Springmeyer, MD, personal communication, 2009).

However, it was also understood that a clinical trial to meet US Food and Drug Administration (FDA) standards for effectiveness would be very difficult because prolonged air-leak cases were sporadic, heterogeneous, and not predictable. For this reason, Spiration defined a select group of postoperative patients after surgical resection

and initiated an application with the FDA in 2003 for humanitarian use device designation. The companies also did preclinical work with air leaks and these provided encouraging results. Wood and colleagues[30] used ex-vivo human and animal tissue to establish proof-of-concept. Fann and colleagues[31] also showed proof-of-concept using thoracotomy and in-vivo lung laceration while giving positive pressure ventilation.

After bronchial valves entered investigational use in patients with emphysema, the possibility arose for treating prolonged air leaks under compassionate use regulations. Case reports using the Emphasys bronchial valve (EBV) first appeared in 2005. Snell and colleagues in Melbourne reported a 53-year-old man with 6 years of bronchio-cutaneous fistula from aspergillosis treated with

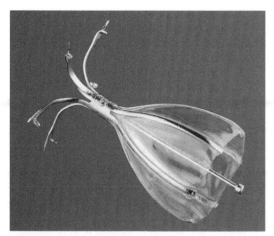

Fig. 3. The IBV Valve used in air leak cases. (*Courtesy of* Spiration, Inc; with permission.)

resection and thoracoplasty. Repeated attempts at muscle transpositions had failed. Four months after placing four EBV valves, the air leak was resolved.[32] In 2006 there were successful reports from five institutions about seven patients. The etiologies for the prolonged air leak were varied and included after segmentectomy for bronchiectasis, LVRS, wedge resection, catheter placement, feeding tube misplacement, thoracentesis, and spontaneous.[33–37] Two more successfully treated cases were published in 2007[26] and a case series was recently published.[38]

The Travaline and colleagues[38] case series summarizes the 4-year experience with 40 subjects from 17 centers using bronchial valves for prolonged air leaks. The subjects had a mean duration of air leak of 119 days (median 20 days) before treatment. The etiology of the air leaks were diverse and included postsurgical, iatrogenic, spontaneous pneumothorax (primary and secondary), trauma, cancer, COPD, and pneumonia. Other treatments before the bronchial valves had been tried in five subjects. After isolation of the feeder airway and bronchial valve placement, there was complete resolution in 48% and partial resolution in an additional 45%, so that 37 of 40 subjects (93%) responded to bronchial valve treatment. A mean of 2.9 (±1.9) valves were used and adverse events occurred in six subjects (15%). One was pneumonia and another was bacterial colonization, whereas two were valve related (expectoration and malpositioning). The authors concluded that bronchial valves are an effective intervention for prolonged air leak.

REGULATORY STATUS AND APPROVALS OF BRONCHIAL VALVES

The Emphasys Medical valve (EBV) and the Spiration IBV Valve System received approval for marketing in the European Union. The IBV valve approval is for treating diseased (emphysema) and damaged (air leak) lung. In the United States, the IBV valve received humanitarian use device designation in 2006, and then approval under the Humanitarian Device Exemption program,[39] which supports the development of medical devices intended to benefit patients in the treatment of diagnosis of diseases or conditions affecting fewer than 4000 people in the United States per year. The FDA approval is for patients who have undergone partial or total removal of a lung lobe or lung volume reduction surgery and who experience prolonged air leaks or significant air leaks that are likely to become prolonged, defined as follows: an air leak still present on the seventh day after surgery is considered prolonged unless it is observed only during forced exhalation or cough, whereas an air leak present on the fifth day after surgery is considered a significant air leak that is likely to become prolonged if the leak is continuous, present during inhalation, or present during exhalation and accompanied by subcutaneous emphysema or respiratory compromise.

In summary, prolonged air leaks are significant clinical problems. In the past, many bronchoscopy approaches to prolonged air leaks have met with limited and inconsistent success, with no widely accepted or established treatment. The recent development of bronchial valves offers a new treatment option. Multiple reports of successful bronchial valve treatment of air leaks along with humanitarian use approval of a bronchial valve for certain postsurgical air leaks suggests there is a role for endobronchial valve treatment of prolonged air leaks. The scope of this role, breadth of indications and contraindications, and overall effectiveness of bronchial valve treatment of air leak requires additional clinical experience that is now possible given the FDA approval of the Spiration IBV Valve System for selected postsurgical patients with prolonged air leaks.

REFERENCES

1. Shrager JB, DeCamp MM, Murthy SC. Intraoperative and postoperative management of air leaks in patients with emphysema. Thorac Surg Clin 2009; 19:223–31.
2. Dines DE, Clagett OT, Payne WS. Spontaneous pneumothorax in emphysema. Mayo Clin Proc 1970;45:481–7.
3. Melton LJ, Hepper NCG, Offord KP. Incidence of spontaneous pneumothorax in Olmstead County Minnesota: 1950–1974. Am Rev Respir Dis 1979; 120:1379–82.

4. Shen KR, Cerfolio RJ. Decision making in the management of secondary spontaneous pneumothorax in patients with severe emphysema. Thorac Surg Clin 2009;19:233–8.

5. George RB, Herbert SJ, Shanes JM, et al. Pneumothorax complicating pulmonary emphysema. JAMA 1975;234:389–93.

6. Videau V, Pillgram-Larsen J, Oyvind E, et al. Spontaneous pneumothorax in COPD; complications, treatment and recurrences. Eur J Respir Dis 1987;71: 365–71.

7. Cerfolio RJ. Advances in thoracostomy tube management. Surg Clin North Am 2002;82:833–48.

8. Jones DR, Stiles BM, Denlinger CE, et al. Pulmonary segmentectomy: results and complications. Ann Thorac Surg 2003;76:343–8.

9. Stolz AJ, Schützner J, Lischke R, et al. Predictors of prolonged air leak following pulmonary lobectomy. Eur J Cardiothorac Surg 2005;27:334–6.

10. Ciccone A, Meyers B, Guthrie T, et al. Long term outcome of bilateral lung volume reduction in 250 consecutive patients with Emphysema. J Thorac Cardiovasc Surg 2003;125:513–25.

11. Cerfolio RJ, Trummala RP, Holman WL, et al. A prospective algorithm for the management of air leaks after pulmonary resection. Ann Thorac Surg 1998;66:1726–31.

12. McKenna RJ, Fischel RJ, Brenner M, et al. Use of the Heimlich valve to shorten hospital stay after lung reduction surgery for emphysema. Ann Thorac Surg 1996;61:1115–7.

13. Cerfolio RJ, Bass CS, Pask AH, et al. Predictors and treatment of persistent air leaks. Ann Thorac Surg 2002;73:1727–31.

14. Cerfolio RJ, Minnich DJ, Bryant AS. The removal of chest tubes despite an air leak or a pneumothorax. Ann Thorac Surg 2009;87:1690–6.

15. Oliveira FH, Cataneo DC, Ruiz RL Jr, et al. Persistent pleuropulmonary air leak treated with autologous blood: results from a university hospital and review of literature. Respiration 2009. [Epub ahead of print].

16. Bardell T, Petsikas D. What keeps post pulmonary resection patients in hospital? Can Respir J 2003; 10:86–9.

17. DeCamp MM, Blackstone EH, Naunheim KS, et al. Patient and surgical factors influencing air leak after lung volume reduction surgery: lessons learned from the National Emphysema Treatment Trial. Ann Thorac Surg 2006;82:197–207.

18. McKenna RJ Jr, Benditt JO, DeCamp M, et al. Safety and efficacy of median sternotomy versus video-assisted thoracic surgery for lung volume reduction surgery. J Thorac Cardiovasc Surg 2004;127: 1350–60.

19. Cerfolio RJ, Bryant AS. The benefits of continuous and digital air leak assessment after elective pulmonary resection: a prospective study. Ann Thorac Surg 2008;82:396–401.

20. Baumann MH, Strange C, Heffner JE, et al. ACCP consensus panel. Management of spontaneous pneumothorax. Chest 2001;119:590–602.

21. Henry M, Arnold T, Harvey J. Pleural Diseases Group, Standards of Care Committee, British Thoracic Society. BTS guidelines for the management of spontaneous pneumothorax. Thorax 2003; 58:ii39–52.

22. Tschopp JM, Rami-Porta R, Noppen M, et al. Management of spontaneous pneumothorax: state of the art. Eur Respir J 2006;28:637–50.

23. Lois M, Noppen M. Bronchopleural fistulas. Chest 2005;128:3955–65.

24. Watanabe Y, Matsuo K, Tamaoki A, et al. Bronchial occlusion with endobronchial Watanabe spigot. J Bronchol 2003;10:264–7.

25. Weinreb N, Riker D, Beamis J, et al. Ease of use of watanabe spigot for alveolopleural fistulas. J Bronchol Intervent Pulmonol 2009;16:130–2.

26. Toma TP, Kon OM, Oldfield W, et al. Reduction of persistent air leak with endoscopic valve implants. Thorax 2007;62:829–32.

27. Springmeyer SC, Bolliger CT, Waddell TK, et al. Treatment of heterogeneous emphysema using the Spiration IBV valves. Thorac Surg Clin 2009;19: 247–53.

28. Toma TP, Hopkinson NS, Hillier J, et al. Bronchoscopic volume reduction with valve implants in patients with severe emphysema. Lancet 2003; 361:931–3.

29. Wood DE, McKenna RJ Jr, Yusen RD, et al. A multicenter trial of an intrabronchial valve for treatment of severe emphysema. J Thorac Cardiovasc Surg 2007;133:65–73.

30. Wood D, Gonzalez X, Sirokman W, et al. Reduction of severe air leaks using an intra-bronchial valve delivered via flexible bronchoscopy. Am J Respir Crit Care Med 2004;169:A480.

31. Fann JI, Berry GJ, Burdon TA. The use of endobronchial valve device to eliminate air leak. Respir Med 2006;100:1402–6.

32. Snell G, Holsworth L, Fowler S, et al. Occlusion of a broncho-cutaneous fistula with endobronchial one-way valves. Ann Thorac Surg 2005;80:1930–2.

33. Feller-Kopman D, Bechara R, Garland R, et al. Use of a removable endobronchial valve for the treatment of bronchopleural fistula. Chest 2006;130: 273–5.

34. Ferguson JS, Sprenger K, Van Natta T. Closure of a bronchopleural fistula using bronchoscopic placement of an endobronchial valve designed for the treatment of emphysema. Chest 2006;129:479–81.

35. Mitchell KM, Boley T, Hazelrigg SR. Endobronchial valves for treatment of bronchopleural fistula. Ann Thorac Surg 2006;81:1129–31.

36. De Giacomo T, Venuta F, Diso D, et al. Successful treatment with one-way endobronchial valve of large air-leakage complicating narrow-bore enteral feeding tube malposition. Eur J Cardiothorac Surg 2006;30:811–2.

37. Anile M, Venuta F, De Giacomo T, et al. Treatment of persistent air leakage with endobronchial one-way valves. J Thorac Cardiovasc Surg 2006;132:711–2.

38. Travaline JM, McKenna RJ, DeGiacomo T, et al. Treatment of persistent pulmonary air leaks using endobronchial valves. Chest 2009;136:355–60.

39. FDA News. FDA approves lung valve to control some air leaks after surgery. Available at: http://www.fda.gov/NewsEvents/Newsroom/Press Announcements/2008/ucm116970.htm. Accessed June 26, 2009.

Bronchial Thermoplasty

Gerard Cox, MB, FRCP(C), FRCP(I)

KEYWORDS

• Asthma • Thermoplasty • Broncoconstriction • Allergy

Airway narrowing is a central event in asthma.[1] Contraction of airway muscles, or bronchoconstriction, is a dynamic process that contributes to airway narrowing in asthma and has long been the target of treatment with drugs that cause muscle relaxation.[1,2] Since inflammatory events underlie asthma, therapy typically includes antiinflammatory agents.[3,4] The current standard-of-care has been defined by a variety of expert groups and evidence-based guidelines for the treatment of asthma have been published.[5] As asthma is most often mild or moderate, it can be appropriately managed provided there is adequate compliance with prescribed measures; typically included in these are bronchodilating and antiinflammatory medications.[5]

Asthma, by definition is a variable disease. When there is greater than normal natural variation in airflow, the illness can be provoked by a wide range of stimuli that include infectious, allergic, and environmental agents.[6] Bronchoconstriction determines much of the short-term variability in airflow that characterizes asthma.[1,6] Development of bronchoconstriction is facilitated because the airways in asthma are hyperresponsive in that they can constrict to a greater degree and are more sensitive than normal.[7]

In chronic asthma, certain characteristic structural abnormalities are found in the airway walls.[8] These changes are collectively termed remodeling. Excessive accumulation of smooth muscle is typical of airway remodeling and has been found in the airways of patients with a range of severity of asthma.[8,9] Such remodeling of the airway wall, with increased smooth muscle along with heightened connective tissue elements and mucus glands may contribute further to the airway narrowing that is fixed and largely resistant to conventional asthma treatment.[1,3,6,8] It is not surprising that airflow obstruction as a result of tissue changes in the airway does not improve with bronchodilators; antiinflammatory therapy that controls cellular changes including eosinophilia has also not been found to reverse remodeling of the airway walls.[8]

Thus, there is evident need for new approaches that target airway smooth muscle. Ideally, such a treatment should address both mechanisms of airway narrowing, that is, preventing bronchoconstriction and reducing the amount of muscle in the remodeled airway. Such an intervention should have a prolonged effect.

DEVELOPMENT OF THE ALAIR SYSTEM FOR BRONCHIAL THERMOPLASTY

Thermoplasty refers to the use of heat to induce structural changes. Bronchial thermoplasty (BT) is performed during bronchoscopy using the Alair system, which comprises a specially designed treatment catheter and a radiofrequency (RF) controller.[10] The energy delivered at each treatment site is about 18 W. This is substantially lower than the energy used in other procedures that use RF for cautery or tissue ablation. For example, the Prosiva system for treating benign prostatic hypertrophy delivers 30 W for 2 to 3 minutes and the COBRA surgical probe delivers up to 150 W. When passed through the working channel of an (adult) bronchoscope, the electrode array at the end of the catheter is expanded to touch the airway wall under direct vision. Once contact is achieved, a 10-second pulse of RF energy is delivered, and the array is collapsed and moved 5 mm proximally to the next treatment site.

Firestone Institute for Respiratory Health, St Joseph's Healthcare Hamilton, 50 Charlton Avenue E, Hamilton, ON L8N 4A6, Canada
E-mail address: coxp@mcmaster.ca

Clin Chest Med 31 (2010) 135–140
doi:10.1016/j.ccm.2009.09.003

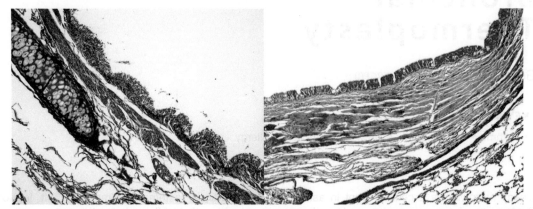

Fig. 1. Histology of canine airway 3 years after treatment, stained with Masson's trichrome. Control airway in the left panel was untreated and shows normal airway wall elements including bundles of smooth muscle. The panel on the right shows a treatment site, which contains reduced amounts of smooth muscle. In addition, the area previously occupied by muscle now contains connective tissue elements with no evidence of excessive collagen deposition or scarring.

The Alair system was developed over a series of preclinical studies and was first applied in the canine airway.[11] The treatment effect was dependent on the temperature reached in the airway wall. During preclinical studies parameters for energy delivery, duration of treatment, and temperature were examined. The optimal parameters that led to stable partial reduction in muscle mass without excessive tissue injury were identified. Histologic examination of treated sites revealed that smooth muscle was replaced with connective tissue elements.[11] Long-term studies of 3 years showed no evidence of scarring and the effect on reducing muscle mass was stable (**Fig. 1**). Functionally, airways treated with BT contracted less following methacholine instillation than untreated sites and this effect was related to the degree to which muscle was reduced (**Fig. 2**).[11,12]

High-resolution computed tomography (HRCT) has been used to examine structural and functional changes in airways over time.[13] After BT, canine airways were significantly less sensitive to challenge with aerosolized methacholine. Bronchoconstriction of treated airways continues to some degree indicating that BT reduces, but does not completely ablate, the mass of airway smooth muscle.[11] Furthermore, there was a detectable increase in the baseline diameter of treated airways consistent with lower tone as a result of the reduced amount of muscle present. That the maximal postbronchodilator diameter was similar in treated and control airways shows that relaxation is not impaired. Treated airways were more distensible suggesting that when muscle is replaced by connective tissue elements the stiffness or elasticity of the airway is not adversely affected.[14] This functional outcome

echoes the histology findings, which showed no evidence of scar formation over 3 years following BT (see **Fig. 1**).

HUMAN STUDIES OF BT

BT was first applied in the human airway in patients who were scheduled for surgery for

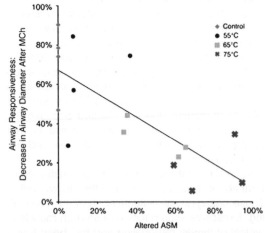

Fig. 2. Relationship between the potential for stimulated bronchoconstriction and the amount of smooth muscle present in the airway wall, expressed as how much of the circumference of the airway contained recognizable muscle bundles. Untreated airways had almost complete circumferential muscle layer and narrowed by 80%. Treatment at increasing temperatures caused dose-dependent reduction in the amount of muscle, which correlated with diminished bronchoconstriction following local instillation of methacholine. (*From* Danek C, Lombard CM, Dungworth DL, et al. Reduction in airway hyperresponsiveness to methacholine by the application of RF energy in dogs. J Appl Physiol 2004;97:1949; with permission.)

suspected lung cancer.[15] At the time of bronchoscopy, which was performed 1 to 3 weeks before surgery, BT was performed in normal-appearing airways in the areas to be removed. Following resection, histologic comparison of treated and untreated sites showed less smooth muscle in airways treated with BT. The extent and nature of the treatment effects in the human airway closely resembled those documented in the canine airway.[11,15] Over an interval of 1 to 3 weeks, there was evidence of resolution of the acute changes that follow treatment. The epithelium, which can be injured mechanically by the catheter and by heat, was largely reconstituted between the second and third weeks. As had been seen in the canine airway, the tissue changes were temperature dependent.

Mayse and colleagues[16] provided a description of how to use the Alair system for performing BT in patients with asthma. Although general anesthetic was used for the very first procedure, local anesthetic and moderate or conscious sedation are now standard.[16,17] This is an outpatient procedure, performed in endoscopy or bronchoscopy units. Typically, it takes 3 separate procedures, usually 3 weeks apart, to treat the entire bronchial tree (except the right middle lobe because of concerns about causing the right middle lobe syndrome). All airways that can be accessed are targeted for treatment. The catheter is deployed only under direct vision; airways outside the bronchoscopic field of view are not treated. Thus, any treated airway can be inspected later in case there are any concerns. The Alair catheter must be partially expanded before it can be activated. Hence, it can treat airways with a diameter between 3 and 10 mm. The treatment begins as distally as possible. The RF energy is delivered at 5-mm intervals, providing continuous treatment to the airway (as the exposed section of the electrode is 5-mm long). In practice, each procedure lasts between 45 and 60 minutes; the duration is determined mainly by the number of treatment activations delivered. Since the endobronchial anatomy and caliber can vary considerably among patients, the number of activations per procedure is quite variable but is expected to average between 40 and 60. At the time of treatment, there is little if any evidence of heat effect. The most common observations are blanching of the airway when there is contact with electrode arms. A buildup of mucus on the electrode array may occur and may need to be removed to prevent the field of view being obscured. As a mechanical device is being deployed, superficial trauma to the airway is inevitable. Minor immediate bleeding, or more often oozing, is observed occasionally, but is minimal and self-limited. Since the energy delivered is modest and the temperature in the tissues reaches 65°C, there is no evidence of tissues burning or of sparking.

TREATING ASTHMA WITH THE ALAIR SYSTEM FOR BT

BT for asthma was first studied in 16 patients with a range of asthma severity.[17] This study showed that it was feasible to perform BT safely in patients with asthma. In addition, certain asthma parameters (numbers of symptom-free days and peak expiratory flows) showed improvements at 3 months. Bronchial hyperresponsiveness was reduced and this effect persisted beyond 12 months. Treatment was well tolerated and adverse events that occurred following bronchoscopy were managed with the same measures used to treat usual exacerbations of asthma symptoms.

The impact of BT in 109 patients with moderate to severe asthma was examined in the Asthma Intervention Research (AIR) trial.[18] Asthma severity was indicated by medication, all subjects were using at least 200 µg/d of inhaled corticosteroids (ICS) for maintenance treatment (**Table 1**). All subjects also required treatment with long-acting β-agonists (LABA) shown by deterioration in asthma control on withholding LABA for 2 weeks.

The group that underwent treatment with the Alair system showed statistically significant reduction in their rates of mild exacerbations. They also enjoyed improvements in a number of other parameters including asthma quality of life, asthma control, use of rescue medication and numbers of symptom-free days (**Table 2**). Performing BT causes temporary worsening of asthma symptoms that usually begins on the day of the procedure. Subjects in the AIR trial had severe asthma to begin with; on occasion, their symptoms were severe enough to require hospital admission soon after treatment, which did not occur in the previous trial (**Table 3**). There were 6 hospitalizations among 55 subjects who had undergone 161 treatment procedures compared with 2 admissions for asthma deterioration in 54 control subjects. Reassuringly, these adverse events following BT are familiar problems that respond typically within 1 week to usual measures for care of asthma exacerbations.

A population with even more severe asthma was enrolled in the Research in Severe Asthma (RISA) trial.[19] The 32 subjects had higher requirements for maintenance medications that included oral corticosteroids (OCS), and had other evidence of more severe asthma than the subjects in either of the 2 previous trials (see **Table 1**). At 22 weeks

Table 1
Comparison of inclusion criteria for clinical trials of BT for asthma

	Feasibility	AIR	RISA	AIR2
Age (y)	18–65	18–65	18–65	18–65
ICS dose (μg/d) (beclomethasone or equivalent)	≤1800	≥200	>1500	>1000
LABA dose (μg/d) (salmeterol)	0–100	≥100	≥100	≥100
OCS dose (mg/d)	0	0	≤30	≤10
Pre-BD FEV$_1$ (% predicted)	>65 (post-BD)	60–85	≥50	≥60
Symptoms	Not required	Worse with LABA withdrawal	Symptoms on ≥10/ 14 d, or rescue med use on ≥8/14 d	≥2/28 d

after treatment, subjects followed an algorithm to taper their steroid dose providing control of their asthma did not deteriorate. This is the only time that reductions in antiinflammatory therapy were advocated in subjects undergoing BT. Because the therapeutic rationale for BT is that it reduces the amount of smooth muscle in the airway, it is expected that following successful treatment patients would still need to take their antiinflammatory medications.[10] The difference in severe asthma is that patients may be taking excessive doses of steroids and that reduction in the dosage may be possible if asthma control is improved by some other means.

According to various parameters, the group treated with the Alair system showed improvement in the control of their asthma.[19] There were significantly greater improvements in asthma quality of life, asthma control questionnaire score, and use of rescue medications (see **Table 2**). Doses of steroids for maintenance treatment were reduced in both groups and the difference between them was not statistically different (the trial had insufficient power to detect this difference as only half of the subjects were taking oral steroids at entry).

There was an increase in the severity of adverse events encountered in the actively treated group compared with previous trials probably related to the severity of asthma of the subjects (see **Table 3**). There were 5 hospital admissions within 1 week of 45 procedures in the BT-treated group.

Even though multiple studies reported benefits following treatment with BT, it should be recognized that there is substantial potential for placebo effect, especially with a novel procedure.[20] Thus, the Asthma Intervention Research 2 (AIR2) trial was designed with a control group that underwent 3 bronchoscopies and sham treatment with the Alair system.[21] This comprised placement of the treatment catheter in targeted airways, expansion of the electrode array but no delivery of RF energy when the controller was activated. The selection of subjects was designed to enroll subjects with asthma of sufficient severity to have large potential for benefit, but not so severe as to be at high risk of requiring hospitalization should asthma symptoms worsen post procedure.[18,19] A total of 297 subjects with severe asthma and persistent symptoms were randomized 2:1 to active and sham control groups. The primary outcome was a

Table 2
Comparison among studies of outcomes indicating benefit from BT

Feasibility	AIR	RISA	AIR2
Well tolerated	Exacerbations	AQLQ	AQLQ
PEF	AQLQ	ACQ	Severe exacerbations
Symptom-free days	Symptom-free days	Rescue medications	ER visits
Hyperresponsiveness	Rescue medications	[Reduced oral steroids $P = .12$]	Time lost from work/ school

Table 3
Comparison among studies of rates of hospitalization in the period following treatment bronchoscopy

	AIR		RISA		AIR2	
	Alair (n = 55)	Control (n = 54)	Alair (n = 15)	Control (n = 17)	Alair (n = 190)	Sham (n = 98)
No. hospitalizations (no. of subjects)	6 (4)	2 (2)	7 (4)	0 (0)	19 (16)	2 (2)
No of bronchoscopies	161	—	45	—	558	292
Events/bronch (%)	3.7	—	15.6	—	3.4	0.7

change in the asthma quality of life questionnaire (AQLQ) score. This improved in both groups, but to a statistically significant greater extent in the BT group compared with the sham group.[22] Secondary outcomes showed trends for benefit from BT that were not statistically significant. Safety was reported by rates of hospitalization and other health care use at 2 time intervals: around the time of treatment and from then to the end of 1 year (see **Table 2**). The selection criteria were successful in excluding subjects at risk of severe asthma exacerbation following the procedure, and this was confirmed by the rate of hospitalization, which approximated that found in the AIR trial and was substantially less than in the RISA trial (see **Table 3**). Use of health care resources, such as unscheduled office or emergency department visits, and admissions were lower in the BT-treated group than the sham control group during the second interval of follow-up (see **Table 2**).[22]

LONG-TERM CLINICAL FOLLOW-UP

There has been speculation from the very outset regarding the possibility of certain adverse outcomes developing late after BT. One specific concern relates to the potential for long-term damage to treated airways because of scar formation or to loss of integrity of the airway wall. It is now possible to begin to address such concerns with data from long-term follow-up of treated patients. HRCT examinations have been performed annually for 5 years in the subjects who participated in the feasibility trial. Treated airways appear normal, without evidence of either airway stenosis or dilation (bronchiectasis). There was also no evidence of damage to the parenchyma adjacent to treated airways indicating the treatment effect is limited to the airways.

Longer term follow-up of subjects who were treated in the Feasibility, AIR, AIR2 and RISA trials

now exceeds 500 patient-years. The majority of subjects report either stable or improved control of their asthma. Pre- and postbronchodilator FEV_1 has remained stable over 3 or more years in subjects who completed the first 3 studies. This experience suggests there are no late developing adverse consequences of treating asthmatic airways with BT.

SUMMARY

Despite major progress in developing medical treatments for asthma, a substantial proportion of patients continue to suffer from inadequate control of their disease.[23] In others, although their disease can be controlled this requires such high doses of medications that side effects are troublesome.[24,25] Current treatments do not redress the excess smooth muscle mass that is present in the remodeled airway in chronic asthma. Thus, it is intriguing to consider the potential contribution of BT (a procedure that involves controlled heat treatment to reduce the mass of the airway smooth muscle) as an effective therapy for poorly controlled asthma. If effective, BT would reverse the excess accumulation of muscle in the airway and reduce the potential for bronchoconstriction. Although the short-term increase in asthma symptoms (requiring hospitalization at times) is evident, these should be weighed against the benefits that are present for a prolonged time (>1 year in all trials to date). Even though the results of 4 clinical trials show benefits following BT in patients with asthma ranging from mild to severe, it is most likely that this treatment will be indicated for patients with severe asthma that is not well controlled by combinations of currently available therapies. These are the patients who most need an additional effective asthma therapy and, based on the results of trials published to date, have the greatest potential to benefit from BT.

REFERENCES

1. Doherty DE. The pathophysiology of airway dysfunction. Am J Med 2004;117(Suppl 12A):11S–23S.
2. Sears MR, Lövtall J. Past, present and future-β_2-adenoreceptor agonists in asthma management. Respir Med 2005;99:152–70.
3. Djukanovic R, Roche WR, Wilson JW, et al. Mucosal inflammation in asthma [State of the art]. Am Rev Respir Dis 1990;142:434–57.
4. Drazen JM. Asthma therapy with agents preventing leukotriene synthesis or action. Proc Assoc Am Physicians 1999;111:547–59.
5. Global Initiative For Asthma. Global strategy for asthma management and prevention. National Heart, Lung, and Blood Institute/World Health Organization. 2002. Publication Number 02-3659. Bethesda (MD): National Institutes of Health.
6. Holgate ST, Polosa R. The mechanisms, diagnosis, and management of severe asthma in adults. Lancet 2006;368:780–93.
7. Cockroft DW, Killian DN, Mellon JJA, et al. Bronchial reactivity to inhaled histamine: a method and clinical survey. Clin Allergy 1977;7:235–43.
8. Bergeron C, Boulet LP. Structural changes in airway diseases: characteristics, mechanisms, consequences, and pharmacologic modulation. Chest 2006;129:1068–87.
9. Carroll N, Elliot J, Morton A, et al. The structure of large and small airways in nonfatal and fatal asthma. Am Rev Respir Dis 1993;147:405–10.
10. Cox PG, Miller J, Mitzner W, et al. Radiofrequency ablation of airway smooth muscle for sustained treatment of asthma: preliminary investigations. Eur Respir J 2004;24:659–63.
11. Danek C, Lombard C, Dungworth D, et al. Reduction in airway hyperresponsiveness to methacholine by the application of RF energy in dogs. J Appl Physiol 2004;97:1946–53.
12. Miller P, Danek CJ, Cox G, et al. Development of a bronchoscopic technique for airway diameter measurement. Chest 2001;120:229S.
13. Brown RH, Wizeman W, Danek C, et al. In vivo evaluation of the effectiveness of bronchial thermoplasty with computed tomography. J Appl Physiol 2005;98:1603–6.
14. Brown RH, Wizeman W, Danek C, et al. Effect of bronchial thermoplasty on airway distensibility. Eur Respir J 2005;26:277–82.
15. Miller JD, Cox G, Vincic L, et al. A prospective feasibility study of bronchial thermoplasty in the human airway. Chest 2005;127:1999–2006.
16. Mayse ML, Laviolette M, Rubin AS, et al. Clinical pearls for bronchial thermoplasty. J Bronchol 2007;14:115–23.
17. Cox G, Miller JD, McWilliams A, et al. Bronchial thermoplasty for asthma. Am J Respir Crit Care Med 2006;173:965–9.
18. Cox G, Thomson NC, Rubin AS, et al. AIR Study Group. Asthma control during the year after bronchial thermoplasty. N Engl J Med 2007;356:1327–37.
19. Pavord ID, Cox G, Thomson NC, et al. RISA Trial. Study Group Safety and efficacy of bronchial thermoplasty in symptomatic, severe asthma. Am J Respir Crit Care Med 2008;176:1185–91.
20. Wechsler ME. Bronchial thermoplasty for asthma: a critical review of a new therapy. Allergy Asthma Proc 2008;29:365–70.
21. Cox G, Israel E, Jarjour N, et al. AIR2 Trial: execution of a sham-controlled double-blind study of a novel device for the treatment of severe asthma. Am J Respir Crit Care Med 2009;179:A2787.
22. Castro M, Rubin AS, Laviolette M, et al. Effectiveness and safety of bronchial thermoplasty in the treatment of severe asthma: a multicenter, randomized, double-blind, sham-controlled clinical trial. Am J Respir Crit Care Med 2009. [Epub ahead of print].
23. Dolan CM, Fraher KE, Bleecker ER, et al. TENOR Study Group. Design and baseline characteristics of the epidemiology and natural history of asthma: outcomes and treatment regimens (TENOR) study: a large cohort of patients with severe or difficult-to-treat asthma. Ann Allergy Asthma Immunol 2004;92(1):32–9.
24. Peters SP, Ferguson G, Deniz Y, et al. Uncontrolled asthma: a review of the prevalence, disease burden and options for treatment. Respir Med 2006;100:1139–51.
25. Beasley R. Unmet need in inadequately controlled asthma. Respirology 2007;12(Suppl 3):S18–21.

Airway Stents

Pyng Lee, MD[a,*], Elif Kupeli, MD[b], Atul C. Mehta, MD[c,d]

KEYWORDS

- Tube stents
- Metal stents
- Airway stenosis
- Aortic allograft

A stent is a hollow, cylindrical prosthesis that maintains luminal patency and provides support. It is named after Charles Stent, a British dentist, who created dental splints in the nineteenth century, and stenting of the airway has been practiced for more than a century. Stents are used for providing a barrier effect by protecting the airway lumen from tumor or granulation tissue ingrowth, for splinting effect by counterbalancing the extrinsic pressure exerted on the airway, or for both.[1] The covering provides the barrier effect, whereas dynamic and static properties determine the splinting effect.[2]

The first stents were implanted surgically by Trendelenburg[3] and Bond[4] for the treatment of airway strictures, which quickly progressed to endoscopic application by Brunings and Albrecht[5] in 1915. In 1965, Montgomery[6] designed a T-tube with an external side limb made of silicone and rubber for the treatment of subglottic stenosis. Since then, silicone has become the most commonly used material for stents. However, the designs of the silicone stents at that time abolished the innate mucociliary mechanisms essential to clear the airway of secretions. The real breakthrough in airway stenting was achieved when Dumon[7] presented a dedicated tracheobronchial prosthesis that could be introduced with the rigid bronchoscope. These straight stents made of silicone, with studs on the outer wall that reduce interference to the ciliary action, are relatively inexpensive and can be easily removed when needed. However, these stents require rigid bronchoscopy for their placement, and only 5% of the pulmonologists surveyed in North America are trained in the procedure.[8] Moreover, the silicone stent is poorly

tolerated in the subglottis, and it tends to migrate when used to treat complex tracheal strictures. These limitations have led to the modification of metal stents that were originally developed for the vascular system for use in the tracheobronchial tree.[9,10] Although metal stents are easy to apply via flexible bronchoscopy, they are fraught with problems, such as tumor or granulation tissue ingrowth around the struts and epithelialization into the airway wall, which makes removal difficult and challenging.[10]

Therefore, the search for an ideal stent that is (1) easy to insert and remove, (2) customized to fit the dimensions and shape of the stricture, (3) able to reestablish the airway and maintain luminal patency with minimum rate of migration, (4) made of an inert material that does not irritate the airway, precipitate infection, or promote granulation tissue formation, (5) able to exhibit similar clearance characteristics like the normal airway so that mobilization of secretions is not impaired, and (6) economically affordable (**Box 1**) has become the holy grail of interventional pulmonologists, radiologists, thoracic surgeons, and otolaryngologists alike.

INDICATIONS FOR AIRWAY STENTING

Approximately 30% of patients with lung cancer present with central airway obstruction, of whom 35% will die as a result of asphyxia, hemoptysis, and postobstructive pneumonia.[11] Airway stenting is a valuable adjunct to the other therapeutic bronchoscopic techniques, which not only results in rapid relief of symptoms and improved quality of life but also gives time for adjuvant

[a] Department of Respiratory and Critical Care Medicine, Singapore General Hospital, Singapore
[b] Department of Pulmonary Medicine, Mesa Hospital, Turkey
[c] Sheikh Khalifa Medical City, Abu Dhabi, UAE
[d] Respiratory Institute, Cleveland Clinic Foundation, Cleveland, OH, USA
* Corresponding author.
E-mail address: lee.pyng@sgh.com.sg (P. Lee).

Clin Chest Med 31 (2010) 141–150
doi:10.1016/j.ccm.2009.08.002

<table>
<tr><td>

Box 1
Characteristics of an ideal stent

1. Easy to insert and economically affordable.
2. Available in different sizes and lengths appropriate to relieve airway obstruction.
3. Reestablish the airway with minimal morbidity and mortality.
4. Sufficient expansive strength to resistive compressive forces and elasticity to conform to airway contours.
5. Maintain luminal patency without causing ischemia or erosion into adjacent structures.
6. Minimal migration but can be easily removed if necessary.
7. Made of inert material that will not irritate the airway, precipitate infection, or promote granulation tissue formation.
8. Preserves mucociliary function of the airway for mobilization of secretions.

</td><td>

Box 2
Indications for airway stenting

Malignant neoplasm

1. Airway obstruction from extrinsic bronchial compression or submucosal disease.
2. Obstruction from endobronchial tumor when patency is less than 50% after bronchoscopic laser therapy.
3. Aggressive endobronchial tumor growth and recurrence despite repetitive ablative treatments.
4. Loss of cartilaginous support from tumor destruction.
5. Sequential insertion of airway and esophageal stents for tracheoesophageal fistulas.

Benign airway disease

1. Fibrotic scar or bottleneck stricture after

    a. Posttraumatic: intubation, tracheostomy, laser, and balloon bronchoplasty

    b. Postinfectious: endobronchial tuberculosis, histoplasmosis-fibrosing mediastinitis, herpes virus, diphtheria, klebsiella rhinoscleroma

    c. Postinflammatory: Wegener granulomatosis, sarcoidosis, inflammatory bowel disease, foreign body aspiration

    d. Post-lung transplantation anastomotic complications

2. Tracheobronchomalacia

    a. Diffuse: idiopathic, relapsing polychondritis, tracheobronchomegaly (Mounier-Kuhn syndrome)

    b. Focal: tracheostomy, radiation therapy, post-lung transplantation

3. Benign tumors

    a. Papillomatosis

    b. Amyloidosis

</td></tr>
</table>

chemoradiotherapy that might lead to prolonged survival.[1,11–14] Chhajed and coworkers[15] have demonstrated no survival difference between those patients without malignant airway obstruction who received palliative chemotherapy (median survival, 8.4 months) and others with airway obstruction who received treatment with laser (25%), stent (25%), or both (50%) followed by chemotherapy (median survival, 8.2 months; $P = .395$). Contrary to previous perception, airway obstruction is not a poor prognostic sign if treated appropriately.

Benign strictures secondary to postintubation injury, inflammatory diseases, and infectious diseases may require stenting if the patient's underlying disease or associated comorbidity prohibits definitive surgical repair. Lung transplant recipients who develop airway dehiscence in the immediate postoperative period may benefit from the placement of endobronchial stents. The Cleveland clinic experience of using uncovered metal stent as an alternative treatment for high-grade anastomotic dehiscence after lung transplantation in 7 patients deemed high risk for second operation demonstrated not only that airway healing is satisfactory but also that stent removal is not difficult if performed within 8 weeks before epithelialization takes place.[16] **Box 2** details the indications for stent placement.

TYPES OF STENTS

A variety of stents are available for application in the tracheobronchial tree, and the biomechanical properties depend on the materials used and how they are constructed (**Box 3, Table 1**). Stents are grouped into (1) tube stents which include Montgomery T-tube (Boston Medical Products, Boston, MA, USA), Dumon (Novatech, France), Polyflex (Boston Scientific, Natick, MA, USA), Noppen (Reynders Medical Supplies, Lennik, Belgium), and Hood (Hood Laboratories, Pembroke, MA, USA); (2) metal covered and uncovered stents, such as Palmaz (Cordis Corp, Miami, FL, USA) and Ultraflex stents (Boston Scientific, Natick, MA, USA); and (3) hybrid stents that are made of silicone and reinforced by metal rings,

Box 3
Characteristics of metallic stents

Balloon expandable

Strecker (Boston Scientific)

   Tantalum monofilament knitted into a wire mesh, most useful in narrow stenoses.

Palmaz (Corning/Johnson & Johnson, NJ, USA)

   Stainless steel tube with rectangular slots along the long axis, may collapse with strong external pressure (eg, vigorous cough).

Self-expandable

Wallstent (Boston Scientific)

   Wire mesh made of cobalt-based alloy filaments and coated with silicone, uncovered metallic ends prevent migration. Rarely used.

Ultraflex

   Cylindrical wire mesh of nitinol, which is available in covered and uncovered form.

for example, Orlowski (Rüsch Incorporated, Duluth, GA, USA) and Dynamic stents (**Figs. 1** and **2**).

Major advantages of tube stents are that they allow repositioning and removal without difficulty and they are relatively inexpensive. Disadvantages include stent migration, granuloma formation, mucous plugging, insufficient flexibility to conform to irregular airways, interference with mucociliary clearance, and a need for rigid bronchoscopy for their placement (**Table 2**). Expertise in rigid bronchoscopy to deploy and remove tube stents poses an obstacle that limits their use because pulmonologists' training in rigid bronchoscopy has dramatically declined worldwide.[8]

TUBE STENTS
Montgomery T-tube

After its introduction in 1965, the Montgomery T-tube has undergone only slight modifications and continues to be used for the treatment of subglottic and tracheal stenosis.[6] Earlier models made of acrylic were later replaced with those made of silicone rubber. They are available in different diameters and variable lengths for the 3 limbs. The prerequisite for this stent is a tracheostomy, and the stent can be placed during operation or via rigid bronchoscopy. The limb protruding out of the tracheostoma is left open for cricoid or glottic stenosis, unplugged transiently for bronchial toilet, or closed to allow speech. Migration is rarely encountered, as 1 limb is fixed in the tracheostomy opening. High mucosal pressure is not required to hold the stent in position and blood and lymphatic flows to the sensitive upper trachea are not compromised, thereby making the Montgomery T-tube especially safe for high tracheal stenosis.

Dumon Stent

Dumon[7] initially described his experience with a new dedicated tracheobronchial prosthesis made of silicone with studs. A multicenter trial[17] followed 1058 patients in whom 1574 stents were performed, of which 698 were for malignant

Table 1
Characteristics of tube stents

Montgomery T-tube	Designed for treatment of subglottic and midtracheal stenosis. Introduced through a tracheostomy with the side tube protruding through the stoma, the proximal limb within the stenosis, and the distal limb into the distal trachea
Dumon	Silicone tube with external studs to prevent migration, most widely used silicone stent. Y shaped and right main bronchus designs are available
Hood	Smooth silicone tube with flanges to prevent migration. L- or Y-shaped designs available
Noppen	Screw-thread cylindrical silicone prosthesis, more rigid than regular silicone tubes. Needs a special introducer, and cannot be folded into an applicator for bronchoscopic insertion
Dynamic	Silicone Y-stent with the anterior and lateral wall reinforced by steel struts to simulate tracheal wall. Requires special forceps with rigid laryngoscope
Polyflex	Self-expandable stent made of polyester wire mesh with a thin layer of silicone.
Alveolus	Hybrid stent that conforms to airway tortuosity without foreshortening on deployment. It can be deployed with the rigid or flexible bronchoscope

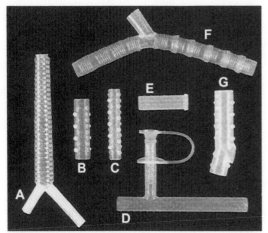

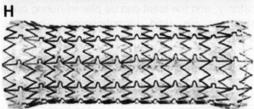

Fig. 1. Types of tube and hybrid stents. (*A*) Rusch stent, (*B*) Dumon tracheal stent, (*C*) Dumon bronchial stent, (*D*) Montgomery T-tube, (*E*) Hood bronchial stent, (*F*) Orlowski stent, and (*G*) Hood custom tracheobronchial stent. (*H*) Hybrid stent (Alveolus) can be deployed with flexible or rigid bronchoscope without foreshortening.

airway obstruction. Stent migration occurred in 9.5% of the patients, granuloma formation in 8%, and stent obstruction by mucus in 4% during a mean follow-up of 4 months for malignant stenoses and 14 months for benign stenoses. In a similar study conducted by Diaz-Jimenez and colleagues,[18] 125 silicone stents were placed in 60 patients with malignant disease and 30 patients with benign tracheobronchial disease. Migration was observed in 13%, granuloma in 6%, and mucous plugging in 2% of the patients. Lower

complication rates were observed by Cavaliere and colleagues,[11] when a series of 393 silicone stents were placed in 306 patients with malignant airway strictures. Stent migration was observed in 5% and granuloma formation in 1%.

After its introduction, the Dumon stent has become the most frequently used stent worldwide and is considered the "gold standard" by many experts. Stents with different diameters and lengths are available for structural stenoses of the trachea, mainstem bronchus, and bronchus intermedius of adults and children. A recent addition is a bifurcated model known as Dumon Y stent (Tracheobronxane Y, Novatech, France) which can be applied to palliate lower tracheal and/or main carinal stenoses. However, because good contact pressure between the airway wall and the studs is required to prevent stent migration, it is not ideal for tracheobronchomalacia or to bridge tracheoesophageal fistula.

Noppen Stent

The Noppen stent is made of Tygon (Reynders Medical Supplies, Lennik, Belgium) and has a corkscrew-shaped outer wall that prevents migration by generating friction between the airway and stent. Results of a study that compared the use of Noppen stents with the Dumon stents demonstrated lower migration rate for benign tracheal stenoses with use of the former.[19]

Polyflex Stent

The Polyflex stent is a self-expanding stent made of cross-woven polyester threads embedded in silicone. Its wall to inner diameter is thinner than the Dumon or Noppen stents. This stent can be used to treat benign and malignant strictures and tracheobronchial fistula. Stents of different lengths and diameters and tapered models are available for sealing stump fistula. Incorporation of tungsten into the stent makes it radiopaque; however, the

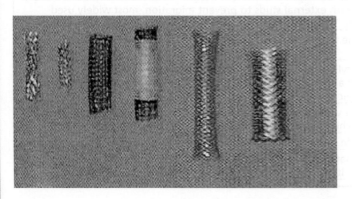

Fig. 2. Types of metallic stents. (*Left to right*) Palmaz stent, Tantalum Strecker stent, uncovered Ultraflex stent, covered Ultraflex stent, uncovered Wallstent, and covered Wallstent.

Table 2
Comparison of the Dumon stent and the covered Ultraflex stent

Characteristics	Dumon Stent	Covered Ultraflex Stent
Mechanical considerations		
High internal to external diameter ratio	−	+++
Resistant to recompression when deployed	+	++
Radial force exerted uniformly across stent	+	++
Absence of migration	−	++
Flexible for use in tortuous airways	−	+++
Removable	+++	−
Dynamic expansion	−	++
Can be customized	+++	−
Tissue-stent interaction		
Biologically inert	++	++
Devoid of granulation tissue	+	−
Tumor ingrowth	++	+
Ease of use		
Can be deployed with flexible bronchoscopy	−	+++
Deployed under local anesthesia with conscious sedation	−	++
Radiopaque for position evaluation	−	+++
Can be easily repositioned	++	−
Cost		
Inexpensive	+	−

−, poor; +, fair; ++, good; +++, best.

outer surface is smooth, which increases the risk for migration. In a small series of 12 patients in whom 16 Polyflex stents were used for benign airway disorders, such as anastomotic stenosis after lung transplantation, tracheal stenosis, tracheobronchomalacia, tracheobronchopathia osteochondroplastica, relapsing polychondritis, and bronchopleural fistula, the reported complication rate was alarmingly high at 75% even though immediate palliation was achieved in most cases (90%). Stent migration was the most common complication that occurred between 24 hours and 7 months after deployment. Notably, all 4 patients with lung transplant–related anastomotic stenoses encountered complications with the Polyflex stents; 2 had significant mucous plugging requiring emergent bronchoscopy, whereas the stents migrated in the other 2 patients. The investigators have since abandoned the use of Polyflex stents in their practice.[20]

Hood Stent

The Hood stent is made of silicone, and it can be dumbbell shaped for bronchial anastomosis or tube shaped with flanges customized to an L- or Y shape.

Dynamic Stent

The dynamic stent (Rüsch Y stent, Rüsch AG Duluth, GA) is a bifurcated silicone stent that is constructed to simulate the trachea. It is reinforced anteriorly by horseshoe-shaped metal rings that resemble tracheal cartilages and a soft posterior wall that behaves like the membranous trachea by allowing inward bulge during cough. Stent fracture from fatigue and retained secretions are rarely encountered, and the stent is used for strictures of the trachea, main carina and/or main bronchi; tracheobronchomalacia; tracheobronchomegaly, and esophageal fistula.

METALLIC STENTS

Metallic stents are gaining popularity because of their ease of insertion. They can be placed at an outpatient setting via flexible bronchoscopy and under local anesthesia.[21,22] They are categorized into 2 by the method of deployment: balloon expandable and self-expanding. A balloon-expandable stent consists of a stent balloon assembly and relies on the balloon to dilate it to its correct diameter at the target site. A self-expanding stent has a shape memory that enables it to assume its predetermined configuration when released from a constraining delivery catheter.

Advantages of metallic stents for the management of malignant tracheobronchial obstruction include their (1) radiopaque nature that allows radiographic identification, (2) greater airway cross-sectional diameters because of thinner walls, (3) ability to conform to tortuous airways, (4) preservation of mucociliary clearance and ventilation when placed across a lobar bronchial orifice, and (5) ease of insertion when compared with tube stents. Major disadvantages include granulation tissue formation within the stent and difficulty in removal or repositioning after stent epithelialization, which usually occurs in 6 to 8 weeks (see **Table 2**).

Palmaz and Strecker Stents

The balloon-expandable stents (Palmaz and Strecker) can be dilated to diameters of 11 to 12 mm, and they are primarily restricted for use in children. The Palmaz stent is not indicated for adults because strong external force from vigorous cough or compression from an enlarging tumor or adjacent vascular structure can cause stent collapse, obstruction, and migration.[23]

The Strecker stents are available in 20- to 40-mm lengths and are used for precise stenting of short-segment stenoses because they do not foreshorten on deployment.[24] Palmaz and Strecker stents are uncovered and are therefore unsuitable for malignant lesions because they do not protect against tumor ingrowth and may become loose when these stenoses improve after chemoradiotherapy.

The Wallstent and Ultraflex stents are self-expanding stents. They do not require hooks to prevent migration because they have outward radial force that is uniformly applied over the bronchial wall, which stabilizes the stent and reduces the risk of perforation. They are easy to deploy and are available in covered forms.

The Wallstent is a self-expandable wire mesh made of cobalt-based superalloy monofilaments (**Fig. 3**). Dasgupta and coworkers[9] used 52 uncovered Wallstents in 37 patients, 20 with malignant airway obstruction and 17 with benign disease. Stent-related obstructive granuloma occurred in 11% of patients; 2 patients developed staphylococcal bronchitis which necessitated stent removal in 1 patient. Stent migration and mucous plugging were, however, not observed.

The Ultraflex is a self-expanding stent made of nitinol (**Fig. 4**). Nitinol is an alloy with shape memory, which deforms at low temperatures and regains its original shape at higher temperatures. Miyazawa and coworkers[25] deployed 54 Ultraflex

stents in 34 patients with inoperable malignant airway stenoses via flexible or rigid bronchoscopy. Immediate relief of dyspnea was achieved in 82% of the patients, who also had corresponding improvements in spirometry. Retained secretions and migration were not observed. Stent removal and repositioning was possible in 1 case of misplacement, and the Ultraflex stent was found to be safe for subglottic stenosis. Herth and colleagues[26] further demonstrated that the Ultraflex stents could be placed satisfactorily without fluoroscopy, thus minimizing radiation exposure to patients and staff.

Long-term outcome of patients with malignant and benign airway strictures treated with Wallstents and Ultraflex stents was analyzed. Median follow-up was 42 days for patients with lung cancer, 329 days for lung transplant recipients, and 336 days for other benign conditions. No cases of mucous plugging, fistulous formation, or fatal hemoptysis were observed. Overall observed complication rate was 0.06 complications per patient-month. The most common complication

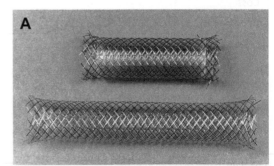

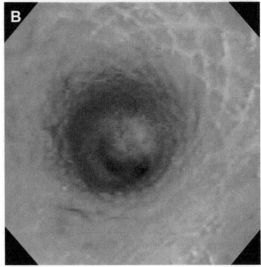

Fig. 3. (A) Covered and uncovered Wallstents. (B) Wall stent in main bronchus.

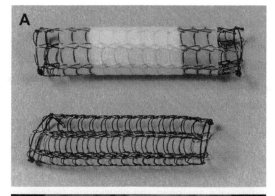

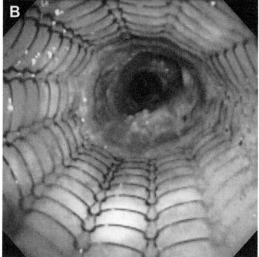

Fig. 4. (*A*) Covered and uncovered Ultraflex stents. (*B*) Ultraflex stent in trachea.

(15.9%) was infectious tracheobronchitis, and 1 patient had the stent removed because of persistent *Staphylococcus aureus* tracheobronchitis. Obstructing granuloma (14.6%) was the second most common complication necessitating multiple interventions to restore airway patency. Tumor ingrowth was seen in 6.1% of patients, early migration in 4 patients treated with Wallstents, and stent fracture in 1 patient after 2 years.[27] Long-term data on the use of Ultraflex stents for complex malignant airway stenoses have demonstrated low complication rates over a median follow-up of 91 days, which included mucous plugging in 8%, stenosing granulation tissue in 5%, tumor ingrowth in 5%, and stent migration in 5% of patients.[28] Ultraflex stent seems to be a good prosthesis for complex malignant airway stricture because of the ease of placement, excellent flexibility, and biocompatibility. In benign airway disease, experience with Ultraflex stent remains scarce, and its use is cautioned against.

Alveolus Stent

Alveolus stent (Alveolus Inc, Charlotte, NC, USA) is a new self-expanding, completely polyurethane-covered metallic stent that has been designed for use even in nonneoplastic airway strictures, as it can be easily removed. Accurate sizing for the stent can be achieved with an Alveolus stent-sizing device (Alveolus Inc), which can be introduced through the working channel of a therapeutic flexible bronchoscope. It consists of a sliding external sheath and an inner wire. The device has a measuring tool on one end and a handle on the other. When the internal wire is retracted from the handle, the wings of the measurement device open and are capable of measuring diameters between 6 and 20 mm. Once contact with tissue is made, the color bars that code for specific lumen diameters appear, which aid the bronchoscopists in the selection of appropriate stents.

The Alveolus stent is laser constructed from a single piece of nitinol, with concentric rings held in position by nitinol strands. Due to its structure, it is amenable to length modification. Because it does not foreshorten with deployment and is completely covered in polyurethane coating, the stent keeps to its trimmed length and structural integrity.[29] Despite its advantages, stent collapse caused hemoptysis and dyspnea in a woman who was treated for postintubation tracheal stenosis.[30]

CHOICE OF STENT

Besides the site, shape, and length of stenosis, presence or absence of malacia or fistula determine the choice of stent; the underlying cause of airway pathology is also an important consideration. Proper sizing of the stent (length and diameter) in relation to the dimensions of the trachea or bronchus is also important to avoid stent-related complications, such as migration, mucous plugging, granulation, and tumor ingrowth.

Tube stent placement requires specialized equipment, training, and competency in rigid bronchoscopy, whereas metal stents can be inserted via flexible bronchoscopy and in an outpatient setting. The ease of placement should not lead to the erroneous choice of the easiest stent over the best one to treat a given condition. Considering the immediate and long-term complications associated with indwelling stents, the endoscopist should run through a checklist: (1) is a stent required? (2) will the patient benefit from stent placement in terms of quality of life or prognosis? (3) does the stent interfere or prohibit a curative surgical procedure later? (4) do I have the expertise, equipment, and team to place the stent? (5) what is the underlying airway pathology and which stent is ideal? (6) is it safe to place a stent in this anatomic site? (7) what are the required stent dimensions (length and diameter)? and (8) do I have the optimal stent or should I order a more appropriate one?

For benign strictures, stents that are easy to remove and replace (eg, tube stent) are preferred to minimize mucosal damage that might otherwise preclude subsequent surgery. For malacia caused by relapsing polychondritis or tracheomegaly syndrome, uncovered wire mesh stents are preferred because they do not interfere with mucociliary clearance and have a low migration rate.[31,32] In expiratory dynamic airway collapse associated with chronic obstructive pulmonary disease, a removable stent is considered for use only after standard therapy, including noninvasive ventilation failures,[33] whereas covered metal and tube stents are indicated in malignant stenoses[11,17,18,21,29] and tracheoesophageal fistulae.[34]

STENT INSERTION TECHNIQUES

Before stent insertion, dilatation of the stricture to its optimal diameter should be attempted using a rigid bronchoscope, bougie, or balloon. Tumor tissue should be removed with either laser or electrocautery. The largest possible prosthesis should be selected, and even if it does not completely unfold, it can be opened with a balloon or forceps.

Special catheters and deployment systems have been developed for metal stents. The Palmaz and Strecker stents are mounted on balloon catheters. These stents are deployed over the stenotic areas and expanded to their specified dimensions by means of balloon inflation. The Ultraflex stent is a self-expanding stent that is mounted on an introduction catheter with crochet knots. Pulling on a thread unravels the knots and releases the stent. The distal release model is easier to deploy than the proximal release design.

The Polyflex stent with its pusher system is deployed with the help of a rigid bronchoscope. Insertion of the Dumon stent is facilitated by the use of the dedicated Dumon-Efer rigid bronchoscope and stent applicator set (Efer, France). Placement of dynamic and other bifurcated stents is facilitated with dedicated forceps.

A stent alert card detailing the type and dimensions of the stent and its location in the tracheobronchial tree should be given to the patient. It should also indicate the appropriate size of endotracheal tube to be used if emergent intubation is required with the stent in situ.

A NOVEL TREATMENT OF TRACHEAL MALIGNANCY WITH AORTIC ALLOGRAFT

Primary tracheal tumors can arise from the respiratory epithelium, salivary glands, and mesenchymal structure of the trachea. Primary tracheal tumors account for up to 0.4% of malignant diseases, with 2.6 new cases per million people every year.[35,36] In adults, 90% are malignant with squamous cell carcinoma, and adenoid cystic carcinoma accounts for two-thirds of these tumors.[36] The adult trachea measures 12 cm in length and is 1.5 to 2.5 cm wide. Depending on an individual's anatomic and physiologic factors, up to 50% of the trachea (ie, not more than 7 cm) can be resected. Tracheal resection with end-to-end anastomosis is the treatment of choice unless the tumor involves more than 50% of trachea, invades mediastinal structures and lymph nodes, or metastasizes to distant sites or the mediastinum has received a maximum radiation of more than 60 Gy.[37,38] In these circumstances, patients do not undergo surgery but receive palliation with endotracheal stents, debridement, external beam radiation, or brachytherapy.[39]

Preliminary animal studies using allogenic aortic allografts to replace the trachea have demonstrated promising results, as there were no occurrences of anastomotic leak, dehiscence, stenosis, or rejection over a period of 1 to 16 months.[40,41] Recipient cells colonized the aortic graft. The tracheal epithelium that developed is composed of basal, secretory, and ciliated cells. A posterior membrane and cartilage rings could also be detected.

Tracheal transplantation is shown to be feasible in humans. Two patients with chemoradiotherapy-resistant mucoepidermoid and adenoid cystic carcinomas underwent tracheal resection and replacement with aortic allografts. Silicone Y-stents were left in place postoperatively to prevent collapse of the aortic grafts. Biopsy specimens of the aortic allografts in both patients at 1 year showed development of respiratory epithelium, although it was unclear if host mesenchymal stem cells had engrafted the aortic allograft and undergone cartilaginous differentiation. No complications of graft ischemia, suture dehiscence, infection, or graft rejection were observed despite notable omission of immunosuppressive therapy.[42]

SUMMARY

Airway stenting is a valuable adjunct to other therapeutic bronchoscopic techniques used for relieving central airway obstruction. Notwithstanding that various stents are available, each has its complications, and the search for the ideal stent continues. Moreover, clinical studies are required to identify patients who will derive the greatest benefit from stenting. Creation of biocompatible stents that can be customized and airway replacement using aortic allograft may offer promise in the future for patients with complex strictures of the tracheobronchial tree.

REFERENCES

1. Bolliger CT, Sutedja TG, Strausz J, et al. Therapeutic bronchoscopy with immediate effect: laser, electrocautery, argon plasma coagulation and stents. Eur Respir J 2006;27:1258–71.

2. Freitag L. Tracheobronchial stents. In: Bolliger CT, Mathur PN, editors, Interventional bronchoscopy, progress in respiratory research, vol. 30. Basel (Switzerland): Karger; 2000. p. 171–86.

3. Trendelenburg F. Beitrage zu den Operationen an den Luftwegen. Langenbecks Arch Chir 1872;13: 335 [in German].

4. Bond CJ. Note on the treatment of tracheal stenosis by a new T-shaped tracheostomy tube. Lancet 1891; 1:539–40.

5. Brunings W, Albrecht W. Direkte Endoskopie der Luft und Speisewege. Stuttgart, Enke (Germany) 1915. p. 134–8.

6. Montgomery WW. T-tube tracheal stent. Arch Otolaryngol 1965;82:320–1.

7. Dumon JF. A dedicated tracheobronchial stent. Chest 1990;97:328–32.

8. Colt HG, Prakash UB, Offord KP. Bronchoscopy in North America: survey by the American Association for Bronchology. J Bronchol 2000;7:8–25.

9. Dasgupta A, Dolmatch BC, Abi-Saleh WJ, et al. Self-expandable metallic airway stent insertion employing flexible bronchoscopy: preliminary results. Chest 1998;114:106–9.

10. Lemaire A, Burfeind WR, Toloza E, et al. Outcomes of tracheobronchial stents in patients with malignant airway disease. Ann Thorac Surg 2005;80: 434–8.

11. Cavaliere S, Venuta F, Foccoli P, et al. Endoscopic treatment of malignant airway obstruction in 2008 patients. Chest 1996;110:1536–42.

12. Colt HG, Harrell JH. Therapeutic rigid bronchoscopy allows level of care changes in patients with acute respiratory failure from central airways obstruction. Chest 1997;112:202–6.

13. Bolliger CT, Probst R, Tschopp K, et al. Silicone stents in the management of inoperable tracheobronchial stenoses. Indications and limitations. Chest 1993;104:1653–9.

14. Lee P, Kupeli E, Mehta AC. Therapeutic bronchoscopy in lung cancer. Laser therapy, electrocautery,

15. brachytherapy, stents, and photodynamic therapy. Clin Chest Med 2002;23:241–56.

15. Chhajed PN, Baty F, Pless M, et al. Outcome of treated advanced non-small cell lung cancer with and without airway obstruction. Chest 2006;130:1803–7.

16. Mughal MM, Gildea TR, Murthy S, et al. Short-term deployment of self-expanding metallic stents facilitates healing of bronchial dehiscence. Am J Respir Crit Care Med 2005;172:768–71.

17. Dumon J, Cavaliere S, Diaz-Jimenez JP, et al. Seven experience with the Dumon prosthesis. J Bronchol 1996;31:6–10.

18. Diaz-Jimenez JP, Farrero Munoz E, Martinez Ballarín JI, et al. Silicone stents in the management of obstructive tracheobronchial lesions: 2 year experience. J Bronchol 1994;1:15–8.

19. Noppen M, Meysman M, Claes I, et al. Screw-thread vs Dumon endoprosthesis in the management of tracheal stenosis. Chest 1999;115:532–5.

20. Gildea TR, Murthy SC, Sahoo D, et al. Performance of a self-expanding silicone stent in palliation of benign airway conditions. Chest 2006;130: 1419–23.

21. Mehta AC, Dasgupta A. Airway stents. Clin Chest Med 1999;20:139–51.

22. Rafanan AL, Mehta AC. Stenting of the tracheobronchial tree. Radiol Clin North Am 2000;38: 395–408.

23. Slonim SM, Razavi M, Kee S, et al. Transbronchial Palmaz stent placement for tracheo-bronchial stenosis. J Vasc Interv Radiol 1998;9:153–60.

24. Strecker EP, Liermann D, Barth KH, et al. Expandable tubular stents for treatment of arterial occlusive diseases: experimental and clinical results. Radiology 1990;175:87–102.

25. Miyazawa T, Yamakido M, Ikeda S, et al. Implantation of ultraflex nitinol stents in malignant tracheobronchial stenoses. Chest 2000;118:959–65.

26. Herth F, Becker HD, LoCicero J, et al. Successful bronchoscopic placement of tracheobronchial stents without fluoroscopy. Chest 2001;119: 1910–2.

27. Saad CP, Murthy S, Krizmanich G, et al. Self-expandable metallic airway stents and flexible bronchoscopy. Chest 2003;124:1993–9.

28. Breitenbücher A, Chhajed PN, Brutsche MH, et al. Long-term follow-up and survival after Ultraflex stent insertion in the management of complex malignant airway stenoses. Respiration 2008;75:443–9.

29. Hoag JB, Juhas W, Morrow K, et al. Predeployment length modification of a self-expanding metallic stent. J Bronchol 2008;15:185–90.

30. Trisolini R, Paioli D, Fornario V, et al. Collapse of a new type of self-expanding metallic tracheal stent. Monaldi Arch Chest Dis 2006;65:56–8.

31. Dunne JA, Sabanathan S. Use of metallic stents in relapsing polychondritis. Chest 1994;105:864–7.

32. Collard PH, Freitag L, Reynaert MS, et al. Terminal respiratory failure from tracheobronchomalacia. Thorax 1996;51:224–6.

33. Murgu SD, Colt HG. Tracheobronchomalacia and excessive dynamic airway collapse. Respirology 2006;11:388–406.

34. Freitag L, Tekolf E, Steveling H, et al. Management of malignant esophago-tracheal fistulas with airway stenting and double stenting. Chest 1996;110:1155–60.

35. Gelder CM, Hetzel MR. Primary tracheal tumors: a national survey. Thorax 1993;48:688–92.

36. Bhattacharyya N. Contemporary staging and prognosis for primary tracheal malignancies: a population-based analysis. Otolaryngol Head Neck Surg 2004;131:639–42.

37. Gaissert HA, Grillo HC, Shadmehr MB, et al. Long-term survival after resection of primary adenoid cystic and squamous cell carcinoma of the trachea and carina. Ann Thorac Surg 2004;78:1889–96.

38. Grillo HC. Development of tracheal surgery: a historical review. Part 2: treatment of tracheal diseases. Ann Thorac Surg 2003;75:1039–47.

39. Macchiarini P. Primary tracheal tumors. Lancet Oncol 2006;7:83–91.

40. Martinod E, Seguin A, Holder-Espinasse M, et al. Tracheal regeneration following tracheal replacement with an allogenic aorta. Ann Thorac Surg 2005;79:942–9.

41. Jaillard S, Holder-Espinasse M, Hubert T, et al. Tracheal replacement with allogenic aorta in the pig. Chest 2006;130:1397–404.

42. Wurtz A, Porte H, Conti M, et al. Tracheal replacement with allogenic aorta. N Engl J Med 2006;355:1938–40.

Radiofrequency Ablation of Lung Tumors

Roberto F. Casal, MD[a], Alda L. Tam, MD[b], George A. Eapen, MD[a],*

KEYWORDS

- Radiofrequency • Lung • Tumor • Ablation
- Thermal • Therapy • RFA • Cancer

Lung cancer continues to be the commonest cause of cancer-related mortality in the United States and throughout the world.[1] Despite recent advances in treatment modalities, the overall 5-year survival rate remains very poor at approximately 16%. Although surgical resection is the preferred treatment in early stages and confers the best outcomes, only a quarter of the patients are diagnosed in the early stages of lung cancer. In general, lung cancer is diagnosed late, presenting with distant metastases in 40% of the cases and locally advanced in 30% to 35%.[2,3] Additionally, many patients who present with potentially surgically resectable early lung cancer are found to have respiratory or cardiac comorbidities that render them medically inoperable. These patients with medically inoperable stage I non–small cell lung cancer (NSCLC) are traditionally offered treatment with conventional external-beam radiotherapy. Whereas the 5-year survival rate after surgery for early-stage NSCLC is about 70%, the 5-year survival rate after external beam radiotherapy for medically inoperable early-stage NSCLC is only 10% to 30% in most series.[4–8] Furthermore, patients who cannot undergo surgical resection because of impaired respiratory function might also be less than optimal candidates for conventional radiotherapy because of the risk of radiation fibrosis. There is therefore a pressing need for loco-regional therapies with similar efficacy to surgery but with less morbidity and mortality in patients with early-stage lung cancer.

After the lymphatic system, the lungs are the second most common organ involved by solid tumor metastases.[9–11] Carefully selected patients have been shown to benefit from surgical resection of lung metastases with improvement in disease-free survival.[9,12–14] Those patients with potentially resectable lung metastases who are not medically fit for surgery or those who have failed surgery, chemotherapy, or radiotherapy may also benefit from loco-regional control therapies such as radiofrequency ablation, radio-embolization, or chemo-embolization.[15]

Radiofrequency ablation (RFA) has recently emerged as an alternative to surgery or radiotherapy for the local control of both primary and secondary lung neoplasms. RFA was originally used to treat hepatic tumors as early as in 1990.[16] It was not until 2000 when Dupuy and colleagues[17] reported the treatment of lung tumors in three patients with the use of percutaneous CT-guided RFA. Since then, more than 120 original articles, review articles, and case reports have been published in major journals worldwide covering well over 1000 patients ablated for primary or secondary lung neoplasms with curative or palliative intent.[18] In December of 2007, the Food and Drug Administration (FDA) issued a warning that RFA had not been specifically evaluated for the treatment of lung tumors; a statement was subsequently issued clarifying that RFA for lung tumors was covered under the indication for soft tissue ablation (Available at: http://www.fda.gov/MedicalDevices/Safety/AlertsandNotices/PublicHealthNotifications/ucm061985.htm). Although additional studies evaluating the clinical applications and benefits

[a] Department of Pulmonary Medicine, The University of Texas M.D. Anderson Cancer Center, 1515 Holcombe Boulevard, Houston, TX 77030, USA
[b] Department of Diagnostic Radiology, Section of Interventional Radiology, The University of Texas M.D. Anderson Cancer Center, 1515 Holcombe Boulevard, Houston, TX 77030, USA
* Corresponding author.
E-mail address: geapen@mdanderson.org (G.A. Eapen).

Clin Chest Med 31 (2010) 151–163
doi:10.1016/j.ccm.2009.08.021

are desirable, RFA for lung tumors is performed widely in the United States and is not considered experimental. In this review we will discuss the technical considerations, post-procedural imaging, indications, outcomes, and complications of RFA for the treatment of lung tumors.

TECHNICAL FEATURES
Basic Principles of RFA

In RFA, a radiofrequency energy generator produces an alternating current of 460 to 480 kHz, which is passed from an active electrode, through tissue, to a ground or to a second electrode if a bipolar technique is used. This rapidly alternating current agitates ions in the tissue surrounding the electrode causing them to fluctuate at high speed. In turn, these high-speed ionic oscillations generate frictional heat.[19,20] Biologic tissues heated to greater than 50°C for more than 5 minutes undergo coagulation necrosis. When tissues are heated to more than 105°C to 115°C they are carbonized and produce gas.[21] Charring and cavitation obtained with overheating can increase tissue impedance, which, in turn, decreases current flow and the amount of coagulation necrosis. A temperature of 60°C to 105°C is thus preferred for RFA.[19] The greatest effect of RFA is achieved in close proximity to the electrode. The current density dissipates with increasing distance from the electrode limiting the damage to surrounding tissues. The area of coagulation necrosis is related to the strength of the radiofrequency energy, the current-carrying time, the diameter and shape of the electrode, and the composition of the surrounding tissues.[19] The large amount of air surrounding lung lesions is thought to provide an "insulating effect" that protects the nearby normal structures while concentrating the RF energy in the tumor, making the lung a particularly suited organ to apply this technique.[20]

Equipment

An RFA system consists of three components: a radiofrequency generator (source of electromagnetic energy), an active electrode (which will be introduced into the target for energy delivery), and ground pads (to dissipate the returning current).[18,19] There are currently three RFA systems approved by the FDA for the ablation of soft tissue. These are the Boston Scientific (BOS; Natick, MA), RITA (RITA Medical Systems, Fremont, CA), and Valleylab (VL; Boulder, CO) systems. The BOS system uses the LeVeen probe (Boston Scientific, Watertown, MA), which is

available in 15-gauge and 17-gauge and has from 8 to 12 tines that deploy laterally and arch backward like the spokes of an umbrella. The RITA system uses the Starburst probe (RITA Medical Systems), available in 14-gauge and 15-gauge, and also expandable with 7 to 9 tines that travel forward and laterally similarly to the stems in a bouquet of flowers.[9] The VL system uses the Cool-tip probe (Valleylab), which is not expandable, and consists of either a single needle or a cluster probe with three parallel needles. The tip of this probe is irrigated with a continuous infusion of iced-water to prevent charring around the probe as the tumor is heated, thereby improving RF energy distribution and increasing the ablation diameter.

The tines of the RFA probe are deployed within the tumor to allow maximal distribution of the thermal energy. To control the volume of ablation and limit the damage to surrounding structures, all three systems have an automatic feedback mechanism that will determine when to terminate the procedure. Most algorithms are provided by the manufacturers. The BOS and VL system algorithms are impedance-based, where the end point of treatment is signaled by a specific increase in impedance. Unlike the BOS and the VL systems, the RITA system is a temperature-based device that relies on raising the tumor's temperature to a specific level during a predetermined period of time.[22]

Technical Procedure

The decision to perform RFA for the treatment of lung tumors should ideally be made by a multidisciplinary team composed of a thoracic surgeon, a thoracic oncologist, a radiation oncologist, a pulmonologist, an anesthesiologist, and an interventional radiologist.[15] The pre-procedural evaluation is very similar to that of a surgical procedure where cardiopulmonary conditions and bleeding risk are thoroughly assessed. In patients with cardiac pacemakers, use of an alternative focal ablative technology such as microwave or cryo-ablation may be preferable, particularly in patients who are constantly dependent on a functioning pacemaker.[9] Some authors suggest that patients who are healthy enough to undergo a CT-guided needle biopsy of the lung are generally good candidates for RFA.[23]

RFA is usually a painful procedure and it should be performed with either the combination of local anesthesia and conscious sedation or with general anesthesia. Advantages of general anesthesia are the absence of pain and improved airway control. General anesthesia also provides the ability to suspend respiration, which can be very helpful during needle placement. On the other hand, it carries disadvantages such as increased cost of the procedure, prolonged duration, and potential exacerbation of pneumothorax with positive-pressure ventilation.[9] A study from Hoffmann and colleagues[24] compared RFA for lung tumors under general anesthesia versus conscious sedation. No differences were found in technical success and feasibility, complication rates and types, and rate of local tumor control. However, this was a small retrospective analysis and prospective randomized studies are required for an accurate comparison.

Although in general RFA is performed percutaneously with imaging guidance, in rare occasions, the RFA electrodes are introduced during thoracotomy.[25,26] The most frequently used imaging modality for guidance is CT.[15,19,23] CT is widely available and it provides a precise location of the pulmonary mass or nodule and its relation to the electrode. One limitation of conventional CT guidance would be the lack of real-time imaging during the advancement of the electrodes into the tumor. When CT fluoroscopy is available and the operator and patient are willing to accept a higher radiation dose, this real-time imaging technique can be of great value for electrode placement.[9]

Patients are brought to the CT scanner where, depending on the RFA system used, one or two ground pads are applied on each leg to allow for current grounding. Of note, poor adhesion of the pads to the skin will concentrate the energy current at the edges of the pads and may cause burn injury.[27] Patients are placed in either supine or prone position to obtain the shortest distance from the chest wall entry point to the target tumor. The skin area is cleaned and draped in a sterile fashion and local anesthesia is applied at the entry site. Before introducing the RFA electrode, a localizing needle (21- or 22-gauge, 10 to 15 cm long) can be introduced into the tumor. After corroborating with CT imaging the correct position of this needle within the target tumor, the RFA electrode is advanced into the target. It is of utmost importance to remove the localizing needle before starting the RFA as it is not electrically insulated.[9] The technical goal of RFA is to achieve coagulation necrosis of the entire tumor and of a rim of 0.5 to 1.0 cm of lung parenchyma surrounding the tumor to obtain a "surgical margin." For lesions smaller than 2 cm in diameter, central and distal positioning of the RFA electrode is preferable for the first ablation, with subsequent more proximal tandem ablation zones.[23] For tumors greater than 2 cm in diameter the options are larger or expandable electrodes, or several overlapping ablation zones. In general, less time and current are required for lung tumors

compared with liver tumors. Each RFA system uses a different algorithm with respect to energy, heating temperature, and time that needs to be set for different lesions. Operators should be familiarized with the owner's manual.

RFA of surrounding air-filled lung parenchyma produces ground-glass attenuation (GGA) on CT imaging. If a rim of at least 0.5 cm of thickness of GGA can be demonstrated in the entire perimeter of the ablated tumor, complete coagulation of the tumor is likely.[9,28,29] Many, but not all authors perform ablation of the needle track in the lung parenchyma while removing the electrode at a low output (around 10 W). The potential advantages of this maneuver are a decreased probability of pneumothorax, bleeding and tumor dissemination.[9,19] When the procedure is complete, complications are usually ascertained with a CT scan.

Following RFA, patients are generally recovered in a post-procedure care unit with pulse oximetry and vital signs monitoring. Pain control is cornerstone, and it can be initially achieved with patient-controlled anesthesia pumps. Chest roentgenograms should be performed 1 to 4 hours later to check for complications. Patients should be warned that a low-grade fever for the initial 48 hours is common as part of the inflammatory response elicited by RFA. Discharge occurs, in most cases, within 1 or 2 days.[9]

ASSESSMENT OF TREATMENT RESPONSE

Rigorous imaging follow-up after ablation is essential to monitor for tumor regression or recurrence. Although a definitive imaging algorithm has yet to be devised, the generally accepted routine is contrast-enhanced CT of the chest at 1, 3, 6, and 12 months following ablation. Positron emission tomography (PET)/CT is recommended at 6, 12, and 24 months. This combination of contrast-enhanced CT and PET/CT probably gives the best sensitivity for detecting tumor recurrence early: contrast-enhanced CT allows for evaluation of the size and morphology of the ablation zone whereas PET/CT can evaluate for metabolic activity. Assessment of treatment response can be difficult because RFA leaves a permanent scar in the lung parenchyma and there is significant variation in the current literature regarding imaging modality or time interval for the evaluation of treatment response. This, in turn, has lead to a wide range of reported response rates in the literature.

Owing to the local inflammation produced by RFA, a rim of GGA around the tumor is evident immediately after the procedure. A study from Anderson and colleagues[30] proposes GGA as an early indicator of treatment success after percutaneous RFA, with receiver operator characteristic curve analysis suggesting a cut-off of 4.5 mm for complete tumor ablation. Cavitation occurs in 25% of the cases and it is more commonly seen in lesions that significantly enlarge their original diameter by more than 200% (**Fig. 1**).[23] Increase in size of the original density seen on CT is the rule during the first three months after ablation. Hence, during this period, size comparison is not an option to assess treatment response.[31] Following this early growth, the lesion progressively shrinks (**Fig. 2**).

Along with tumor size, CT densitometry is currently one of the preferred methods to follow-up lung tumors after RFA.[15,32–34] This technique measures the degree of contrast enhancement of lung nodules, based on the difference in blood supply of malignant versus benign lesions.[35] Both tumor size and contrast enhancement, when available, are generally followed every 3 months for the first year and twice a year thereafter.

18F-fluoro-2-deoxy-D-glucose PET with and without CT imaging fusion has been shown to have a very high sensitivity and specificity for the evaluation of response to RFA in lung tumors.[36–38] A comparison of PET with CT[38] and CT densitometry[36] revealed its superiority, particularly shortly after the procedure. Furthermore, in their 2006 article, Okuma and colleagues[39] demonstrated that follow-up PET at 2 months postablation may predict tumor regrowth at the RFA site on CT at 6 months or later. Residual uptake or less than 60% reduction of uptake relative to baseline at 2 months may be associated with tumor recurrence. Having this early assessment potentially allows for earlier reintervention should it be required.

The crucial question for imaging follow-up is whether the residual imaging abnormality contains viable tumor.[9] Unfortunately, the results of most of the previously mentioned studies on follow-up were not corroborated with pathology or cytology samples.

Response Evaluation Criteria In Solid Tumors (RECIST) is a widely accepted system that allows objective measurement of treatment response to chemotherapy.[40] This system is based on changes in diameter of the lesions either by CT or magnetic resonance imaging (MRI). In the case of RFA, this system would be suboptimal to evaluate a response, as it cannot differentiate viable from nonviable tumor or adjacent devitalized tissue.[9] As a result, Herrera and colleagues[26] have described a modified RECIST using the size and density of the lesions on CT and the metabolic activity on PET scanning to assess tumor response to RFA. World Health Organization (WHO) criteria for determining recurrent/progressive disease following RFA are the following: growth at the ablation site after 3 to 6 months, increasing contrast enhancement at the RFA site as defined by greater than 50% baseline enhancement after 180 seconds, nodular enhancement of more than 15 mm, and any central enhancement greater than 15 Hounsfield units (HU). Regional or distant lymph node enlargement and new sites of intra- or extrathoracic disease are also felt to represent progression.

INDICATIONS
Lung Cancer

Although patients who present with stage I and II NSCLC will benefit from surgical resection with approximately 70% survival after 5 years, many patients in this group are not medically operable because of comorbidities. These patients are

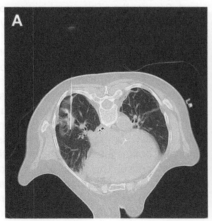 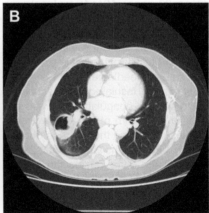

Fig.1. (A) CT scan showing radiofrequency ablation of right lower lobe colorectal metastasis. (B) Follow-up CT scan 2 months post ablation demonstrates a large cavitary lesion at the site of ablation. The patient was asymptomatic and no additional interventions were performed.

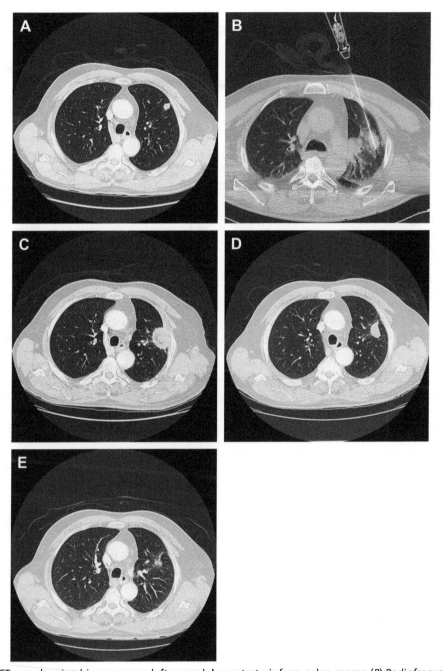

Fig. 2. (*A*) CT scan showing biopsy-proven left upper lobe metastasis from colon cancer. (*B*) Radiofrequency abla-tion of the lesion with adjacent parenchymal hemorrhage and ground glass changes. (*C*) Follow-up CT scan 1 month post ablation demonstrates an enlarged ablation zone that gradually regresses at the 6-month follow-up CT scan (*D*) and at the 1-year follow-up study (*E*).

typically offered external beam radiotherapy, although its outcome has in general been poor. Fractionated radiation with 60 to 65 Gy results in a 19% to 34% survival rate after 3 years, with local recurrence as the main cause of treatment failure.[7,41] In addition, postradiation pneumonitis could significantly affect individuals who originally did not undergo surgery owing to lack of respira-tory reserve.[15] These patients with medically inop-erable stage I NSCLC are potential candidates for RFA. Those with stage II NSCLC should not receive RFA alone, as it provides only local tumor control without addressing nodal metastases.[42] In general, tumors of up to 3 cm in diameter and located in the periphery of the lung are the ideal candidates for RFA. The rate of complete ablation in tumors larger than 3 cm in diameter has been shown to be poor in several studies.[26,34,36,43–48] Additionally, tumors larger than 3 cm in diameter are more likely to have nodal metastases that would not be controlled by RFA. Although there are no absolute contraindications for RFA in lung tumors, tumor contact with a permeable vessel of more than 3 mm in diameter are thought to create a heat sink effect that may make coagulation necrosis less successful. Also, a distance of less than 1 cm from the hilum might result in damage to nearby organs.[49] Of note however, Iguchi and colleagues[50] safely performed RFA in 42 lung tumors located less than 10 mm from the aorta or heart without any complications related to the proximity of these structures.

Another potential role of RFA in the management of NSCLC is the palliation of symptoms in advanced stages. Improvement of pain, cough, hemoptysis, and dyspnea has been reported by several authors.[34,51–53]

Pulmonary Metastases

Because of the anatomic location of the lungs, they are commonly affected by metastatic spread from solid tumors. In fact, as mentioned previously, they constitute the second most common place for solid tumor metastases after the lymphatic system. In the International Registry of Lung Metastases trial with 5206 patients undergoing pulmonary metastasectomy, 42% had sarcoma, 14% had colorectal cancer, 9% breast cancer, 8% renal cancer, 7% germ-cell tumor, 6% melanoma, and 5% head and neck cancer.[54] Unlike breast cancer and melanoma, which tend to metastasize to multiple organs, sarcoma, renal cell carcinoma, and head and neck cancers have a preferential spread to the lungs as the only site of metastases.[55] Several retrospective studies have demonstrated survival benefit after resection of pulmonary metastases.[12,56,57] In general, patients whose primary tumor is under control, who have no extrapulmonary metastases, and who have a small pulmonary metastatic burden, will benefit the most from surgical resection.[42] The previously mentioned International Registry of Lung Metastases trial reported a 5-year survival of 45%, with a disease-free period of 36 months or more.[54]

As with NSCLC, RFA has a role for the management of pulmonary metastases in medically inoperable patients. Additionally, patients who have recurrent metastatic disease after surgical resection or radiotherapy could also benefit from this treatment modality.

RESULTS

Since 2000, a large number of studies have investigated the use of RFA for the treatment of lung tumors. The inclusion of heterogeneous populations of primary lung cancers with metastatic disease of different origins, and the use of various end points evaluated with different methodologies, makes a comparison of the results of these studies extremely difficult. Additionally, many of the studies are retrospective, with small sample populations. To aid further analysis, we will describe those studies that report local tumor control separately from those that report survival results. It is beyond the scope of this review to analyze each and every study in detail; as such we will tend to briefly describe the main findings of the most relevant studies.

Local Tumor Control

After the initial feasibility studies of RFA in human beings for the treatment of lung tumors performed by Dupuy and colleagues[17] and Nishida and colleagues,[58] several other larger efficacy series have been published.

Herrera and colleagues[26] used their modified RECIST criteria to assess tumor response in 18 patients who underwent ablation of 33 tumors, including 5 patients with NSCLC and 13 with metastatic disease. With a mean follow-up of 6 months (range 1–14 months), complete or partial response was achieved in 67% of tumors smaller than 5 cm in diameter, and in only 33% of tumors larger than 5 cm.

Steinke and colleagues[59] treated a total of 52 lesions in 23 patients with pulmonary metastases from colorectal carcinoma. Tumor diameter ranged from 0.3 to 4.2 cm. All cases were done under conscious sedation. Four patients had bilateral tumors treated within the same session, and six patients had a second procedure for new metastases. Overall, tumor control assessed by CT was reported in 65% of the lesions.

Lee and colleagues[34] performed RFA with cool-tip electrode and CT guidance in 26 patients with NSCLC and 4 patients with five lung metastases. The procedure was performed with the intent to cure in 10 patients with stage I NSCLC and for palliation in the remaining 20 patients (67%). Follow-up with contrast-enhanced CT demonstrated complete ablation in 38% of the patients and partial response in 62%. Of note, mean survival for patients with complete ablation was 19.7 months versus only 8.7 months in patients with partial response ($P<.01$). Once again, tumor size was predictive of response to RFA. All 6 tumors smaller than 3 cm achieved complete necrosis, whereas only 6 (23%) of 26 tumors larger than 3 cm demonstrated a complete response. The authors also reported on symptom palliation with improvement of hemoptysis in 80% (4 of 5), chest pain in 36% (5 of 14), and cough in 25% (2 of 8).

Belfiore and colleagues[51] reported on 33 patients with unresectable primary lung cancer who underwent 35 CT-guided ablation sessions. Contrast-enhanced CT at 6 months post procedure showed 4 cases of complete and 13 cases of partial treatment response, 11 cases of stabilized lesion size, and 1 case of lesion enlargement. CT-guided fine-needle biopsy of 19 treated lesions was performed at 6 months. Strikingly, 42% (5 of 12) of patients who had decrease in tumor size by CT at 6 months were found to have tumor cells in biopsies of the low-density zone evidenced by CT. The authors therefore emphasized the inadequacy of CT as the sole method of follow-up after RFA of lung tumors, suggesting that studies that have relied on this method alone might have overestimated the efficacy of RFA.

Akeboshi and colleagues[36] ablated 54 lesions in 31 patients and used contrast-enhanced CT and PET scanning to evaluate for residual tumor. Complete ablation occurred in 69% of tumors smaller than 3 cm in diameter, and in 39% of tumors greater than 3 cm in diameter. In cases of discordant imaging results between CT and PET, histologic sampling revealed that PET scanning is slightly more sensitive and specific than contrast-enhanced CT for the detection of residual tumor. The use of PET scanning after RFA was also studied by Kang and colleagues,[38] who obtained pre- and posttreatment images of 50 patients with primary or metastatic lung tumors treated with RFA. Of the 50 patients, 17 had a single lesion and the rest had multiple lesions. All tumors smaller than 3.5 cm in diameter completely disappeared after treatment. Although CT showed an increase in tumor size within the first 2 weeks, PET scanning demonstrated tumor destruction in 70% of the cases, compared with 38% by CT. The authors concluded that PET scanning is superior to CT in evaluating response shortly after ablation. One of the major limitations of this study is the lack of additional follow-up or serial imaging.

VanSonnenberg and colleagues[53] reported their initial experience in 30 patients who underwent ablation of 36 lesions. Eighteen patients had primary lung cancer, 11 had lung metastases, 1 had mesotheliomas, and 5 had secondarily eroded painful ribs. Twenty-six of the 29 patients with lung tumors had more than 90% necrosis seen on postprocedure contrast-enhanced CT or MRI studies. Pain was ameliorated in 11 of 11 patients, with total relief in 4 and partial in 7 patients.

Survival

One of the initial reports on survival was a study from Fernando and colleagues,[25] who treated 21 NSCLC tumors in 18 patients. Nine patients had stage I, two had stage II, three had stage III, and four had stage IV. Median tumor diameter was 2.8 cm (range 1.2–4.5 cm). RFA was performed percutaneously in 16 patients and through a minithoracotomy in 2 cases. At a median follow-up of 14 months, 15 patients (83%) were alive. Mean progression-free interval was 16.8 months for the entire group, and 17.6 months for stage I NSCLC.

Ambrogi and colleagues[44] reported their experience with the use of RFA for 64 lesions on 54 patients. Forty lesions were NSCLC, and 24 were metastatic disease. The mean tumor size was 2.4 cm (range 1–5 cm). The overall median survival was 28.9 months. For patients with NSCLC the median survival was 18.9 months, and, at a mean follow-up of 23.7 months, the median survival had not yet been reached for patients with lung metastases. Unfortunately, clear stage groupings were not reported by the authors. Interestingly, this study also investigated the effect of RFA on pulmonary function tests (PFT). Forced vital capacity and forced expiratory volume in the first second were slightly decreased 1 month after the procedure, and almost returned to baseline at 3 months post-procedure. More recently, the same authors updated their data on RFA for NSCLC with a slightly longer follow-up period.[45] A total of 50 patients were treated, 36 with stage I NSCLC and 14 with advanced stages. Overall, the median follow-up period was 31 months, the radiological complete response rate was 29%, and the median survival was 25 months. For patients with stage I NSCLC, the median survival was 28.9 months.

Yan and colleagues[60] studied 55 patients who underwent RFA for medically inoperable lung metastases from colorectal carcinoma, with overall survival as their primary end point. Median overall survival was 33 months, with actuarial 1-, 2-, and 3-year survival of 85%, 64%, and 46% respectively. Multivariate analysis demonstrated that largest size of lung metastases greater than 3 cm was independently associated with decreased overall survival (P<.003).

de Baère and colleagues[61] prospectively enrolled 51 patients with lung metastases and 9 patients with NSCLC to evaluate the efficacy of RFA. At 18 months of follow-up he found an overall survival of 71% and a lung disease-free survival of

34%. PFT performed before and 2 months after RFA were unchanged.

One of the initial reports on long-term survival was the one from Simon and colleagues.[52] She retrospectively evaluated a large mixed cohort of 153 patients with either NSCLC or lung metastases. The overall 1-, 2-, 3-, 4-, and 5-year survival rates, respectively, for stage I NSCLC (n = 75) were 78%, 57%, 36%, 27%, and 27%; rates for colorectal pulmonary metastases were 87%, 78%, 57%, 57%, and 57%. Survival was longer for tumors smaller than 3 cm in diameter (P<.002).

A multicenter retrospective study from Japan performed by Yamakado and colleagues[48] evaluated the efficacy of RFA for lung metastases from colorectal cancer. Seventy-one patients with 155 lesions were treated. Maximum tumor size was 3.1 cm in 61 patients, and from 3 to 6 cm in 10 patients. The estimated 3-year survival rate was 46% for all patients. In multivariate analysis, tumor size and the presence of extrapulmonary metastases were independently associated with worse survival. Thirty-six patients with small lung metastases (≤3 cm) and no extrapulmonary metastases had a 3-year survival rate of 78%.

Table 1 summarizes some of the retrospective articles that have described survival for stage I NSCLC following RFA. **Table 2** summarizes the retrospective survival data for the patients who have undergone RFA for pulmonary metastases related to colorectal cancer.

A large prospective, multicenter study known as the Radiofrequency Ablation of Pulmonary Tumors Response Evaluation (also known as "the RAPTURE study") conducted by Lencioni and colleagues[62] was recently published. This was a prospective, intention-to-treat, single-arm, multicenter clinical trial from seven countries in Europe, the United States, and Australia. One hundred and six patients with 183 lung tumors who were unsuitable for surgery or unfit for chemotherapy or radiotherapy were enrolled. Thirty-three NSCLC, 55 lung metastases from colorectal cancer, and 20 lung metastases from other origins were included. RFA was performed percutaneously under CT guidance. A complete response of target tumor at 1 year was confirmed in 75 (88%) of 85 assessable patients. Patients with NSCLC having 1- and 2-year survival rates were 70% (CI 51%–83%) and 48% (CI 30%–65%), respectively. Those with colorectal lung metastases having 1- and 2-year survival rates were 89% (CI 76%–95%) and 66% (CI 53%–79%), respectively. Unfortunately, most of the patients included in this study were high risk because of respiratory or cardiac comorbidities and they died of noncancer-related causes. Patients with stage I NSCLC (n = 13) had a 2-year survival rate of 75% (CI 45%–92%) and a 2-year cancer-specific survival rate of 92% (CI 66%–99%). Additionally, PFT were performed at baseline, 1, 3, 6, and 12 months from ablation showing no statistically significant changes.

A potential synergistic effect of conventional external beam radiotherapy and RFA has been recently proposed. External beam radiotherapy is thought to reduce the number of cancer cells, alter cell cycle kinetics, and change the tumor microenvironment, thereby potentiating the effects of RFA. Dupuy and colleagues[63] treated 24 patients with medically inoperable stage I NSCLC with RFA followed by radiotherapy at a dose of 66 Gy. The median follow-up was 26.7 months (range, 6 to 65

Table 1
Outcomes following radiofrequency ablation in stage I non–small-cell lung cancer

	No. of Patients (Tumors)	Mean Size, cm	Follow-up, Mo	Local Tumor Control Rate	1-year Survival	2-year Survival
Lee (2004)[34]	10 (10)	4.1 ± 1.1	6.9 ± 5.8	60%	80%	NA
Fernando (2005)[25]	18 (9 stage I)	2.8	14 (median)	62%	83%	83%
Laganà (2006)[75]	9 (10)	3.7 ± 1.1	5.5 ± 4.4	80%	NA	NA
Rossi (2006)[76]	15 (15)	2.2 ± 0.8	11.4 ± 7.7	80%	NA	NA
Simon (2007)[52]	75 (80)	3.0	29 (median)	83% <3 cm, 45% >3 cm	78%	57%, 27% 5-year survival rate
Ambrogi (2007)[45]	36 (36)	2.4	31	61%	NA	NA

Abbreviation: NA, not available.

Table 2
Outcomes following radiofrequency ablation of pulmonary metastases from colorectal cancer

	No. of Patients (Tumors)	Maximum Size, cm	Survival			
			1-year (%)	2-year (%)	3-year (%)	5-year (%)
Steinke (2004)[59]	23 (52)	4.2	78	—	—	—
Yan (2006)[60]	55 (NR)	5	85	64	46	—
Yamakado (2007)[48]	71 (155)	6	84	62	46	—
Simon (2007)[52]	18 (28)	8.5	87	78	57	57

Abbreviations: NR, not reported; —, data not available.

months). They reported cumulative survival rates of 83%, 50%, and 39% at 1, 2, and 5 years, respectively. Combination therapy was also used by Grieco and colleagues.[46] His group reported on the treatment of 41 patients with medically inoperable stages I (n = 38) and II (n = 3) NSCLC. Ablation was the initial procedure and it was performed with RF in 37 cases and with microwaves in another 4 patients. Within 90 days of the ablation, patients received standard-fraction external beam radiotherapy (n = 27) or brachytherapy (n = 14). The median follow-up was 19.5 months. The overall survival rates were 87%, 70%, and 57% at 1, 2, and 3 years

respectively. Outcomes in the conventional radiotherapy and brachytherapy groups did not differ significantly. Compared with RFA alone, combination therapy seems to have a significant survival benefit, although head-to-head trials would be required to corroborate this assumption.

COMPLICATIONS

The Society of Interventional Radiology has defined "major complications" as those adverse events that result in death, permanent disability, increased level of care, or prolonged hospitalization.[64] Sano

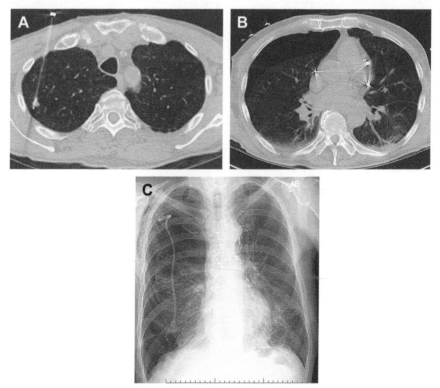

Fig. 3. (*A*) Radiofrequency ablation of biopsy-proven right upper lobe NSCLC. (*B*) Immediate post-procedural pneumothorax seen on CT scan. (*C*) Chest x-ray demonstrating residual pneumothorax and subcutaneous emphysema following chest tube insertion.

and colleagues[65] published the safety data from more than 200 ablations of lung tumors in which they found a major morbidity rate of 17.1%, slightly larger than most series. With regard to procedure-specific mortality, rates vary from less than 1.0% to 2.6%.[52,65]

The most common complication of RFA is pneumothorax, which typically occurs in 30% to 60% of the procedures (**Fig. 3**).[48,52,60,66–69] The need for aspiration or chest tube placement is usually less than 30%. Factors associated with the development of pneumothorax after RFA have been evaluated by several authors. Hiraki and colleagues[66] found risk factors for post RFA pneumothorax to include male sex, no history of lung surgery, greater number of tumors ablated, involvement of middle or lower lobe, and increased length of aerated lung parenchyma traversed by the electrode. Gillams and Lees[67] also demonstrated on multivariate analysis that the length of the trajectory of the needle or electrode through aerated lung was independently associated with the risk of pneumothorax. Persistent air leak owing to broncho-pleural fistula has been reported.[70] It is thought to occur more often

in lesions that are close to the pleura once they undergo necrosis.

Small pleural effusions are seen often and they are felt to develop as a sympathetic response to thermal injury. The incidence of pleural effusions that need to be evacuated with either thoracentesis or chest tube ranges between 1% and 7%.[31,61,66] Hiraki and colleagues[66] studied the risk factors for development of large pleural effusions after RFA. Use of internally cooled cluster electrodes, large tumor size, proximity of tumor to the pleura (<10 mm) and total ablation time have been described as risk factors. Although hemothorax is extremely rare, rapidly accumulating fluid on intraprocedural CT scanning, with or without signs of hypovolemia, should prompt further investigation to rule out this potentially lethal complication.

As RFA implies the introduction of a sharp instrument into the lung parenchyma, local complications should be expected. Parenchymal hemorrhage occurs in approximately 7% to 8% of the procedures.[31,71] Fortunately, it is only associated with hemoptysis in a minority of the patients.[65] As long as the target lesion is not obscured with

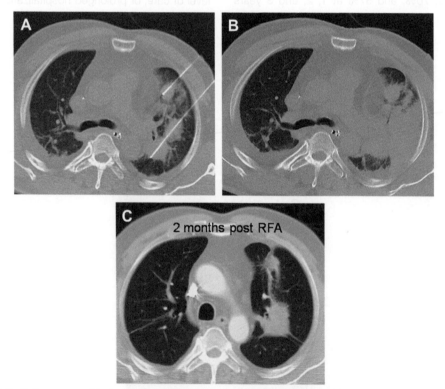

Fig. 4. (*A*) Radiofrequency ablation of two pulmonary metastases in the left upper lobe. Parenchymal hemorrhage is seen anterior to the more posterior lesion but did not preclude radiofrequency probe insertion. (*B*) Pulmonary hemorrhage in the left upper lobe seen immediately following ablation. (*C*) Follow-up CT scan 2 months after ablation demonstrates interval resolution of the parenchymal hemorrhage.

the hemorrhage, and the patient is stable, the procedure can be continued (**Fig. 4**).[18] Pneumonia, lung abscess, exacerbation of chronic obstructive pulmonary disease, and acute lung injury have all been reported following RFA.[34,36,46,48,52,53]

Although the production of air micro-emboli that pass from the pulmonary veins to the systemic circulation has been described, it is not clear if this can cause cerebral ischemia.[72,73] One case of massive stroke immediately after RFA has been reported.[74]

SUMMARY

Radiofrequency ablation may play a useful role in the management of patients with medically inoperable early-stage lung cancer, and in a selected group of patients with lung metastases. Being a minimally invasive technique, it can provide local tumor control with negligible mortality and low morbidity. Appropriate patient selection is critical, and it is fairly clear that lesions smaller than 3.5 cm have a much higher rate of response. Follow-up imaging for assessment of treatment response remains very challenging, and further studies are needed in this area.

REFERENCES

1. Jemal A, Thomas A, Murray T, et al. Cancer statistics, 2002. CA Cancer J Clin 2002;52(1):23–47.
2. Rami-Porta R, Ball D, Crowley J, et al. The IASLC lung cancer staging project: proposals for the revision of the T descriptors in the forthcoming (seventh) edition of the TNM classification for lung cancer. J Thorac Oncol 2007;2(7):593–602.
3. Smith RA, Glynn TJ. Epidemiology of lung cancer. Radiol Clin North Am 2000;38(3):453–70.
4. Jeremic B, Classen J, Bamberg M. Radiotherapy alone in technically operable, medically inoperable, early-stage (I/II) non-small-cell lung cancer. Int J Radiat Oncol Biol Phys 2002;54(1):119–30.
5. Sibley GS, Jamieson TA, Marks LB, et al. Radiotherapy alone for medically inoperable stage I non-small-cell lung cancer: the Duke experience. Int J Radiat Oncol Biol Phys 1998;40(1):149–54.
6. Kaskowitz L, Graham MV, Emami B, et al. Radiation therapy alone for stage I non-small cell lung cancer. Int J Radiat Oncol Biol Phys 1993;27(3):517–23.
7. Kupelian PA, Komaki R, Allen P. Prognostic factors in the treatment of node-negative nonsmall cell lung carcinoma with radiotherapy alone. Int J Radiat Oncol Biol Phys 1996;36(3):607–13.
8. Zierhut D, Bettscheider C, Schubert K, et al. Radiation therapy of stage I and II non-small cell lung cancer (NSCLC). Lung Cancer 2001;34(Suppl 3): S39–43.
9. Rose SC. Radiofrequency ablation of pulmonary malignancies. Semin Respir Crit Care Med 2008; 29(4):361–83.
10. Burt M, Martini N, Grinsberg R. Surgical treatment of lung carcinoma. In: Baue AE, editor. Glenn's thoracic and cardiovascular surgery. Stamford (CT): Appleton and Lange; 1996. p. 421–43.
11. Willis R. Secondary tumors of the lungs. In: Willis RA, editor. The spread of tumors in the human body. London: Butterworth; 1973. p. 167–74.
12. Friedel G, Pastorino U, Ginsberg RJ, et al. Results of lung metastasectomy from breast cancer: prognostic criteria on the basis of 467 cases of the International Registry of Lung Metastases. Eur J Cardiothorac Surg 2002;22(3):335–44.
13. Mountain CF, McMurtrey MJ, Hermes KE. Surgery for pulmonary metastasis: a 20-year experience. Ann Thorac Surg 1984;38(4):323–30.
14. Saito Y, Omiya H, Kohno K, et al. Pulmonary metastasectomy for 165 patients with colorectal carcinoma: a prognostic assessment. J Thorac Cardiovasc Surg 2002;124(5):1007–13.
15. Gomez FM, Palussiere J, Santos E, et al. Radiofrequency thermocoagulation of lung tumours. Where we are, where we are headod. Clin Transl Oncol 2009;11(1):28–34.
16. McGahan JP, Browning PD, Brock JM, et al. Hepatic ablation using radiofrequency electrocautery. Invest Radiol 1990;25(3):267–70.
17. Dupuy DE, Zagoria RJ, Akerley W, et al. Percutaneous radiofrequency ablation of malignancies in the lung. AJR Am J Roentgenol 2000;174(1):57–9.
18. Steinke K. Radiofrequency ablation of pulmonary tumours: current status. Cancer Imaging 2008;8: 27–35.
19. Matsuoka T, Okuma T. CT-guided radiofrequency ablation for lung cancer. Int J Clin Oncol 2007; 12(2):71–8.
20. White DC, D'Amico TA. Radiofrequency ablation for primary lung cancer and pulmonary metastases. Clin Lung Cancer 2008;9(1):16–23.
21. Kruskal JB, Oliver B, Huertas JC, et al. Dynamic intrahepatic flow and cellular alterations during radiofrequency ablation of liver tissue in mice. J Vasc Interv Radiol 2001;12(10):1193–201.
22. Pennathur A, Luketich JD, Abbas G, et al. Radiofrequency ablation for the treatment of stage I non-small cell lung cancer in high-risk patients. J Thorac Cardiovasc Surg 2007;134(4):857–64.
23. McTaggart RA, Dupuy DE. Thermal ablation of lung tumors. Tech Vasc Interv Radiol 2007;10(2): 102–13.
24. Hoffmann RT, Jakobs TF, Lubienski A, et al. Percutaneous radiofrequency ablation of pulmonary tumors—is there a difference between treatment

under general anaesthesia and under conscious sedation? Eur J Radiol 2006;59(2):168–74.

25. Fernando HC, De Hoyos A, Landreneau RJ, et al. Radiofrequency ablation for the treatment of non-small cell lung cancer in marginal surgical candidates. J Thorac Cardiovasc Surg 2005;129(3):639–44.

26. Herrera LJ, Fernando HC, Perry Y, et al. Radiofrequency ablation of pulmonary malignant tumors in nonsurgical candidates. J Thorac Cardiovasc Surg 2003;125(4):929–37.

27. Goldberg SN, Solbiati L, Halpern EF, et al. Variables affecting proper system grounding for radiofrequency ablation in an animal model. J Vasc Interv Radiol 2000;11(8):1069–75.

28. Yamamoto A, Nakamura K, Matsuoka T, et al. Radiofrequency ablation in a porcine lung model: correlation between CT and histopathologic findings. AJR Am J Roentgenol 2005;185(5):1299–306.

29. Yasui K, Kanazawa S, Sano Y, et al. Thoracic tumors treated with CT-guided radiofrequency ablation: initial experience. Radiology 2004;231(3):850–7.

30. Anderson E, Lees W, Gillams A. Early indicators of treatment success after percutaneous radiofrequency of pulmonary tumors. Cardiovasc Intervent Radiol 2009;32(3):478–83.

31. Steinke K, King J, Glenn D, et al. Radiologic appearance and complications of percutaneous computed tomography-guided radiofrequency-ablated pulmonary metastases from colorectal carcinoma. J Comput Assist Tomogr 2003;27(5):750–7.

32. Jin GY, Lee JM, Lee YC, et al. Primary and secondary lung malignancies treated with percutaneous radiofrequency ablation: evaluation with follow-up helical CT. AJR Am J Roentgenol 2004;183(4):1013–20.

33. Suh RD, Wallace AB, Sheehan RE, et al. Unresectable pulmonary malignancies: CT-guided percutaneous radiofrequency ablation—preliminary results. Radiology 2003;229(3):821–9.

34. Lee JM, Jin GY, Goldberg SN, et al. Percutaneous radiofrequency ablation for inoperable non-small cell lung cancer and metastases: preliminary report. Radiology 2004;230(1):125–34.

35. Swensen SJ, Viggiano RW, Midthun DE, et al. Lung nodule enhancement at CT: multicenter study. Radiology 2000;214(1):73–80.

36. Akeboshi M, Yamakado K, Nakatsuka A, et al. Percutaneous radiofrequency ablation of lung neoplasms: initial therapeutic response. J Vasc Interv Radiol 2004;15(5):463–70.

37. Higaki F, Okumura Y, Sato S, et al. Preliminary retrospective investigation of FDG-PET/CT timing in follow-up of ablated lung tumor. Ann Nucl Med 2008;22(3):157–63.

38. Kang S, Luo R, Liao W, et al. Single group study to evaluate the feasibility and complications of radiofrequency ablation and usefulness of post treatment position emission tomography in lung tumours. World J Surg Oncol 2004;2:30.

39. Okuma T, Okamura T, Matsuoka T, et al. Fluorine-18-fluorodeoxyglucose positron emission tomography for assessment of patients with unresectable recurrent or metastatic lung cancers after CT-guided radiofrequency ablation: preliminary results. Ann Nucl Med 2006;20(2):115–21.

40. Therasse P, Arbuck SG, Eisenhauer EA, et al. New guidelines to evaluate the response to treatment in solid tumors. European Organization for Research and Treatment of Cancer, National Cancer Institute of the United States, National Cancer Institute of Canada. J Natl Cancer Inst 2000;92(3):205–16.

41. Qiao X, Tullgren O, Lax I, et al. The role of radiotherapy in treatment of stage I non-small cell lung cancer. Lung Cancer 2003;41(1):1–11.

42. Fernando HC. Radiofrequency ablation to treat non-small cell lung cancer and pulmonary metastases. Ann Thorac Surg 2008;85(2):S780–4.

43. Simon CJ, Dupuy DE. Current role of image-guided ablative therapies in lung cancer. Expert Rev Anticancer Ther 2005;5(4):657–66.

44. Ambrogi MC, Fontanini G, Cioni R, et al. Biologic effects of radiofrequency thermal ablation on non-small cell lung cancer: results of a pilot study. J Thorac Cardiovasc Surg 2006;131(5):1002–6.

45. Ambrogi MC, Dini P, Melfi F, et al. Radiofrequency ablation of inoperable non-small cell lung cancer. J Thorac Oncol 2007;2(Suppl 5):S2–3.

46. Grieco CA, Simon CJ, Mayo-Smith WW, et al. Percutaneous image-guided thermal ablation and radiation therapy: outcomes of combined treatment for 41 patients with inoperable stage I/II non-small-cell lung cancer. J Vasc Interv Radiol 2006;17(7):1117–24.

47. Nguyen CL, Scott WJ, Goldberg M. Radiofrequency ablation of lung malignancies. Ann Thorac Surg 2006;82(1):365–71.

48. Yamakado K, Hase S, Matsuoka T, et al. Radiofrequency ablation for the treatment of unresectable lung metastases in patients with colorectal cancer: a multicenter study in Japan. J Vasc Interv Radiol 2007;18(3):393–8.

49. Steinke K, Haghighi KS, Wulf S, et al. Effect of vessel diameter on the creation of ovine lung radiofrequency lesions in vivo: preliminary results. J Surg Res 2005;124(1):85–91.

50. Iguchi T, Hiraki T, Gobara H, et al. Percutaneous radiofrequency ablation of lung tumors close to the heart or aorta: evaluation of safety and effectiveness. J Vasc Interv Radiol 2007;18(6):733–40.

51. Belfiore G, Moggio G, Tedeschi E, et al. CT-guided radiofrequency ablation: a potential complementary therapy for patients with unresectable primary lung cancer—a preliminary report of 33 patients. AJR Am J Roentgenol 2004;183(4):1003–11.

52. Simon CJ, Dupuy DE, DiPetrillo TA, et al. Pulmonary radiofrequency ablation: long-term safety and efficacy in 153 patients. Radiology 2007;243(1): 268–75.

53. VanSonnenberg E, Shankar S, Morrison PR, et al. Radiofrequency ablation of thoracic lesions: part 2, initial clinical experience—technical and multidisciplinary considerations in 30 patients. AJR Am J Roentgenol 2005;184(2):381–90.

54. Friedel G, Pastorino U, Buyse M, et al. [Resection of lung metastases: long-term results and prognostic analysis based on 5206 cases—the International Registry of Lung Metastases]. Zentralbl Chir 1999; 124(2):96–103 [in German].

55. Davidson RS, Nwogu CE, Brentjens MJ, et al. The surgical management of pulmonary metastasis: current concepts. Surg Oncol 2001;10(1-2):35–42.

56. Pastorino U. History of the surgical management of pulmonary metastases and development of the International Registry. Semin Thorac Cardiovasc Surg 2002;14(1):18–28.

57. Pfannschmidt J, Hoffmann H, Muley T, et al. Prognostic factors for survival after pulmonary resection of metastatic renal cell carcinoma. Ann Thorac Surg 2002;74(5):1653–7.

58. Nishida T, Inoue K, Kawata Y, et al. Percutaneous radiofrequency ablation of lung neoplasms: a minimally invasive strategy for inoperable patients. J Am Coll Surg 2002;195(3):426–30.

59. Steinke K, Glenn D, King J, et al. Percutaneous imaging-guided radiofrequency ablation in patients with colorectal pulmonary metastases: 1-year follow-up. Ann Surg Oncol 2004;11(2):207–12.

60. Yan TD, King J, Sjarif A, et al. Percutaneous radiofrequency ablation of pulmonary metastases from colorectal carcinoma: prognostic determinants for survival. Ann Surg Oncol 2006;13(11): 1529–37.

61. de Baère, Palussiere J, Auperin A, et al. Midterm local efficacy and survival after radiofrequency ablation of lung tumors with minimum follow-up of 1 year: prospective evaluation. Radiology 2006;240(2): 587–96.

62. Lencioni R, Crocetti L, Cioni R, et al. Response to radiofrequency ablation of pulmonary tumours: a prospective, intention-to-treat, multicentre clinical trial (the RAPTURE study). Lancet Oncol 2008;9(7): 621–8.

63. Dupuy DE, DiPetrillo T, Gandhi S, et al. Radiofrequency ablation followed by conventional radiotherapy for medically inoperable stage I non-small cell lung cancer. Chest 2006;129(3):738–45.

64. Sacks D, McClenny TE, Cardella JF, et al. Society of Interventional Radiology clinical practice guidelines. J Vasc Interv Radiol 2003;14(9 Pt 2):S199–202.

65. Sano Y, Kanazawa S, Gobara H, et al. Feasibility of percutaneous radiofrequency ablation for intrathoracic malignancies: a large single-center experience. Cancer 2007;109(7):1397–405.

66. Hiraki T, Tajiri N, Mimura H, et al. Pneumothorax, pleural effusion, and chest tube placement after radiofrequency ablation of lung tumors: incidence and risk factors. Radiology 2006;241(1):275–83.

67. Gillams AR, Lees WR. Analysis of the factors associated with radiofrequency ablation-induced pneumothorax. Clin Radiol 2007;62(7):639–44.

68. Yamagami T, Kato T, Hirota T, et al. Pneumothorax as a complication of percutaneous radiofrequency ablation for lung neoplasms. J Vasc Interv Radiol 2006;17(10):1625–9.

69. Okuma T, Matsuoka T, Yamamoto A, et al. Frequency and risk factors of various complications after computed tomography-guided radiofrequency ablation of lung tumors. Cardiovasc Intervent Radiol 2008;31(1):122–30.

70. Sakurai J, Hiraki T, Mukai T, et al. Intractable pneumothorax due to bronchopleural fistula after radiofrequency ablation of lung tumors. J Vasc Interv Radiol 2007;18(1 Pt 1):141–5.

71. Steinke K, King J, Glenn D, et al. Pulmonary hemorrhage during percutaneous radiofrequency ablation: a more frequent complication than assumed? Interact Cardiovasc Thorac Surg 2003;2(4):462–5.

72. Ahrar K, Stafford RJ, Tinkey PT, et al. Evaluation of cerebral microemboli during radiofrequency ablation of lung tumors in a canine model with use of impedance-controlled devices. J Vasc Interv Radiol 2007;18(7):929–35.

73. Rose SC, Fotoohi M, Levin DL, et al. Cerebral microembolization during radiofrequency ablation of lung malignancies. J Vasc Interv Radiol 2002;13(10): 1051–4.

74. Jin GY, Lee JM, Lee YC, et al. Acute cerebral infarction after radiofrequency ablation of an atypical carcinoid pulmonary tumor. AJR Am J Roentgenol 2004;182(4):990–2.

75. Laganà D, Carrafiello G, Mangini M, et al. Radiofrequency ablation of primary and metastatic lung tumors: preliminary experience with a single center device. Surg Endosc 2006;20(8):1262–7.

76. Rossi S, Dore R, Cascina A, et al. Percutaneous computed tomography-guided radiofrequency thermal ablation of small unresectable lung tumours. Eur Respir J 2006;27(3):556–63.

Current Status of Medical Pleuroscopy

Andrew R.L. Medford, BS, MD, DM, MRCP, Dip(Clin Risk Mgt)[a,b,*],
Jonathan A. Bennett, BS, MD, DM, FRCP[a],
Catherine M. Free, MD, DM, MRCP[a],
Sanjay Agrawal, MD, FCCP[a]

KEYWORDS
- Medical pleuroscopy • Pleural effusion • Pleural infection
- Pneumothorax • Malignancy • Pleurodesis

Pleural conditions comprise approximately 25% of cases presenting to pulmonologists. Hence, there has been an increasing interest in novel investigations by pulmonologists in pleural disease. Medical pleuroscopy (MP)—also referred as medical thoracoscopy, local anesthetic thoracoscopy, or video-assisted thoracoscopy—can be performed by nonsurgeons, as distinct from video-assisted thoracoscopic surgery (VATS).

Thoracoscopy was first described by Jacobaeus using rigid instruments in 1910, although the first thoracoscopy was actually performed in 1865 in Dublin.[1,2] The term, MP, describes a different procedure that is similar to VATS.[3] There are differences, however, in that MP is performed by a pulmonologist on (usually) spontaneous breathing patients commonly via a single port whereas VATS is performed via several ports by a thoracic surgeon on an intubated patient with a double-lumen tube. MP is most often a diagnostic procedure (especially for pleural effusion), occasionally for poudrage, whereas VATS is primarily performed with a therapeutic intent. MP and VATS should be regarded as invasive procedures.

PROCEDURAL ISSUES
Patient Selection

Patients with unexplained pleural effusion, pleural infection, and pneumothorax may potentially be suitable for MP. Contraindications include a World Health Organization performance status[4] of greater than 2 unless related to the effusion, uncontrolled coughing, hypoxemia unrelated to the effusion, pulmonary hypertension, unstable myocardial status or function, or a bleeding diathesis. The only absolute contraindication is lack of a pleural space due to adhesions, as a partially collapsed lung is required to safely introduce the pleuroscope into the pleural cavity.

Preprocedure

Detailed history and physical examination are prerequisites as is accurate assessment of functional status of patients. Recent chest radiograph, pleural CT, or pleural ultrasound scan are highly desirable prior to performing an MP along with an electrocardiogram, clotting profile, and complete blood count. The international normalized ratio should ideally be below 1.5 for performing the pleural biopsy and a platelet count greater than 60,000 per μL of blood. Aspirin prolongs the bleeding time but is not a contraindication. Clopidogrel, however, can result in significant bleeding and should be with held 1 week before MP. Efforts to optimize lung function in those with pre-existing obstructive lung disease are helpful. Coughing should also be minimized preprocedure.

MP can be performed in an appropriately sterile endoscopy suite or an operating room. In many institutions, decubitus pleural ultrasound is performed on the day of the procedure, which may

[a] Department of Respiratory Medicine, Glenfield Hospital, University Hospitals of Leicester NHS Trust, Leicester LE3 9QP, Leicestershire, UK
[b] North Bristol Lung Centre, Southmead Hospital, Westbury-on-Trym, Bristol BS10 5NB, Avon, UK
* Corresponding author. North Bristol Lung Centre, Southmead Hospital, Westbury-on-Trym, Bristol BS10 5NB, Avon, United Kingdom.
E-mail address: andrewmedford@hotmail.com (A.R.L. Medford).

Clin Chest Med 31 (2010) 165–172
doi:10.1016/j.ccm.2009.10.001

be particularly helpful if loculations are suspected, to optimize the site of entry and avoid potential technical challenges.[5,6] Alternatively, operators may use a Boutin needle or a similar device to artificially create a pneumothorax and collapse the lung, creating a space for trocar insertion. After placing an intravenous cannula, patients are usually premedicated with an opiate, atropine (intramuscular), and intravenous crystalloid infusion. Routine antibiotic prophylaxis is not indicated provided the environment is sterile and an aseptic technique is used.

Technique

Patients lie in the lateral decubitus position with the abnormal hemithorax uppermost and the arm raised above the head to allow access to the insertion point along the anterior axillary line and to maximize the space between the ribs. Essential monitoring includes respiratory rate, heart rate, blood pressure, oxygen saturations, and electrocardiogram monitoring. Patients usually are breathing spontaneously, without intubation, under conscious sedation with a combination of midazolam and fentanyl or propofol infusion and laryngeal mask airway. Occasionally, assisted ventilation using a propofol infusion via a single lumen endotracheal tube is used for better analgesia; an anesthesiologist's input may be needed in such a scenario. MP thus can avoid the need for more than one port, general anesthesia, or assisted ventilation via a double-lumen endotracheal tube, as is required in VATS.

After infiltration of the skin and the chest wall with a mixture of local anesthetic and adrenaline, blunt dissection to the pleural space is performed in the anterior axillary line (or as guided by lateral decubitus ultrasound) in the same manner as inserting an Argyle intercostal chest tube, typically between the fourth and seventh intercostal spaces. The trocar is inserted with the release valve open. MP can be performed with one or two ports typically and using a rigid or a semirigid scope or a minithoracoscope (discussed later). A single port is used for diagnostic MP and talc instillation whereas the two-port technique may be used if need for diathermy is anticipated. The latter is used to overcome adhesions causing parts of the hemithorax to be inaccessible via a single port, to drain complex effusions, or for more advanced applications, such as lung biopsy.

The effusion is completely drained under direct visualization and then the pleural surfaces are inspected thoracoscopically for optimal biopsy sites and the presence of any evidence of trapped lung. If there are thin adhesions obscuring view, they can be carefully severed but with vigilance for bleeding (very thick fibrous adhesions may often require surgical decortication). Targeted parietal pleural biopsies are taken under direct vision, avoiding the visceral pleura and intercostal vessels, and over a rib if possible. A long sweeping motion is used to obtain the pleura rather than a snap-and-grasp technique. If there is no evidence of a trapped lung with no obvious visceral pleural thickening or adhesions, then a talc poudrage is performed, especially if there is clear evidence of pleural malignancy. At the end of the procedure, a 24-gauge (or larger, especially in cases of pleural infection) chest drain is inserted and removed within a few hours to 3 days, depending on re-expansion of the lung and drainage of the pleural fluid. If the lung is trapped, options are to try a normal chest drain with or without suction or to place a tunneled chest drain for outpatient management. If no talc has been instilled and the lung has re-expanded with the patient stable, the patient could be discharged the same day.

Equipment

Rigid MP uses a light source, endoscopic camera, video monitor, and image capture device with a trocar of between 5 and 10 mm diameter and 5-mm rigid forceps (**Figs. 1** and **2**). Direct or oblique rigid 7-mm pleuroscopes are available, which

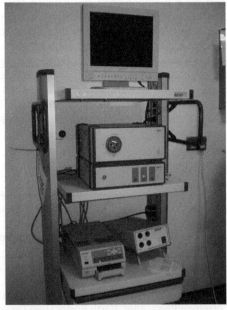

Fig. 1. Rigid pleuroscopy stack system: monitor (*top level*), light source (*top second level*), pleuroscope power supply (*lower second level*), image capture device (*bottom level left*).

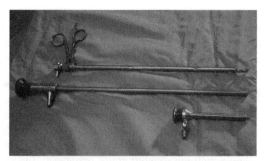

Fig. 2. Rigid biopsy forceps (*upper*), rigid pleuroscope (*middle*) and trocar (*lower*).

provide more panoramic view of the pleural space (**Fig. 3**). Other essentials include sterile drapes and gowns, standard instruments for chest tube insertion, a talc atomizer system, a chest tube (usually 24F–32F), and a negative suction drainage system.

Variants of rigid MP exist. A minirigid MP 3.3-mm telescope with 3-mm biopsy forceps has been used for small loculated effusions inaccessible to the standard size rigid MP scope and larger nonloculated effusions. The diagnostic yield is still favorable at more than 93%.[7] Some operators prefer to use a semirigid thoracoscope in preference to the rigid scope on the basis that pulmonologists find this system easier to learn as it is close to a flexible bronchoscope in its maneuverability.[8,9] The outer diameter of this instrument is 7 mm and it has a 2.8-mm working channel that can accommodate conventional flexible biopsy forceps. It is also compatible with existing processors and light sources used for flexible bronchoscopy, reducing costs. Despite concerns that semirigid thoracoscopy may lead to inferior biopsies that are significantly smaller in size compared with the rigid system, available data suggest that good yields (93%) can be obtained.[10] Comparative studies are awaited. Semirigid MP is probably best reserved for assessment of indeterminate pleural effusions, where the suspicion of malignant mesothelioma is lower, until further data are available. In all other cases, rigid MP is the procedure of choice. Finally, a flexible

bronchoscope has been used as a flexible MP but experience has found the rigid MP superior with bigger samples and better yield.[11,12]

Complications

MP is a safe procedure when performed by a trained operator. Mortality rates with rigid MP are 0.8% or less in published series, including centers where it has been recently established.[13–15] Complications are few, with reported rates of between 2% and 6%.[16] These include postoperative fever, subcutaneous emphysema, persistent air leak (>7 days), re-expansion pulmonary edema, cardiac arrhythmia, myocardial ischemia, bleeding, empyema, wound infection, and seeding of the chest wall by the neoplastic cells.[17,18] With the semirigid MP scope, complications are expectedly rarer with no reported mortality in published studies to date.[8–10]

INDICATIONS FOR MEDICAL PLEUROSCOPY
Pleural Malignancy—Undiagnosed Pleural Effusion

The main benefits of MP in malignancy are diagnosing pleural metastasis by guided biopsy under direct vision (**Fig. 4**) and providing large amounts of tissue to allow histologic confirmation,[14] histologic differentiation (especially mesothelioma from adenocarcinoma), hormone receptor analysis, and assessment of lung expandability. MP also allows for complete drainage of the effusion, removal of adhesions, and talc pleurodesis, if appropriate, during one procedure in a controlled environment and optimizing chest tube placement.

MP is often needed because of the limitations of less invasive diagnostic techniques. Thoracentesis is the first investigation into unexplained pleural effusions but pleural cytology is diagnostic

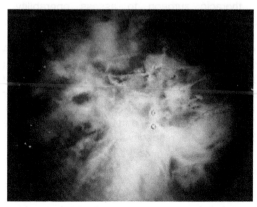

Fig. 4. Metastatic lung adenocarcinoma on parietal pleura viewed at MP.

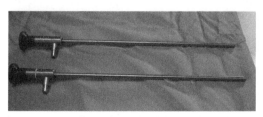

Fig. 3. Direct (*upper*) and oblique (*lower*) rigid pleuroscopes.

only in approximately 62% of cases for malignancy, with a much lower yield in mesothelioma and in early cancers, as positive cytology requires malignant cell exfoliation from the pleura into the pleural fluid and adequate cytologic characteristics.[19] Even after further sampling with larger volumes, at least 25% of suspected malignant effusions remain undiagnosed. If there is a high pretest probability of pleural malignancy, then MP is normally indicated at this stage, unless there is an ipsilateral shifting or midline mediastinum in the presence of an effusion, which would suggest main bronchus obstruction, which may require bronchoscopy as an initial diagnostic test.

Closed (ie, not image-guided, using an Abrams needle) pleural biopsy only increases the yield for malignancy over cytology by 7% to 27%.[19] Pleural malignant deposits tend to predominate near the midline and the diaphragm, accounting for the lower yield of closed pleural biopsy compared with CT-guided pleural biopsy or MP.[20] CT-guided pleural biopsy can achieve yields of 87% to 88% for malignancy and 86% for mesothelioma.[20–22] The yield of MP is superior at 90% to 95%.[23,24] MP offers a superior diagnostic option to closed pleural biopsy and advantages (described previously), resulting in a short duration of hospital stay.[14] Although CT-guided pleural biopsy gives a better yield than closed pleural biopsy (87% vs 44%),[20] MP is superior as it allows combined diagnostic and therapeutic options (drainage and pleurodesis) in a single visit, if indicated, with a larger tissue sample for analysis.

Metastatic pleural disease in non–small cell lung cancer precludes surgery and has recently been reclassified from T4 to M1 disease, taking into account the abysmal prognosis for patients with malignant pleural effusion.[25] MP can assess accurately whether or not the effusion is paramalignant or due to metastases, although in clinical practice, VATS may often be performed in this setting by a thoracic surgeon to assess operability.[26] Changes in practice and an increased drive to reduce inpatient hospital stay have resulted in increasing use of MP by the pulmonologists. A recent United Kingdom survey demonstrated that 37 centers now offer an MP service; 15 (41%) of these perform fewer than 20 procedures per year (Dr N. Downer, personal communication, 2009). There have been 218% and 336% increases since 2004 and 1999, respectively.[27]

Pleurodesis

Although low pleural pH due to large tumor burden predicts failure of pleurodesis,[28] MP talc poudrage can be 88% effective even when the pleural pH is less than 7.3.[29] MP talc poudrage (**Fig. 5**) has been shown superior to talc slurry (relative risk of nonrecurrence 1.19) via a normal chest drain in a recent Cochrane systematic review.[30] Although a recent randomized trial did not show an overall superiority for thoracoscopic talc poudrage over talc slurry via chest drain, a subgroup of patients with lung and breast cancer had greater success with talc poudrage (82% vs 67% success at 30 days).[31] In the same study, the proportion of patients with talc-related acute respiratory failure was slightly higher in the poudrage group than the slurry group (8% vs 4%, respectively).

Pleural Tuberculous

For tuberculous (TB) pleural effusion, closed pleural biopsy has a much higher yield than in pleural malignancy due to the more diffuse nature of the pleuritis with combined yield of histology, tissue culture, pleural fluid smear, and culture varying between 80% and 90%.[19] MP remains superior to closed pleural biopsy (100% vs 80% yield), however, in areas with a high TB prevalence.[32] If MP is not locally available, however, closed pleural biopsy is a reasonable first-line investigation in this situation. CT-guided pleural biopsy may be performed yet requires interventional radiologic expertise and a pleural CT.

MP has the advantage over closed and CT-guided pleural biopsy of obtaining a greater amount of tissue, which may be relevant when the diagnosis is in doubt or when there is a need to obtain anti-TB drug sensitivity profiling for suspected drug-resistant cases. MP also allows the simultaneous opportunity to break down adhesions and drain the effusion in a safe, sterile, and controlled fashion, which may be necessary for larger effusions while waiting for response to anti-TB treatment.

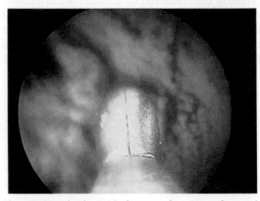

Fig. 5. Standard rigid forceps for MP after talc poudrage.

Pleural Infection and Empyema

In pleural infection, loculations may impede drainage via a conventional chest tube and intrapleural fibrinolysis is not recommended in this context.[33] The exact timing and role of MP remains an area of ongoing debate. Guidelines from the American College of Chest Physicians and the British Thoracic Society do not refer to MP but focus on the role of VATS under such circumstances.[34,35]

MP can be useful early in the course of empyema where thin fibrinous adhesions can be broken down and the fluid and the infected material can be removed to allow lung expansion, providing an opportunity to take targeted biopsies to exclude occult undiagnosed infection or malignancy.[34,36] Further research is ongoing to assess the potential of pleural lavage in pleural infection, which is also possible at MP.

In the later phase of empyema, when there are thick fibrous adhesions (**Fig. 6**),[37] trapped lung, or a pleural peel, early VATS decortication may be required using classic multiport intervention under general anesthesia with double-lumen intubation.[38,39] Expert medical pleuroscopists can also perform MP in empyema in the fibrinopurulent stage, however, and this may be a preferred option in frail or elderly patients, where conventional chest drainage has not been successful and patients are at a high risk for VATS.[40,41] Existing data on MP in pleural infection are sparse but a 93% primary success rate in avoiding surgical intervention has been achieved in early-stage pleural infection.[42]

Pneumothorax

MP can visualize blebs and bullae in patients with spontaneous pneumothorax. Pleural abrasion or

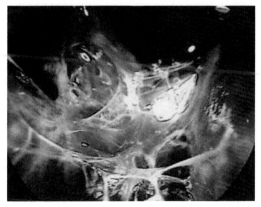

Fig. 6. Chronic sterile empyema at MP with thick fibrous septations and pleural peel.

talc pleurodesis can be performed or even coagulation of such blebs. MP with talc poudrage may be particularly helpful in the setting of patients with significant comorbidity and advanced lung disease that may not be suitable for VATS[43] and is superior to standard pleurodesis via a chest tube.[44] For suitable patients, VATS or thoracotomy detects blebs or bullae better than MP. VATS bullectomy, pleural abrasion, or pleurectomy is superior to MP for recurrent pneumothoraces.[45] Autofluorescence MP has been used recently to detect areas of potential air leak, which are macroscopically normal on white light MP using inhaled fluorescein.[46]

Other Benign Pleural Disease

If thoracocentesis is unhelpful, MP can also help diagnose other benign pleural disorders in certain settings. The parietal pleura can have a gritty appearance in rheumatoid effusion[47] and asbestos pleural plaques have a characteristic smooth, white, but hard consistency that is difficult to biopsy as a result.

ADVANCED TECHNIQUES AND THE FUTURE

Advanced applications of MP include visceral pleural and lung biopsy and sympathectomy. Other potential applications for the future are being researched.

Visceral Pleural and Lung Biopsy

Visceral pleural biopsy and peripheral lung biopsy can be undertaken at the same time as parietal pleural biopsy at MP, especially when there is coexistence of a pleural effusion with lung disease. This may be important for detecting a synchronous tumor or altering prognosis of a known tumor. Often coagulating forceps may be used via a two-port technique, although a single-port technique is possible with optical forceps without coagulation or using minithoracoscopy.[7]

Lung biopsy via MP for diffuse or localized lung disease is less commonly performed with the advent of VATS wedge lung biopsy and improvement of high-resolution CT.[48] International guidelines from several continents on interstitial lung disease have recommended the use of VATS lung biopsy in particular when indicated.[49,50] VATS wedge biopsies contain more vascular structures than forceps biopsies, with less crush artifact and greater size.[51] Therefore, for pulmonary disorders where vascular integrity is important, forceps biopsy via MP is not recommended.

MP is still occasionally used for diffuse lung disease by some interventional pulmonologists when bronchoalveolar lavage and transbronchial biopsy have not yielded a diagnosis with good rates of high quality biopsies.[52] For localized lung disease, yields with MP forceps lung biopsy are lower, at less than 50%[53] and this method is no longer used.

Complications with MP lung biopsy are low, the most common are air leaks, but are at similar rates to VATS lung biopsy.[54,55] Bleeding or tissue coagulation is minimal and mortality is extremely low.

Sympathectomy

Sympathectomy has been used for the treatment of hyperhidrosis or chronic pancreatic pain in particular but percutaneous methods are not very effective with high complication rates.[56] Although generally performed by thoracic surgeons at VATS,[57] advanced pleuroscopists have described a single-port technique via a single lumen endotracheal tube using electrocautery.[58,59] Complications of MP for this indication are rare (usually <1%) but include Horner's syndrome, pneumothorax, and hemorrhage.

Future Research Areas

The applications of MP are evolving. Pleuroscopic lavage is under evaluation in the treatment of pleural infection. Autofluorescence pleuroscopy may potentially have an application in detection of early pleural malignancy as autofluorescence bronchoscopy has been utilized for early detection of malignant lesions in the bronchial tree.[60]

FINANCE AND TRAINING ISSUES
Cost Analysis

There are no published cost analyses of MP. A recent United Kingdom tertiary center theoretic cost analysis, however, which compared Abrams or CT-guided pleural biopsies to MP, calculated cost savings of $2198 (£1527) per patient.[14] The cost savings over Abrams needle biopsy, CT-guided pleural biopsy, and VATS are likely to be a combination of reduced need to repeat the procedure, shorter hospital stay, avoidance of thoracic operating room costs, and allowing increased patient flow through interventional radiology and thoracic surgery services. In health care systems operating by tariff-based revenue, accurate coding is essential to allow correct remuneration. Coding errors occur for a variety of reasons and are well described in MP and other specialties.[61,62]

Competency

The American Thoracic Society and European Respiratory Society guidelines on interventional pulmonology do not address MP,[63] although the procedure is regarded as easier to learn than flexible bronchoscopy.[40] The American College of Chest Physicians interventional pulmonology guidelines recommend 20 supervised MP procedures for training and a minimum of 10 per year to maintain skills.[64] The British Thoracic Society is currently revising training guidelines for MP but many centers suggest at least 25 to 30 supervised MP procedures to achieve competency pending the development of formal guidelines. To deliver a robust training program, there needs to be an appropriate service demand in terms of procedures performed per year, which suggests this would not be a procedure for all pulmonologists. Significant demand can occur in tertiary centers despite having thoracic surgery on site.[14]

SUMMARY

MP offers pulmonologists an opportunity to take multiple pleural biopsies to diagnose malignant and nonmalignant pleural diseases. In addition, operators may drain large pleural effusions, break down adhesions, and perform an effective pleurodesis with talc poudrage under direct vision, using conscious sedation. Advanced operators may treat pneumothorax and take lung parenchymal or visceral pleural biopsies.

Close collaboration between the pleuroscopist, thoracic surgeon, and thoracic radiologist is key, as MP remains an invasive procedure requiring training and careful patient selection.

REFERENCES

1. Jacobaeus HC. The practical importance of thoracoscopy in surgery of the chest. Surg Gynecol Obstet 1922;34:289–96.
2. Cruise FR. The endoscope as an aid to the diagnosis and treatment of disease. BMJ 1865;8:345–7.
3. Rao A, Bansal A, Rangraj M, et al. Video-assisted thoracic surgery (VATS). Heart Lung 1999;28(1): 15–9.
4. Oken MM, Creech RH, Tormey DC, et al. Toxicity and response criteria of the Eastern Cooperative Oncology Group. Am J Clin Oncol 1982;5(6): 649–55.
5. Hersh CP, Feller-Kopman D, Wahidi M, et al. Ultrasound guidance for medical thoracoscopy: a novel approach. Respiration 2003;70(3):299–301.
6. Medford AR. The utility of thoracic ultrasound before local anesthetic video-assisted thoracoscopy in patients with suspected pleural malignancy. J Clin Ultrasound 2009. DOI:10.1002/jcu.20635. [Epub ahead of print].

7. Tassi G, Marchetti G. Minithoracoscopy: a less invasive approach to thoracoscopy. Chest 2003;124(5): 1975–7.

8. McLean AN, Bicknell SR, McAlpine LG, et al. Investigation of pleural effusion: an evaluation of the new Olympus LTF semiflexible thoracofiberscope and comparison with Abram's needle biopsy. Chest 1998;114(1):150–3.

9. Ernst A, Hersh CP, Herth F, et al. A novel instrument for the evaluation of the pleural space: an experience in 34 patients. Chest 2002;122(5):1530–4.

10. Wang Z, Tong ZH, Li HJ, et al. Semi-rigid thoracoscopy for undiagnosed exudative pleural effusions: a comparative study. Chin Med J 2008;121(15): 1384–9.

11. Oldenburg FA Jr, Newhouse MT. Thoracoscopy. A safe, accurate diagnostic procedure using the rigid thoracoscope and local anesthesia. Chest 1979; 75(1):45–50.

12. Davidson AC, George RJ, Sheldon CD, et al. Thoracoscopy: assessment of a physician service and comparison of a flexible bronchoscope used as a thoracoscope with a rigid thoracoscope. Thorax 1988;43(4):327–32.

13. Viskum K, Enk B. Complications of thoracoscopy. Poumon Coeur 1981;37(1):25–8.

14. Medford AR, Agrawal S, Free CM, et al. A local anaesthetic video-assisted thoracoscopy service: prospective performance analysis in a UK tertiary respiratory centre. Lung Cancer 2009. DOI:10.1016/j.lungcan.2009.02.023. [Epub ahead of print].

15. Colt HG. Thoracoscopy. A prospective study of safety and outcome. Chest 1995;108(2):324–9.

16. Menzies R, Charbonneau M. Thoracoscopy for the diagnosis of pleural disease. Ann Intern Med 1991; 114(4):271–6.

17. Parker C, Neville E. Lung cancer * 8: management of malignant mesothelioma. Thorax 2003;58(9): 809–13.

18. Boutin C, Rey F, Viallat JR. Prevention of malignant seeding after invasive diagnostic procedures in patients with pleural mesothelioma. A randomized trial of local radiotherapy. Chest 1995;108(3): 754–8.

19. Maskell NA, Butland RJ. BTS guidelines for the investigation of a unilateral pleural effusion in adults. Thorax 2003;58(Suppl 2):ii8–17.

20. Maskell NA, Gleeson FV, Davies RJ. Standard pleural biopsy versus CT-guided cutting-needle biopsy for diagnosis of malignant disease in pleural effusions: a randomised controlled trial. Lancet 2003;361(9366):1326–30.

21. Adams RF, Gleeson FV. Percutaneous image-guided cutting-needle biopsy of the pleura in the presence of a suspected malignant effusion. Radiology 2001;219(2):510–4.

22. Adams RF, Gray W, Davies RJ, et al. Percutaneous image-guided cutting needle biopsy of the pleura in the diagnosis of malignant mesothelioma. Chest 2001;120(6):1798–802.

23. Antony VB, Loddenkemper R, Astoul P, et al. Management of malignant pleural effusions. Eur Respir J 2001;18(2):402–19.

24. Harris RJ, Kavuru MS, Rice TW, et al. The diagnostic and therapeutic utility of thoracoscopy. A review. Chest 1995;108(3):828–41.

25. Goldstraw P, Crowley J, Chansky K, et al. The IASLC Lung Cancer Staging Project: proposals for the revision of the TNM stage groupings in the forthcoming (seventh) edition of the TNM classification of malignant tumours. J Thorac Oncol 2007;2(8):706–14.

26. British Thoracic Society and Society of Cardiothoracic Surgeons of Great Britain and Ireland Working Party. BTS guidelines: guidelines on the selection of patients with lung cancer for surgery. Thorax 2001; 56(2):89–108.

27. Burrows NJ, Ali NJ, Cox GM. The use and development of medical thoracoscopy in the United Kingdom over the past 5 years. Respir Med 2006; 100(7):1234–8.

28. Rodriguez-Panadero F, Lopez Mejias J. Low glucose and pH levels in malignant pleural effusions. Diagnostic significance and prognostic value in respect to pleurodesis. Am Rev Respir Dis 1989;139(3): 663–7.

29. Aelony Y, King RR, Boutin C. Thoracoscopic talc poudrage in malignant pleural effusions: effective pleurodesis despite low pleural pH. Chest 1998; 113(4):1007–12.

30. Shaw P, Agarwal R. Pleurodesis for malignant pleural effusions. Cochrane Database Syst Rev 2004;(1):CD002916.

31. Dresler CM, Olak J, Herndon JE 2nd, et al. Phase III intergroup study of talc poudrage vs talc slurry sclerosis for malignant pleural effusion. Chest 2005; 127(3):909–15.

32. Diacon AH, Van de Wal BW, Wyser C, et al. Diagnostic tools in tuberculous pleurisy: a direct comparative study. Eur Respir J 2003;22(4):589–91.

33. Maskell NA, Davies CW, Nunn AJ, et al. UK controlled trial of intrapleural streptokinase for pleural infection. N Engl J Med 2005;352(9): 865–74.

34. Colice GL, Curtis A, Deslauriers J, et al. Medical and surgical treatment of parapneumonic effusions: an evidence-based guideline. Chest 2000;118(4): 1158–71.

35. Davies CW, Gleeson FV, Davies RJ. BTS guidelines for the management of pleural infection. Thorax 2003;58(Suppl 2):ii18–28.

36. Cameron RJ. Management of complicated parapneumonic effusions and thoracic empyema. Intern Med J 2002;32(8):408–14.

37. Medford AR, Bennett JA. Chronic sterile empyema. QJM 2009. DOI:10.1093/qjmed/hcp131. [Epub ahead of print].

38. Waller DA. Thoracoscopy in management of post-pneumonic pleural infections. Curr Opin Pulm Med 2002;8(4):323–6.

39. Waller DA, Rengarajan A. Thoracoscopic decortication: a role for video-assisted surgery in chronic postpneumonic pleural empyema. Ann Thorac Surg 2001;71(6):1813–6.

40. Loddenkemper R. Thoracoscopy—state of the art. Eur Respir J 1998;11(1):213–21.

41. Soler M, Wyser C, Bolliger CT, et al. Treatment of early parapneumonic empyema by "medical" thoracoscopy. Schweiz Med Wochenschr 1997;127(42):1748–53.

42. Tassi GF, Davies RJ, Noppen M. Advanced techniques in medical thoracoscopy. Eur Respir J 2006;28(5):1051–9.

43. Lee P, Yap WS, Pek WY, et al. An audit of medical thoracoscopy and talc poudrage for pneumothorax prevention in advanced COPD. Chest 2004;125(4):1315–20.

44. Tschopp JM, Boutin C, Astoul P, et al. Talcage by medical thoracoscopy for primary spontaneous pneumothorax is more cost-effective than drainage: a randomised study. Eur Respir J 2002;20(4):1003–9.

45. Schramel FM, Postmus PE, Vanderschueren RG. Current aspects of spontaneous pneumothorax. Eur Respir J 1997;10(6):1372–9.

46. Noppen M, Dekeukeleire T, Hanon S, et al. Fluorescein-enhanced autofluorescence thoracoscopy in patients with primary spontaneous pneumothorax and normal subjects. Am J Respir Crit Care Med 2006;174(1):26–30.

47. Faurschou P, Francis D, Faarup P. Thoracoscopic, histological, and clinical findings in nine case of rheumatoid pleural effusion. Thorax 1985;40(5):371–5.

48. Mack MJ, Hazelrigg SR, Landreneau RJ, et al. Thoracoscopy for the diagnosis of the indeterminate solitary pulmonary nodule. Ann Thorac Surg 1993;56(4):825–30 [discussion: 30–2].

49. American Thoracic Society, European Respiratory Society. American Thoracic Society/European Respiratory Society International Multidisciplinary Consensus Classification of the Idiopathic Interstitial Pneumonias. This joint statement of the American Thoracic Society (ATS), and the European Respiratory Society (ERS) was adopted by the ATS board of directors, June 2001 and by the ERS Executive Committee, June 2001. Am J Respir Crit Care Med 2002;165(2):277–304.

50. Bradley B, Branley HM, Egan JJ, et al. Interstitial lung disease guideline: the British Thoracic Society in collaboration with the Thoracic Society of Australia and New Zealand and the Irish Thoracic Society. Thorax 2008;63(Suppl 5):v1–58.

51. Colt HG, Russack V, Shanks TG, et al. Comparison of wedge to forceps videothoracoscopic lung biopsy. Gross and histologic findings. Chest 1995;107(2):546–50.

52. Vansteenkiste J, Verbeken E, Thomeer M, et al. Medical thoracoscopic lung biopsy in interstitial lung disease: a prospective study of biopsy quality. Eur Respir J 1999;14(3):585–90.

53. Newhouse MT. Thoracoscopy: diagnostic and therapeutic indications. Pneumologie 1989;43(2):48–52.

54. Dijkman JH, van der Meer JW, Bakker W, et al. Transpleural lung biopsy by the thoracoscopic route in patients with diffuse interstitial pulmonary disease. Chest 1982;82(1):76–83.

55. Ayed AK. Video-assisted thoracoscopic lung biopsy in the diagnosis of diffuse interstitial lung disease. A prospective study. J Cardiovasc Surg 2003;44(1):115–8.

56. Wilkinson HA. Radiofrequency percutaneous upper-thoracic sympathectomy. Technique and review of indications. N Engl J Med 1984;311(1):34–6.

57. Hashmonai M, Assalia A, Kopelman D. Thoracoscopic sympathectomy for palmar hyperhidrosis. Ablate or resect? Surg Endosc 2001;15(5):435–41.

58. Noppen M, Herregodts P, D'Haese J, et al. A simplified T2-T3 thoracoscopic sympathicolysis technique for the treatment of essential hyperhidrosis: short-term results in 100 patients. J Laparoendosc Surg 1996;6(3):151–9.

59. Noppen M, Meysman M, D'Haese J, et al. Thoracoscopic splanchnicolysis for the relief of chronic pancreatitis pain: experience of a group of pneumologists. Chest 1998;113(2):528–31.

60. Moghissi K, Dixon K, Stringer MR. Current indications and future perspective of fluorescence bronchoscopy: a review study. Photodiagnosis Photodyn Ther 2008;5(4):238–46.

61. Medford AR, Agrawal S, Free CM, et al. Retrospective analysis of Healthcare Resource Group coding allocation for local anaesthetic video-assisted 'medical' thoracoscopy in a UK tertiary respiratory centre. QJM 2009;102(5):329–33.

62. Audit Commission. PbR Data assurance framework 2007/08: findings from the first year of the national clinical coding audit programme. Available at: http://www.audit-commission.gov.uk/Products/NATIONAL-REPORT/CD8608E5-A7D9-4a5a-B0F3-C161B76DE630/PbRreport.pdf. Accessed September 22, 2009.

63. Bolliger CT, Mathur PN, Beamis JF, et al. ERS/ATS statement on interventional pulmonology. European Respiratory Society/American Thoracic Society. Eur Respir J 2002;19(2):356–73.

64. Ernst A, Silvestri GA, Johnstone D. Interventional pulmonary procedures: guidelines from the American college of chest physicians. Chest 2003;123(5):1693–717.

Index

Note: Page numbers of article titles are in **boldface** type.

Clin Chest Med 31 (2010) 173–177
doi:10.1016/S0272-5231(10)00009-2

chestmed.theclinics.com

Moving?

Make sure your subscription moves with you!

To notify us of your new address, find your **Clinics Account Number** (located on your mailing label above your name), and contact customer service at:

Email: journalscustomerservice-usa@elsevier.com

800-654-2452 (subscribers in the U.S. & Canada)
314-447-8871 (subscribers outside of the U.S. & Canada)

Fax number: 314-447-8029

Elsevier Health Sciences Division
Subscription Customer Service
3251 Riverport Lane
Maryland Heights, MO 63043

*To ensure uninterrupted delivery of your subscription, please notify us at least 4 weeks in advance of move.

Printed and bound by CPI Group (UK) Ltd, Croydon, CR0 4YY

03/10/2024

01040353-0019